T0256066

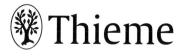

Illustrated Handbook of Toxicology

Edited by

Prof. Dr. Dr. Franz-Xaver Reichl

Department of Operative/Restorative Dentistry,
Periodontology and Pedodontics
Ludwig-Maximilians-University, Munich
Walther Straub Institute of Pharmacology and Toxicology
Ludwig-Maximilians-University, Munich
Germany

Prof. Leonard Ritter

School of Environmental Sciences
University of Guelph
Guelph, Ontario
Canada

With contributions by

Jochen Benecke, Monika Benecke, Herbert Desel,
Juergen Durner, Klaus-Gustav Eckert, Barbara Erber,
Ines C. Golly, Kai Kehe, Helmut Kreppel,
Bernhard Liebl, Harald Mueckter, Ladislaus Szinicz,
Horst Thiermann, Thomas Zilker

150 color plates

Thieme
Stuttgart · New York

Library of Congress Cataloging-in-Publication Data is available from the publisher.

This book is an authorized and revised translation of the 3rd German edition published and copyrighted 2009 by Georg Thieme Verlag, Stuttgart, Germany.
Title of the German edition: Taschenatlas Toxikologie.

Translator: Ursula Vielkind, PhD, CTran, Dundas, Canada

Illustrators: Epline, Ruth Hammelehle, Kirchheim, Germany; BITmap, Mannheim, Germany

© 2011 Georg Thieme Verlag,
Rüdigerstrasse 14, 70469 Stuttgart, Germany
http://www.thieme.de
Thieme New York, 333 Seventh Avenue,
New York, NY 10001, USA
http://www.thieme.com

Cover design: Thieme Publishing Group
Typesetting by Druckhaus Götz GmbH,
    Ludwigsburg, Germany
Printed in Germany by Grafisches Centrum Cuno,
    Calbe

ISBN 978-3-13-126921-8   1 2 3 4 5 6

List of Contributors

Prof. Dr. Jochen Benecke
Sollner Institute
Munich, Germany

Monika Benecke
Sollner Institute
Munich, Germany

Dr. Herbert Desel
Poisons Information Center
Göttingen, Germany

Dr. Dr. Juergen Durner
Department of Operative/Restorative
Dentistry, Periodontology and Pedodontics
Ludwig-Maximilians-University, Munich
Walther Straub Institute of Pharmacology
and Toxicology
Ludwig-Maximilians-University, Munich
Germany

PD Dr. Dr. Klaus-Gustav Eckert
Walther Straub Institute of Pharmacology
and Toxicology
Ludwig-Maximilians-University
Munich, Germany

Dr. Barbara Erber
Pediatric Clinic and Outpatient Clinic
Dr. von Hauner Children's Hospital
Munich, Germany

Prof. Dr. Dr. Ines C. Golly
Walther Straub Institute of Pharmacology
and Toxicology
Ludwig-Maximilians-University
Munich, Germany

PD Dr. Kai Kehe
Institute of Pharmacology and Toxicology
of the Medical and Healthcare Academy
of the Federal Defence Forces
Garching, Germany

Prof. Dr. Dr. Helmut Kreppel
Office for Military Sciences
Bavaria Barracks
Munich, Germany

Prof. Dr. Dr. Bernhard Liebl
Bavarian State Ministry for Health, Nutrition,
and Consumer Protection (StMGEV)
Munich, Germany

PD Dr. Dr. Harald Mueckter
Walther Straub Institute of Pharmacology
and Toxicology
Ludwig-Maximilians-University
Munich, Germany

Prof. Dr. Ladislaus Szinicz
Institute of Pharmacology and Toxicology
of the Medical and Healthcare Academy
of the Federal Defence Forces
Garching, Germany

Prof. Dr. Dr. Horst Thiermann
Institute of Pharmacology and Toxicology
of the Medical and Healthcare Academy
of the Federal Defence Forces
Garching, Germany

Prof. Dr. Thomas Zilker
Klinikum Rechts der Isar
Munich Technical University
Toxicology Department
Munich, Germany

■ Acknowledgements

We would like to thank the following publishers, institutions, and individuals for kindly granting permission to reproduce some of the photos:

Blackwell Verlag, Berlin (plant photos from the book *Giftpflanzen in Natur und Garten* by W. Buff and K. von der Dunk).

German Museum Munich, picture archive (historical illustrations).

F.K. Schattauer Verlagsgesellschaft mbH, Stuttgart, New York (clinical photos from the book *Der diagnostische Blick* by F.W. Tischendorf).

Gräfe and Unzer Verlag GmbH, Munich (photos of mushrooms from the book *Kompaß Pilze* by Edmund Garweidner.

Harenberg Verlag, Dortmund (historical illustrations) from the book *Personenlexikon zur Weltgeschichte* by Bodo Harenberg.

Parey Buchverlag, Berlin (plant photos from the book *Giftpflanzen* by W. Buff and K. von der Dunk).

Wissenschaftliche Verlagsgesellschaft mbH, Stuttgart (photos of mushrooms from *Giftpilze* by Bresinsky and Best; of animals from *Gifttiere* by Dietrich Mebs; and of plants from *Giftpflanzen* by Dietrich Frohne and Hans-Juergen Pfander).

Henkel, Düsseldorf (pictures of the HET-CAM test).

Dr. Alfred Czarnetzki, Osteological collection, Tübingen University (picture of amalgam dental filling).

Professor K.-H. Schulz, MD, Hamburg, emeritus director of the university dermatology clinic ("Chloracne" illustration).

Professor Dieter Szadkowski, MD, and Professor Dennis Nowak, MD, Central Institute for Occupational Medicine of Hamburg University (photos of mineral fibers).

Professor Hartmut Rabes, Pathology Institute of Munich University (pictures of diethylnitrosamine-induced liver tumors in rats).

The diagram "Composition of municipal waste" was produced from data from Professor E. Thomanetz of the Institute for Sanitary Engineering, Water Quality and Solid Waste Management of Stuttgart Technical University.

The illustrations "Lifespan of organic compounds in the atmosphere" and "Emission concentrations in Germany" were produced from the examples in slide series no. 22 (Environment: the air) of the Chemical Industry Fund, Frankfurt, and expanded.

The illustration "Reduction of harmful substances in Germany" was produced from the example in *Environmental Data 2006* of the German Federal Environmental Agency, E. Schmidt Verlag, Berlin 2007.

Preface

Toxicology is the science of the harmful effects of substances and factors on living organisms. The *toxicity* of a substance usually depends on the quantity or concentration of that substance, as well as the duration and frequency of exposure; not all living things are equally sensitive to all toxic substances. Many substances are essential for humans at low doses but may be toxic at higher doses. The famous maxim of *Theophrastus Bombastus von Hohenheim* (1493–1541), known as Paracelsus, that *"Only the dosage makes something a poison or a remedy,"* was undisputed until quite recently. However, this maxim is now being challenged as, for example, in the case of gene-altering substances where only one molecule is thought to suffice, theoretically, to cause a cell to degenerate and thus initiate tumor formation. The same principle may also apply to where a single molecule might be enough to trigger an allergic reaction.

The *Illustrated Handbook of Toxicology* includes a full discussion of threshold and non-threshold toxicology, modern toxicological methods (omics techniques) such as genomics, proteomics and metabolomics, and biological weapons. In addition, the effects of relevant toxicants on the environment and human health are explained and richly illustrated. Additional expert risk assessments provided along with updated (hazardous substance) exposure thresholds for those affected add another important dimension to the utility of the Handbook. These expert assessments are very helpful in providing meaningful context to complex toxicological concepts to the interested reader.

The first part (General Toxicology) provides updated fundamental information on toxicology.

The second part (Special Toxicology) deals with the different groups of harmful and poisonous substances, including the effects of radiation and noise. The full-color toxicological illustrations bring to life various toxicological phenomena. All the chemical formulas are in line with Römpp's Dictionary of Chemistry. This *Illustrated Handbook of Toxicology* is the book of first choice for students of medicine, dentistry, veterinary medicine, pharmacy, biology, chemistry, food chemistry, and other sciences. It is also an invaluable resource for practicing physicians, pharmacists, and scientists. The easy-to-read text, clear tables, and full color illustrations further enhance the utility and accessibility of this handbook to a broad audience.

This *Illustrated Handbook of Toxicology* provides the interested reader with a broad range of topics that will be useful not only for students but also for toxicologists, environmental physicians, political decision-makers and their advisers, whose work is directed toward protection of the environment and human health.

Our thanks go to the authors and our colleagues for their suggestions; to Dr. Juergen Durner and Dr. Mario Seiss for reviewing the chemical formulae; Dr. Tanja Huesch and Mr. Stefan Schulz for the research; in particular Dr. Christina Schoeneborn and Dr. Bettina Hansen of Georg Thieme Verlag; the illustrators Ms. Ruth Hammelehle and Mr. Thomas Heinemann for their outstanding work in producing the color plates for this book.

Franz-Xaver Reichl, Munich, Germany
Leonard Ritter, Guelph, Ontario, Canada

User Instructions

Certain color coding is used for constantly recurring terms (e.g., absorption, toxicity, treatment) so that the content can be viewed and grasped even faster.

The following terms are always shown with the same color coding:

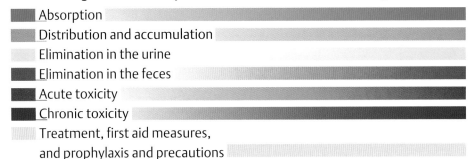

Absorption

Distribution and accumulation

Elimination in the urine

Elimination in the feces

Acute toxicity

Chronic toxicity

Treatment, first aid measures, and prophylaxis and precautions

Characteristic symptoms are shown as follows:

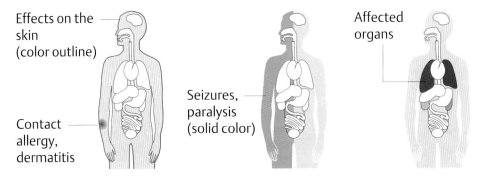

Effects on the skin (color outline)

Contact allergy, dermatitis

Seizures, paralysis (solid color)

Affected organs

If a biochemical reaction is stimulated by a substance, this is marked with a green arrow (➤), and if it is inhibited, by a red bar (⊥).

The following symbols are used for frequently recurring terms:

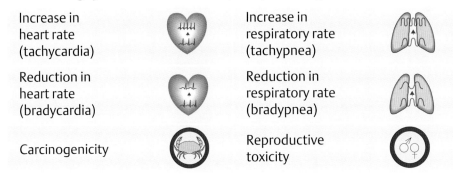

Increase in heart rate (tachycardia)

Increase in respiratory rate (tachypnea)

Reduction in heart rate (bradycardia)

Reduction in respiratory rate (bradypnea)

Carcinogenicity

Reproductive toxicity

The following colors are used for atoms:

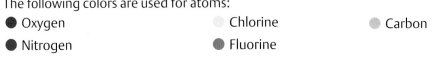

● Oxygen ● Chlorine ● Carbon

● Nitrogen ● Fluorine

▦ Contents

Contents

General Toxicology

History of Toxicology

The term toxicology is derived from the Greek *toxikon* (poison) and *logos* (word, reason) and was coined in the 17th century, although the use of medicinal remedies (e.g., plants) for healing purposes dates back much further.

Even early humans recognized the danger of poisons (e.g., snake bites). In China, the specific poisonous effects of monkshood (*Aconicum*), arsenic, and opium have been known for more than 3000 years. The poisonous effect of the saffron plant (*Crocus sativus*) was recorded in the *Ebers papyrus*, an ancient Egyptian medical document dating from 1500 BC. Harvesting the opium sap dripping from fresh cuts on poppy seedpods was a technique known to the ancient Greeks in 1400 BC. A terracotta statue found in 1936 near Heraklion on the Aegean island of Crete shows a female face in a state of trance, and the head is adorned with scratched poppy seed capsules. The figure is therefore known to archeologists as the *Poppy Goddess* (**A**).

Socrates (470–399 BC). Fellow Athenians accused him of refusing to recognize the gods. He was sentenced to death by drinking a cup of *poison hemlock* (*Conium maculatum*).

Hippocrates (460–355 BC). The oath attributed to this Greek physician states, among other things, that no deadly poison must be prescribed to anyone, and that poison must not be used to destroy unborn life.

Dioscurides of Anazarbos (AD 40–90). In AD 60, this Roman physician described the toxic effects of mandrake (*Mandragora officinarum*) in his encyclopedia *De materia medica* (**B**). The atropine-containing roots of this "love plant" were used in the past as a narcotic and sedative.

Pliny the Elder (AD 23–79) (**C**) and **Galen** (AD 129–199) described the poisonous effects of opium, henbane (*Hyoscyamus* sp.), poison hemlock, and mercury.

The history of medical toxicology is closely connected with the history of forensic toxicology (the study of human deaths by poisoning, including judicial aspects). The proper diagnosis of poisoning always has been, and still is, linked to the detection and identification of the poison. In antiquity, autopsies were generally forbidden for religious and spiritual reasons. It was only in the 15th century that the Roman Catholic church no longer objected to them.

Theophrastus Bombastus von Hohenheim (1493–1541), also called Paracelsus (**D**). He integrated toxicology into medicine, and is regarded as one of the first representatives of scientific thinking. Based on his studies on the amount of a substance that is required to produce an effect in humans, he developed the paradigm of allopathy (conventional medicine): *dosis sola facit venenum*—only the dose makes the poison.

Georgius Agricola (Georg Bauer, 1494–1555). In his work *De re metallica*, published posthumously in 1556, he described the toxicology and prevention of lead poisoning, which is the oldest known occupational disease (**E**).

Alchemy (**F**), which originated in Arabia and was a pseudoscientific precursor of chemistry in medieval times, was concerned with finding the *elixir of life*. Potions consisting mainly of metal salts and various other ingredients were used for treating all kinds of diseases.

In the subsequent early modern period, the development of new methods made it possible to conduct more accurate experiments, and this contributed to the acceptance of scientific approaches. From this point on, analysis and chemistry formed the pillars of toxicology.

James Marsh (1794–1846) was the inventor of the *Marsh apparatus* (**G**), which was first used in 1832 for detecting arsenic poisoning in a murder trial in England.

The importance of research into the relationship of cause and effect was recognized by Justus von Liebig (1803–1873), who discovered chloroform in 1831. Rudolf Buchheim (1820–1879) introduced animal experiments to medicine in 1847. Max von Pettenkofer (1818–1901) studied the effects of gases and introduced the first guidance values (*tolerance values*).

Louis Levin (1850–1929) was concerned with the prevention of industrial poisoning. He is considered to be the founder of health care protection and industrial hygiene.

Marie Curie (1867–1934) fell victim to damage caused by ionizing radiation from her own experiments on radioactivity.

Independent toxicology departments were not established in German universities until the 1960s.

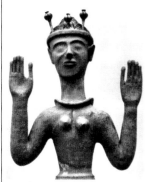

Female terracotta figure, 1400 BC; Museum of Heraklion, Crete, Greece. The smiling face with lifeless lips resembles that of a person under the influence of a narcotic (opium).

A. Poppy Goddess

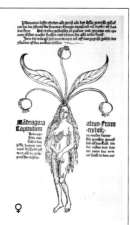

Illustration from *Hortus Sanitatis* by Peter Schoeffer, Mainz 1485; Bavarian State Library, Munich, Germany

B. The mandrake or "love plant" *(Mandragora officinarum)*

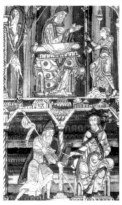
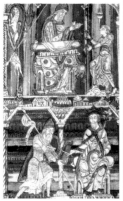

Miniature from a French manuscript (ca. 1150) of Pliny the Elder's *Naturalis Historia* (Natural History). Top: Pliny writing; bottom: Pliny offering his encyclopedia to the emperor.

C. Pliny the Elder

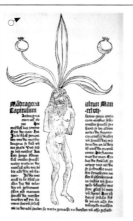

Dosis sola facit venenum

(1493–1541)

D. Paracelsus

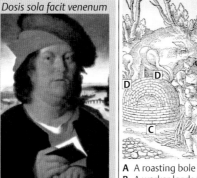

A A roasting bole with lead ore
B A worker loads the lead ore
C A roasting hearth
D Openings from which smoke escapes   (Etching, ca. 1150)

E. Medieval lead smelting

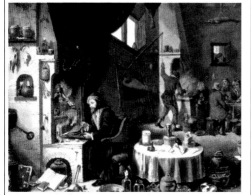

(Photograph of a painting, Deutsches Museum, Munich, Germany)

F. The Alchemist's Kitchen

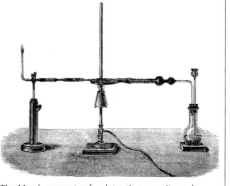

The Marsh apparatus for detecting arsenite and arsenate salts (Photograph, Deutsches Museum, Munich, Germany)

G. Marsh apparatus

▧ General

Objectives of Toxicology

Toxicology is concerned with the harmful or undesirable effects of substances or environmental factors on living organisms, especially humans. Such effects are mostly caused by substances that do not normally occur in the organism (xenobiotics) or that have an effect only at higher, nonphysiological concentrations. Toxicologists also study interactions of substances with sound, electromagnetic waves, and ionizing radiation. Toxicology characterizes the causes of toxic effects, noting their extent and the danger they pose, explaining mechanisms of action, and developing rational countermeasures. For these purposes, toxicology uses methods drawn from other sciences (**A**).

Poison, Exposure, Intoxication, Danger, and Risk

Poison. There is no generally accepted definition of a poison. Traditionally, a poison is a substance that may be harmful to living organisms, particularly humans. The effect of a poison is always species-specific and dose-dependent. We distinguish between *synthetic poisons* and *natural poisons* (toxins), depending on their origin. The latter are derived from microorganisms, plants, or animals (**B**).

Exposure. Every case of poisoning is preceded by exposure. *External exposure* is the action of a poison derived from environmental media (water, soil, air) or food. The poison must first be released from a matrix, or mixture of substances, or it must be dissolved (**C**). The rate of release is increased by large specific surface areas, and it is influenced by the solubility of the poison in aqueous or lipophilic phases. Good solubility in lipids promotes the permeability of a poison through biological membranes and accelerates its distribution.

External exposure is followed by uptake of the poison through the skin (*subcutaneous uptake*), the gastrointestinal tract (*ingestion*), or the respiratory tract (*inhalation*), and is defined by the length of time the poison is retained in the organism. It is important to distinguish between the dose taken up and the dose that is biologically active and causes damage (see also p. 9, **A**).

Intoxication. This term is used for the uptake of poison as well as for the clinically manifest poisoning. The potential of a substance to cause poisoning is defined by the sum of all properties essential for intoxication. *Sensitivity* is the reaction of the organism to the substance.

Danger. The presence of a harmful substance in a specific situation constitutes a *danger* or *hazard*. For example, alcohol abuse endangers one's health, and residues from pesticides may, at certain concentrations, be hazardous to the environment.

Risk. This is the probability per time unit with which a toxic effect is expected to occur after exposure to, and uptake of, a poison under specific conditions. It is expressed as a percentage or as the *unit risk* (one per 1 million).

Haber Rule

The effects of most toxic substances depend on their dose or concentration and the length of exposure time. The Haber rule states that, for a given toxic effect of a substance, the product of the *concentration* (C) and the *exposure time* (t) is a constant (k). The $C \times t$ diagram takes the form of a *hyperbola*. The greater the intensity of the effect, the further the apex of the curve lies from the origin of the graph (**D**). For some substances, no effect can be induced below a certain concentration, even after extended exposure times. This concentration is called the *threshold concentration* (C_T). The $C \times t$ diagram of such a substance shows a shift of the hyperbolic curve in the y direction.

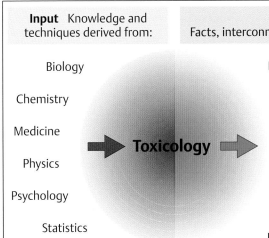

Input Knowledge and techniques derived from:	**Output** Facts, interconnections, guidelines, measures used in:
Biology	Drug toxicology
Chemistry	Biocide toxicology
Medicine	Industrial toxicology
Physics	Epidemiological toxicology
Psychology	Experimental toxicology
Statistics	Clinical toxicology
	Cosmetics toxicology
	Food toxicology
	Risk assessment
	Environmental toxicology

A. The interdisciplinary character of toxicology

Natural poisons	Origin	Minimum lethal dose (µg/kg)
Botulinum toxin A	*Clostridium botulinum*	0.00003
Tetanus toxin	*Clostridium tetani*	0.0001
Ricin	Ricinus plant	0.02
Tetrodotoxin	Pufferfish	10
Aflatoxin B1	Molds	10
Strychnine	Poison nut tree	500
Nicotine	Tobacco plant	1000

B. Lethal dose in humans

Type of mixture		Example
Gas mixture	(gas/gas)	Town gas
Fog	(liquid/gas)	Tin(IV) in the air
Dust	(solid/gas)	Asbestos dust
Emulsion	(liquid/liquid)	Tensides
Suspension	(solid/liquid)	Hydrated iron oxide
Powder	(solid/solid)	Soot

C. Mixtures and their components

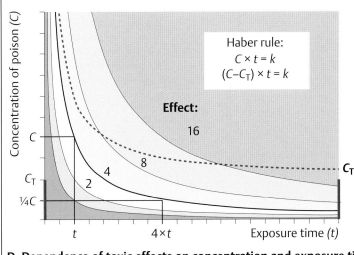

Haber rule:
$$C \times t = k$$
$$(C - C_T) \times t = k$$

Effect:

16

8

4

2

Explanation

The effect of a poison (which in this diagram has an arbitrary intensity of 4) is the product of the concentration C and the exposure time t. The same effect can be achieved by one-quarter of the concentration and four times the exposure time, or by four times the concentration and one-quarter of the exposure time. For materials with a reaction threshold, no effect can be generated below the threshold concentration C_T.

D. Dependence of toxic effects on concentration and exposure time

◾ Toxicity

Acute and Chronic Toxicity

There are different types of toxicity, depending on the length of time for which exposure has occurred (**A**). The dose range of interest differs accordingly (see Haber Rule, p. 5, **D**).

Acute toxicity. This term refers to all specific effects of a substance that occur soon after its application, usually after a single dose.

Chronic toxicity. This term is less accurately defined; it usually implies the application of multiple nonlethal doses, and typically is taken to mean exposure over a substantial portion of the expected lifetime.

The hazard of a substance depends not only on the dose and exposure time but also on the type of application and the species exposed to it. For a given dose, the expected effect may occur immediately or be delayed. In the latter case there is a latency period between the application of the poison and the manifestation of its effect. This latency period plays an important role, especially in the development of cancer, and may last for several decades (e.g., skin cancer after exposure to arsenic). The observation time may thus be limited by the life expectancy of the individual (**B**).

Toxicity Studies

Special tests are available for characterizing the toxicity of a substance. Typical end points include death following a single high-dose exposure (e.g., LD_{50} test) or the presence/absence of a specific effect. Tests for acute toxicity in an experimental animal usually take from approximately 24 h to 14 days. By contrast, testing a substance for safety (e.g., no observed effect level, NOEL) requires long observation times. In addition to testing for acute and chronic toxicity, there are tests for *genotoxicity* (mutagenicity), *reproductive toxicity*, and specific *organ toxicities* (the latter include tests for skin and eye irritation and for contact sensitization). Testing for carcinogenicity is complex and typically involves exposure of the test animals for at least 90 % of their anticipated lifespan. Genotoxicity studies are often used to gain an understanding of the mechanism of carcinogenesis, although some substances that promote tumor formation are not genotoxic (phenobarbital → liver tumors; ascorbate, saccharin → bladder tumors).

Mutagenicity tests are performed both in vivo and in vitro, although predominantly in vitro. The detection of mutagenic properties in these systems is often just a hint that there may also be some danger of genotoxicity, since some models do not cover the multiple possibilities for repair and compensation in complex organisms. On the other hand, a negative result in a mutagenicity test does not rule out the possibility that a substance may indeed contribute to an increased tumor incidence in humans. Some substances are not directly mutagenic but are converted into active metabolites, or interfere with the repair of mutations. Carcinogenicity is investigated in addition to mutagenicity when significant human exposure is expected (e.g., with pesticide residues and medicines).

Teratogenicity studies (which include tests for embryotoxicity and fetotoxicity) and multigeneration studies assess adverse reproductive impact as fertility toxicity (e.g., azoospermia after exposure to 1,2-dibromo-3-chloropropan) and as perinatal and postnatal toxicity. Teratogenic effects occur only during defined developmental periods (**C**).

Organ Toxicity

Several substances are known to have selective effects on organs (**D**). Organ toxicity can be dose-limiting for therapeutically used cytotoxins (e.g., cytostatics). The cause of organ toxicity may lie in the specific sensitivity of specialized structures that are absent in other organs, or in physiologically induced stress to the organ (e.g., renal stress caused by substances excreted by the kidneys).

Testing for	Dose	Test period	Example	End point
Acute toxicity	Single	24 h–14 d	LD$_{50}$ test	Death
			Draize test	Irritation
Subacute toxicity	Multiple	<1 month		Organ damage
Subchronic toxicity	Multiple	<10% LE*	NOEL	
Chronic toxicity	Multiple	>10% LE*	Carcinogenicity test	Neoplasm

*LE, life expectancy

A. Important terms of toxicity testing

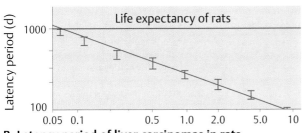

B. Latency period of liver carcinomas in rats

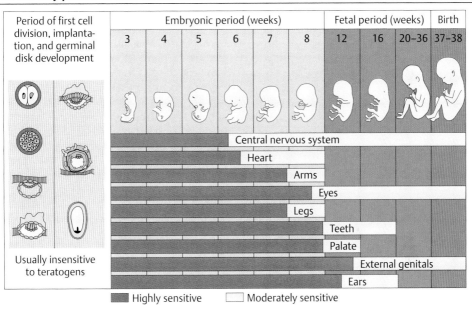

Highly sensitive ▢ Moderately sensitive

C. Teratogenic sensitivities of the human embryo and fetus

Organ toxicity	Target organ	Example of poison
Hepatotoxicity	Liver	Carbon tetrachloride
Immunotoxicity	Immune system	Organotin compounds
Cardiotoxicity	Heart	Digitalis glycosides
Myelotoxicity	Bone marrow	Platinum cytostatics
Ototoxicity	Inner ear	Aminoglycosides
Nephrotoxicity	Kidney	Cadmium salts
Neurotoxicity	Nervous system	Acrylamide
Pulmonary toxicity	Lung	Paraquat

D. Important organ toxicities

▪ Toxicodynamics I

The different phases of poisoning cover the time from the release of a poison to the induction of a toxic effect (**A**). In case of poisoning by xenobiotics, the source of the poison is exogenous, and environmental factors (temperature, humidity) play a role in the exposure. Biotransformation is an essential component of detoxification, although it may occasionally contribute to the toxicity (e.g., conversion of the pesticide parathion into its more toxic metabolite paraoxon).

Dose–Response Relationship

To characterize the (acute) toxicity of a substance, quantitative dose–response relationships are established. A wide dose range is used to illustrate the relationship between the active concentration of a substance and the intensity or frequency of the effect investigated. The resulting curve can provide informative parameters (e.g., LD_{50} values). Typical dose–response curves—plotted linearly and after *logit* or *probit transformation*—are shown in (**B**). The higher the uncertainty of the data-adjusted dose–response curve, the greater the 95 % confidence interval (in which the parameter is found with 95 % probability). To deduce the *benchmark* dose from the confidence interval (risk assessment), go from the 5 % mark of the probit straight line toward the lower doses up to the line of the 95 % confidence interval and read the corresponding dose at the intersection.

In addition to the lethal dose (LD_x), the following parameters are commonly used: lethal concentration (LC_x), effective dose or concentration (ED_x or EC_x), and inhibiting concentration (IC_x). Although the 50 % values have the smallest confidence interval in the regression analyses, and hence the greatest confidence, other levels are also used (e.g., LD_5, ED_{95}).

Mixed Intoxication

When two or more substances act on the same cell or organ system, their effects may be diminished or enhanced. (For example, muscle spasms are caused by DDT and sedation by barbiturates; administration of pentobarbital after DDT intoxication leads to sedation.) This rela-

tionship is illustrated by an isobologram (isobole: curve of doses with similar effects) (**C**). An enhancement may be additive or (in rare cases) potentiating (synergistic). It is recommended that the term *potentiation* should be used instead of *synergism* because simple additive properties are sometimes also called synergism.

Biochemical Mechanisms

At the molecular level, toxic effects are often described as disturbances of vital reactions (**D**). Inhibition of cell proliferation may result from the inhibition of protein synthesis, nucleic acid synthesis, energy metabolism, homeostasis (electrolyte balance), and membrane-associated structures. The prime sites of attack for toxic substances are enzymes and other functional proteins (carrier molecules, receptors) that are reversibly or irreversibly blocked or activated. Uncoupling of sequential biochemical reactions (ATP production, glutathione supply, photosynthesis) by the dissipation of gradients or depletion of cofactors (metal ions, ATP, NAD[P], etc.) may endanger the vitality of cells. The reaction of toxic substances with nucleic acids may lead to cytostatic effects (immunosuppression) and also to mutations and malignant tumors. Also important are disturbances of the dynamics at boundary layers, such as those induced by lipophilic substances (solvents) or surface-active substances (detergents) in the cell membrane and intracellular membranes.

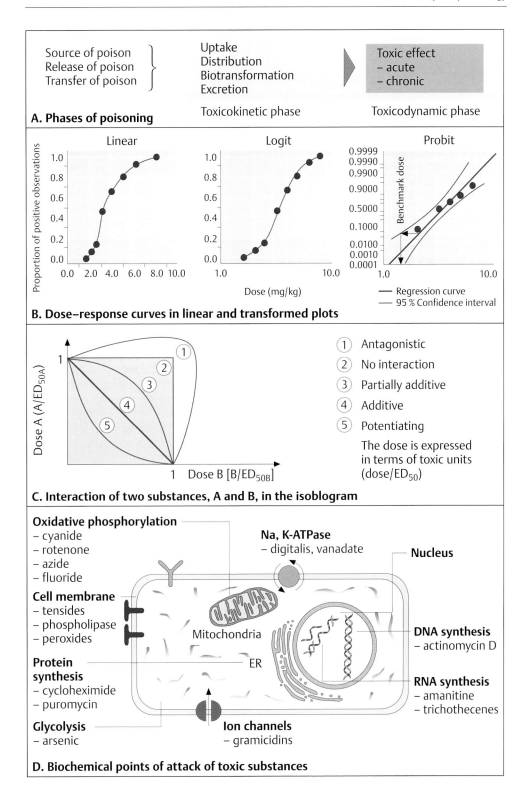

A. Phases of poisoning

Source of poison
Release of poison
Transfer of poison

Uptake
Distribution
Biotransformation
Excretion

Toxic effect
– acute
– chronic

Toxicokinetic phase

Toxicodynamic phase

B. Dose–response curves in linear and transformed plots

Linear Logit Probit

Proportion of positive observations

Dose (mg/kg)

Benchmark dose

— Regression curve
— 95 % Confidence interval

C. Interaction of two substances, A and B, in the isoblogram

Dose A (A/ED$_{50A}$)

① Antagonistic
② No interaction
③ Partially additive
④ Additive
⑤ Potentiating

The dose is expressed in terms of toxic units (dose/ED$_{50}$)

1 Dose B [B/ED$_{50B}$]

D. Biochemical points of attack of toxic substances

Oxidative phosphorylation
– cyanide
– rotenone
– azide
– fluoride

Cell membrane
– tensides
– phospholipase
– peroxides

Protein synthesis
– cycloheximide
– puromycin

Glycolysis
– arsenic

Na, K-ATPase
– digitalis, vanadate

Mitochondria

ER

Ion channels
– gramicidins

Nucleus

DNA synthesis
– actinomycin D

RNA synthesis
– amanitine
– trichothecenes

▨ Toxicodynamics II

Cellular Effects

At the cellular level, toxic effects are frequently recognized as an **inhibition of cell proliferation**. Above a certain concentration, practically all poisons have an inhibitory effect on cellular growth and division. However, this does not allow us to draw any conclusions about the mechanisms involved.

Tissues with high cell turnover—such as bone marrow, the stem cells of which mature into erythrocytes, leukocytes (granulocytes and lymphocytes), and thrombocytes—are especially susceptible to a **disturbance in cellular differentiation or maturation** (**A**). Stem cells are very sensitive to ionizing radiation and chemicals. Any damage to the respective clones may lead to cell death or to the uncontrolled growth of cells where differentiation has been disturbed (leukemia). In mature blood cells, the immunological selection caused by circulating antigen/antibody complexes may lead to a decreased lifespan, or the complete extinction, of certain clones or precursors. A well-known example is the impaired maturation of blood cells by folic acid antagonists (e.g., methotrexate), which leads to erythropenia or aplastic anemia. Rare cases of agranulocytosis may be associated with exposure to phenothiazine and thyreostatics, while thrombocytopenia may be caused by thiazide diuretics or antiphlogistics, for example.

Other poisons produce functional disturbances in cell clusters by **inhibition of cell adhesion** or **cell aggregation**. At a biochemical level, the mechanical and electrochemical coupling of cells with one another occurs by means of proteins, which are either anchored in the cell membrane (cadherins, ICAMs, connexins, selectins, integrins) or undergo dynamic restructuring in the cytosol as components of the cytoskeleton (microfilaments, microtubules) (**B**). Calcium ions also play an essential role in the aggregation of cells and in the organization of the cytoskeleton. Any disturbance of calcium balance can jeopardize cell adhesion, cell polarity, or even the viability of individual cells. Some well-known examples are components of animal poisons, e.g., hydrolytic activities in snake poison (collagenases, hyaluronidases), whose complex-forming substances disturb the calcium balance. Amanitin, cadmium, and thalidomide act on the cytoskeleton or the adhesion of cells.

Some toxic effects are best described as **inhibition of signal transmission** (**C**): communication between neighboring cells is either paracrine (by mediators, cytokines) or takes place by means of gap junctions, while communication between distant organs is either endocrine (by hormones) or synaptic (by transmitter substances). The mechanisms of signal transmission differ with respect to the selectivity, range, spreading rate, and duration of the toxic effect. Gap junctions provide direct continuity between the transmitting and receiving cells; this type of transmission is therefore only possible between directly adjacent cells. Many cellular messengers bind as a *first messenger* to special structures (receptors) on the cell membrane of the recipient cell, from where signal transmission into the cell takes place. The binding of a messenger to receptors may influence the function of ion channels, G-proteins, or enzymes (**D**). Signal transmission into the cell is mediated by a *second messenger*, e.g., cyclic AMP (cAMP) or calcium ions. Other messengers—such as steroid hormones, thyroxin, nitric oxide (NO), and carbon monoxide (CO)—pass directly through the cell membrane and act inside the cell. Poisons can interfere at many levels of signal transmission, by blocking or falsifying the signal. Examples include ouabain, curare, forskolin, nicotine, and calcimycin.

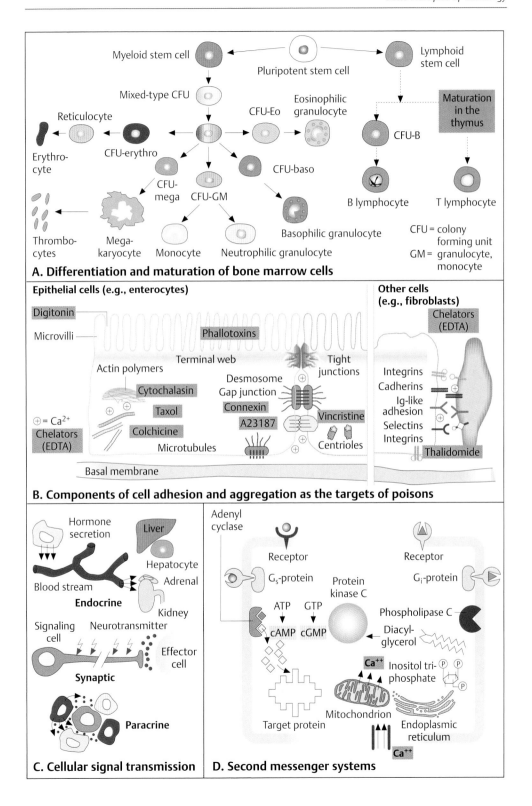

A. Differentiation and maturation of bone marrow cells

Myeloid stem cell

Pluripotent stem cell

Lymphoid stem cell

Mixed-type CFU

Eosinophilic granulocyte

CFU-Eo

Maturation in the thymus

Reticulocyte

CFU-B

Erythro-cyte

CFU-erythro

CFU-baso

CFU-mega CFU-GM

B lymphocyte

T lymphocyte

Thrombo-cytes

Mega-karyocyte Monocyte Neutrophilic granulocyte

Basophilic granulocyte

CFU = colony forming unit
GM = granulocyte, monocyte

B. Components of cell adhesion and aggregation as the targets of poisons

Epithelial cells (e.g., enterocytes)

Other cells (e.g., fibroblasts)

Digitonin

Chelators (EDTA)

Microvilli

Phallotoxins

Terminal web

Tight junctions

Integrins
Cadherins
Ig-like adhesion
Selectins
Integrins

Actin polymers

Desmosome
Gap junction

Cytochalasin

$\oplus$ = Ca^{2+}

Taxol

Connexin

Vincristine

Chelators (EDTA)

Colchicine

A23187

Microtubules

Centrioles

Thalidomide

Basal membrane

C. Cellular signal transmission

Hormone secretion

Liver

Hepatocyte

Blood stream

Adrenal

Endocrine

Kidney

Signaling cell Neurotransmitter

Effector cell

Synaptic

Paracrine

D. Second messenger systems

Adenyl cyclase

Receptor

G$_s$-protein

Protein kinase C

Receptor

G$_i$-protein

ATP GTP

Phospholipase C

cAMP cGMP

Diacyl-glycerol

Ca^{++} Inositol tri-phosphate

Target protein

Mitochondrion

Endoplasmic reticulum

Ca^{++}

11

■ Toxicokinetics I

The effect of a toxic substance depends on the extent and rate of its occurence at the site of its action (receptor) in the organism. Toxicokinetics provides a quantitative (temporal and local) description of the important processes involved: **uptake, distribution, interaction, biotransformation**, and **excretion.** For practical reasons, the concentration of the substance is determined in the blood, plasma and other body fluids, because it cannot be determined accurately at the site of action. Plasma levels measured after uptake by mouth of the poison are usually presented as an exponential function, characterized by the values C_{max} and t_{max} and by the area under the curve (AUC) of the $C \times t$ plot (**A**).

Elimination means the removal of a poison from the organism by metabolic restructuring (biotransformation) and excretion. Distribution of the poison into different compartments (redistribution) takes place at the same time as absorption and elimination.

In terms of kinetics, the **bioavailability** of a poison is the extent and rate at which the unchanged poison appears at the site of action following absorption. In practical terms, this is the absorbed portion of the ingested amount of poison; it can be determined in the plasma or blood. Strictly defined, a substance is 100% bioavailable after IV injection. Hence, bioavailability can be expressed simply as the ratio of the AUC after extravascular administration (oral, SC, etc.) to the AUC after IV application, given as a percentage. This percentage is also called the *absolute* bioavailability. In ecology, however, the term bioavailability can also mean the portion of a poison that has been released from its matrix and is thus available for absorption. Finally, the term is also used in the context of functional groups or atoms of a substance that are available for biosynthetic reactions.

Absorption

The uptake of xenobiotics can take place by ingestion (via the oral mucosa or gastrointestinal tract), by inhalation (via the respiratory tract), or through the skin (percutaneously). The rate of absorption is largely influenced by the physical state (liquid or dissolved > solid), the degree of dispersion (small particulate > coarse particulate), and the solubility of the active substance. Other factors include the degree of ionization (pH value), particle size, rate of passage through the gastrointestinal tract, and concomitant uptake of food. The organism itself influences absorption by the area of the absorbing surfaces of various organs (lungs, gastrointestinal tract) (**B**).

The passage of lipophilic substances through the cutaneous and mucosal epithelia is predominantly by passive diffusion (**C**). For several substances there are carrier systems that clearly speed up the diffusion along a concentration gradient. Active transport against a concentration gradient either uses metabolic energy, or another energetically promoted reaction is coupled with the uphill transport. Larger particles are taken up by *phagocytosis* or *pinocytosis* (liquids) or reach the other side of the epithelial barrier by *persorption* (e.g., coal dust, iron oxide particles).

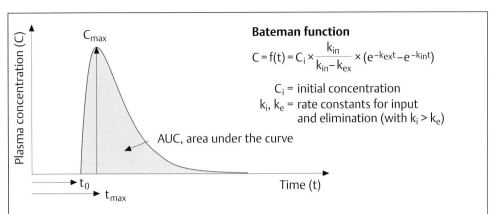

Bateman function

$$C = f(t) = C_i \times \frac{k_{in}}{k_{in} - k_{ex}} \times (e^{-k_{ex}t} - e^{-k_{in}t})$$

C_i = initial concentration
k_i, k_e = rate constants for input and elimination (with $k_i > k_e$)

AUC, area under the curve

A. Time course of the plasma level of a pharmaceutical after oral application

Point of entry	Surface (m²)	Point of entry	Surface (m²)
Oral cavity	0.02	Alveolar space	100–140
Stomach	0.1–0.2	Skin	1.5–2.0
Small intestine	100–200		
Large intestine	0.5–1.0	For comparison:	
Rectum	0.04–0.07	Capillaries	6000–8000

B. Absorption surfaces of important points of entry

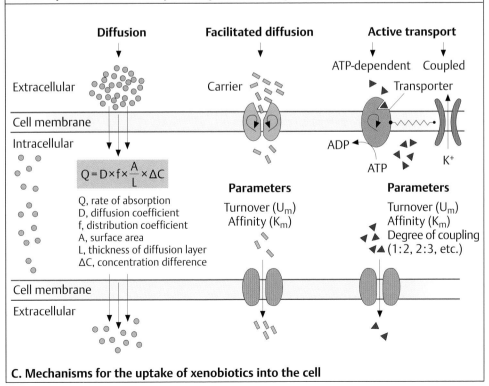

$$Q = D \times f \times \frac{A}{L} \times \Delta C$$

Q, rate of absorption
D, diffusion coefficient
f, distribution coefficient
A, surface area
L, thickness of diffusion layer
ΔC, concentration difference

Parameters
Turnover (U_m)
Affinity (K_m)

Parameters
Turnover (U_m)
Affinity (K_m)
Degree of coupling
(1:2, 2:3, etc.)

C. Mechanisms for the uptake of xenobiotics into the cell

13

Toxicokinetics II

Distribution

The absorption of a poison is followed by its distribution in the organism. Some substances largely dissolve freely in the blood, plasma, or lymph; others are predominantly bound to protein molecules or lipoproteins that serve as a vehicle for them, or else they accumulate in the lipophilic phase. The state of equilibrium (free $\rightleftarrows$ bound) influences the rate of mass transfer (**A**). Stable binding to plasma proteins does not serve only as a depot in the intravascular space; many cells also internalize plasma proteins. The *kinetic distribution volume* (V_k) is the volume calculated from the amount of substance present in the body and the plasma concentration measured in the steady state. V_k may reach high values for substances that accumulate in tissues. A comparison of these values with the actual distribution spaces (**B**) shows that some substances do not seem to leave the plasma, whereas others spread throughout the body's water. Transport by blood into the capillary area of the tissues offers a huge exchange surface (in humans, $\sim 6000–8000\,m^2$ for the total vascular length of $\sim 95\,000\,km$). Some capillary areas possess selective permeability for certain substances and may act as barriers (e.g., the blood–brain barrier). Others are relatively permeable because of openings in the basal membrane. In some places the components of the blood can pass freely into the tissues because the endothelial cells do not form a closed cell layer (e.g., the hepatic sinusoid). Poison is rapidly distributed to some highly vascularized organs, but arrives much more slowly in other organs. If capillaries are damaged by toxic effects, the poison enters the tissue much faster than when the endothelium is intact.

Biotransformation

Biotransformation is the metabolic conversion of xenobiotics. It takes place largely in the liver, and partly also in the kidneys, lungs, skin, and plasma. Many substances are already completely metabolized during absorption into the intestinal mucosa and especially in the liver (first pass effect). We distinguish phase I reactions (functionalization) and phase II reactions in which the substances obtain additional functional groups or hydrophilic adducts (conjugation); the latter makes the substances more polar and also more readily excreted (**C**). Although biotransformation often results in detoxification, phase I reactions may activate seemingly harmless substances by creating reactive intermediates. The main catalysts of such transformations are enzymes of the cytochrome P450 family. An increase in enzyme activity due to enhanced synthesis of the enzyme is called *enzyme induction*. Conjugation has the additional effect of increasing the molecular weight, thus facilitating passage of the conjugation product into the bile. Conjugation with glutathione creates *mercapturic acids* through further enzymatic steps. Methylation or acylation normally does not make compounds more soluble in water, but their reactivity is reduced by masking their SH, OH, and NH groups.

Polymorphisms and Defects

Metabolic competence may differ considerably between species and also between individuals of the same species. If the frequency of deviation from the norm is less than 1%, it is called a genetic defect; otherwise it is called a polymorphism. Polymorphisms are known for alcohol dehydrogenase, glutathione *S*-transferase μ, and acetyltransferase AT 2.

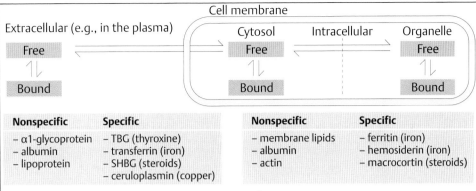

Nonspecific	Specific	Nonspecific	Specific
– α1-glycoprotein – albumin – lipoprotein	– TBG (thyroxine) – transferrin (iron) – SHBG (steroids) – ceruloplasmin (copper)	– membrane lipids – albumin – actin	– ferritin (iron) – hemosiderin (iron) – macrocortin (steroids)

A. States of equilibrium that affect mass transfer

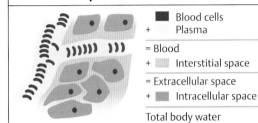

■ Blood cells	4% (2.8% BW)	
+ ░ Plasma	6% (4.2% BW)	
= Blood	10% (7.0% BW)	
+ ░ Interstitial space	25% (18.0% BW)	
= Extracellular space	35% (25.0% BW)	
+ ▒ Intracellular space	65% (45.0% BW)	
Total body water	100% (70.0% BW)	

Substance	V_d (L/kg BW)
Acetylsalicylic acid	0.15
Cocaine	0.54
Paracetamol	0.95
Quinine	1.8
Ethanol	2.0
Morphine	3.3

B. Actual distribution spaces and distribution volumes (V_d)

Phase I reactions (transformation)

Oxidation	(benzene → epoxide) $R-CH_2OH \longrightarrow R-CHO$	Cytochrome P450 families Aldehyde and alcohol dehydrogenases
Reduction	$(H_3C)_3C-OOH \longrightarrow (H_3C)_3COH + H_2O$	Glutathione peroxidase Glucosidases
Hydrolysis	$R^1-\overset{O}{\underset{H}{N}}-R^2 \longrightarrow R^1-NH_2 + R^2-COOH + H_2O$	Peptidases Esterases

Phase II reactions (conjugation)

Glucuroni-dation	(quinoline-OH + UDP-glucuronic acid → conjugate)	UDP-glucuronyl transferases
Sulfation	phenol$-OH \longrightarrow$ phenol$-OSO_3^-$	Sulfotransferases
Glutathiony-lation	O_2N-Ar$-Cl + GSH \longrightarrow O_2N-Ar-SG + HCl$ (with NO_2)	Glutathione S-transferases
Methylation	catechol$-OH + SAM \longrightarrow -O-CH_3$	Catechol O-methyltransferase
Acetylation	H_2NSO_2-Ar$-NH_2 \longrightarrow H_2NSO_2-Ar-\overset{O}{\underset{H}{N}}-C-CH_3$	Acetyltransferases 1 and 2
Aminoacety-lation	Ar$-COOH + H_2N-CH_2-COOH \longrightarrow$ Ar$-\overset{O}{C}-NHCH_2COOH$	Amino acid N-acetyltransferase

C. Important biotransformation reactions

■ Toxicokinetics III

Excretion

Although some substances can leave the organism through the skin (by exudation or desquamation) or via the respiratory tract (by exhalation), most are eliminated with the urine or feces. Renal excretion plays an important role mainly for water-soluble substances and is initially a passive process called **ultrafiltration** (free filtration up to a molecular weight of ~5000 Da, with an exclusion limit at ~6 nm ≈ 60 kDa). The composition of the ultrafiltrate is profoundly altered by reabsorption processes, and in some cases also by the secretion efficiency of the tubular epithelium (**A**).

For substances with a molecular weight of more than 300–500 Da (depending on the species), biliary excretion is important. The substances then either leave the body with the feces or are reabsorbed in distal sections of the intestine, possibly after bacterial biotransformation. The reappearance of a substance in the bile for elimination is called **enterohepatic cycling** (**B**).

Elimination by means of the respiratory tract plays a role for volatile substances, e.g., chlorofluorohydrocarbons (CFCs) and organic selenium compounds.

Clearance and Half-life

Clearance is a measure of the elimination efficiency of the organism. Total body clearance— defined as the sum of renal clearance (excretion by the kidneys) and extrarenal clearance (other routes of elimination, e.g., in feces and sweat)— describes the rate at which a foreign substance is eliminated at a given plasma concentration. The half-life of a substance corresponds to the time in which its concentration (e.g., in the plasma) declines to 50% of the original value. The half-life is independent of the original concentration only for processes that can be described by first-order kinetics (**C**). This condition is met in most cases, at least for concentrations within a certain range. Zero-order kinetics exist when only a constant amount of substance can be eliminated per time interval (e.g., when the rate-determining enzyme or transport system is working at maximum output).

Compartment Models

Compartment models are employed to describe the temporal course of the concentration of a xenobiotic substance in the blood, plasma, etc. (**D**). The simplest model uses an open compartment with a defined volume V and known rate constants k_a and k_e for absorption and elimination of the substance. There is good agreement for substances that remain almost exclusively in the intravascular space (e.g., heparin). If there is mass transfer from the plasma to tissues, a two-compartment model is usually adopted: in addition to the central compartment (with inflow and outflow), a peripheral compartment with its own rate constants is taken into account. In this case, the elimination rate is influenced by excretion and redistribution, and typically two half-lives are obtained (the initial half-life α and the terminal half-life β). Such an analysis is of practical importance for the description of substances that accumulate in the fatty tissue and therefore usually remain in the organism for a long time (e.g., DDT persists for about 1 year, and retinoids for about 100 days).

Mathematical relationships. A few simple mathematical relationships usually are sufficient to describe the toxicokinetics of a substance. The most important equations are listed in (**E**); they show the connections between dose D, plasma concentration C, AUC, half-life $t_{1/2}$, and clearance Cl.

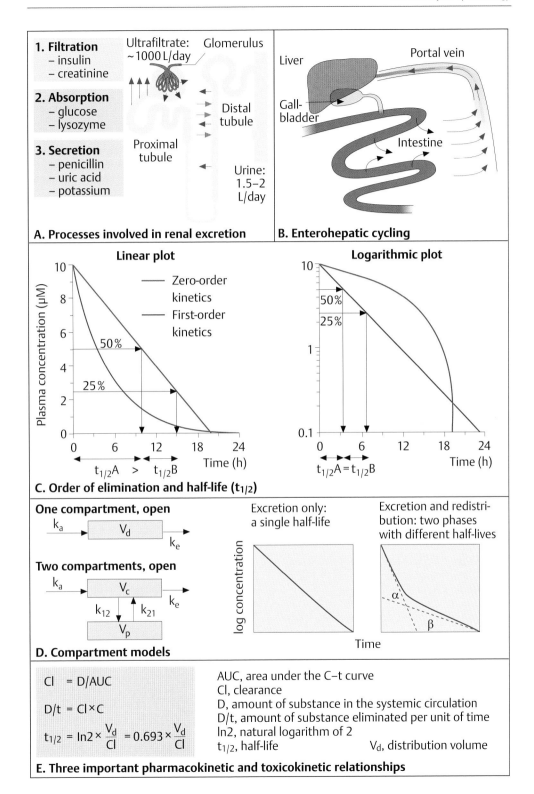

1. Filtration
 – insulin
 – creatinine

2. Absorption
 – glucose
 – lysozyme

3. Secretion
 – penicillin
 – uric acid
 – potassium

Ultrafiltrate: ~1000 L/day   Glomerulus

Proximal tubule

Distal tubule

Urine: 1.5–2 L/day

A. Processes involved in renal excretion

Liver   Portal vein

Gall-bladder

Intestine

B. Enterohepatic cycling

Linear plot

Plasma concentration (µM)

—— Zero-order kinetics

—— First-order kinetics

50%

25%

Time (h)

$t_{1/2}A \; > \; t_{1/2}B$

Logarithmic plot

50%

25%

Time (h)

$t_{1/2}A = t_{1/2}B$

C. Order of elimination and half-life ($t_{1/2}$)

One compartment, open

k_a V_d k_e

Two compartments, open

k_a V_c k_e

k_{12} k_{21}

V_p

D. Compartment models

Excretion only: a single half-life

log concentration

Excretion and redistribution: two phases with different half-lives

α

β

Time

$Cl = D/AUC$

$D/t = Cl \times C$

$t_{1/2} = \ln 2 \times \dfrac{V_d}{Cl} = 0.693 \times \dfrac{V_d}{Cl}$

AUC, area under the C–t curve
Cl, clearance
D, amount of substance in the systemic circulation
D/t, amount of substance eliminated per unit of time
ln2, natural logarithm of 2
$t_{1/2}$, half-life V_d, distribution volume

E. Three important pharmacokinetic and toxicokinetic relationships

■ Biometrics

Biometrics is the application of mathematics and statistics to biological problems.

Correctness and Accuracy

The question of how reliable measurements are is often compared with shooting at a target (**A**).

Correctness and accuracy. Even though these should always be the aim, *systematic* and *random errors* impose practical limitations. Although it is possible to estimate errors based on the range obtained by repeated measurements (see below), the correctness of a mean value or median cannot be decided by purely statistical methods; rather, it requires the aid of reference values or reference methods.

Descriptive Statistics

At the beginning of every statistical analysis the data must be described by stating the average value (median, mean value) and the range (semiquartile distance, variance, or standard deviation). The selection of statistical tests (**B**) is based on the nature of the data, which may be continuous (e.g., length), discrete (e.g., number of deaths), or categorical (e.g., color).

Hypothesis Testing

Once the analysis of an experiment has yielded a plausible answer to the problem, the validity of the test result must always be questioned. To do this, the result for the test population is compared with that for the reference or control population.

Null hypothesis. The basic premise is that there is no significant difference between the two populations.

Alternative hypothesis. In this case a significant difference is assumed to exist. Normally, a statistical test is used to test the null hypothesis. If it is refuted, the alternative hypothesis is then accepted, with a previously fixed probability of error. The proper test procedure depends not only on the type of measurements or test data but also on their distribution (normal, log-nor-mal, non-normal), the number of test groups, and the homogeneity of variances in the test groups (**B**). It is always possible to use distribution-free statistical tests, but they require larger sample sizes.

Type I and Type II Errors

For practical purposes it is important to know whether an observed difference is only statistically significant or has true biological significance. The following two cases are problematic:

(a) The test finds a significant difference when in truth there is none. This **type I error** (*false positive*) is called the producer's risk because the consequences of the assertion (error, false statement, false alarm) are the onus of the originator.

(b) The test does not find a significant difference when in truth there is one. This **type II error** (*false negative*) represents the consumer's risk because the consequences of this misjudgment affect the consumer.

In practice one should therefore carefully consider whether it is more important to keep the type I error or the type II error as small as possible. Reduction of either type I or type II errors requires a larger sample size.

Sensitivity, Specificity

Statistical testing is often used for making predictions. However, there is sometimes a discrepancy between the result of toxicological random tests and the actuality. A truth table of possible outcomes is shown in (**C**).

Sensitivity. This is the proportion of existing markers correctly detected in the test, expressed as a percentage.

Specificity. This is the proportion of nonexistent markers recognized as negative, also expressed as a percentage.

An ideal method would have a sensitivity of 100% (i.e., no false-negative results) and a specificity of 100% (i.e., no false-positive results).

Furthermore, a reliable method is expected to yield a *predictive value*: the method should always correctly detect existing markers and not yield false-positive results.

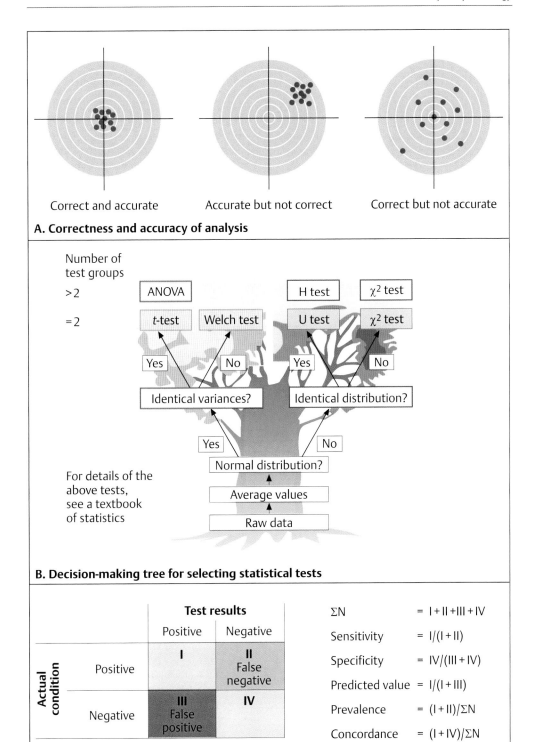

Correct and accurate Accurate but not correct Correct but not accurate

A. Correctness and accuracy of analysis

Number of test groups

>2   ANOVA   H test χ^2 test

=2   *t*-test   Welch test   U test χ^2 test

Yes   No   Yes   No

Identical variances?   Identical distribution?

Yes   No

Normal distribution?

Average values

Raw data

For details of the above tests, see a textbook of statistics

B. Decision-making tree for selecting statistical tests

		Test results	
		Positive	Negative
Actual condition	Positive	**I**	**II** False negative
	Negative	**III** False positive	**IV**

ΣN = I + II + III + IV

Sensitivity = I/(I + II)

Specificity = IV/(III + IV)

Predicted value = I/(I + III)

Prevalence = (I + II)/ΣN

Concordance = (I + IV)/ΣN

C. Truth table for the discrepancy between test results and reality

19

Basics

The study of toxic effects in *animal models*, or *in-vivo models* (Latin: *vivus*, living), has for a long time been the foundation of experimental toxicology. Today, animal experiments are being supplemented by procedures aiming more at the biochemical causes of toxic effects. Rather than using a complex organism, these *in-vitro models* (Latin: *vitrum*, glass) employ isolated organs or tissues, isolated cells, cell extracts, or cell components (organelles, enzymes). Studies on microorganisms also come into this category. (The terminology is not uniform: a geneticist might, for example, regard intact bacterial cells, as opposed to cell extracts, as an in-vivo model.) The use of in-vitro models is based on the assumption that all toxic effects occur at the cellular level.

Some in-vitro assays have been used effectively as a supplement or replacement of specific in-vivo tests. For some effects (e.g., on circulation, behavior), however, there are no accepted in-vitro models. Furthermore, long-term effects cannot, at least thus far, be reliably tested in cell cultures.

In-Vivo Methods

In-vivo methods require living organisms. Legislation demands that toxicological studies are carried out in experimental animals before a new drug can be approved for use in humans. The preferred test animals are inbred mice, rats, guinea pigs, and rabbits, and in some cases other mammals. International concern for the welfare of experimental laboratory animals initially resulted in declines in the number of animals used; however, the use of animals is now on the rise again (**A**).

LD$_{50}$ (Lethal Dose) Test

The LD$_{50}$ test was developed in 1927. According to its modern definition, LD$_{50}$ is the single dose of a substance that is expected to kill 50% of the experimental animals. Apart from the fact that large numbers of animals are required for statistically sound determinations (e.g., > 400 at ± 20% accuracy), interlaboratory tests (round-robin tests) have revealed poor agreement and reproducibility. By using a modified form of the test, the sorting of test results into *three poison classes* (harmful, toxic, very toxic) can be achieved with 25 animals.

Acute Toxicity Class Test

Testing for *acute toxicity* is done sequentially (**B**). First, an orientation dose of the substance is administered to three animals; the effect determines the next dosage level. If fewer than two animals die, the second step involves a 10-fold increase in dose, otherwise the dose is reduced. Classification is often possible at this step; hence, seven to eight animals usually suffice.

Draize Test

The Draize test was developed in 1944 for the identification of irritants (*irritation test*). Irritants cause typical reactions when applied to the skin of rabbits (redness, weal or blister formation, necrosis) or when introduced into the conjunctival sac of a rabbit's eye (clouding of the cornea, iris reactions, infiltration of the conjunctiva, and lacrimation) (**C**). Assessment is by means of a point scale using five degrees of severity: not irritating, mildly irritating, moderately irritating, very irritating, extremely irritating. Here, too, round-robin tests have revealed considerable uncertainties with regard to the grading. Moreover, the lack of a tear duct in the rabbit eye has raised important questions regarding the applicability of this test model for predicting eye irritancy effects in humans.

Hen's Egg Test

This test, too, is used for the detection of *irritants* (**D**). Incubated hen's eggs are opened at the blunt end, and the test substance is applied in dissolved or solid form to the chorioallantoic membrane (CAM). After a few minutes, the reactions of the egg white are evaluated, and typical vascular changes in the CAM are recorded, such as hemorrhage and necrosis. The test is now undergoing trials as a supplement to the Draize test (see above).

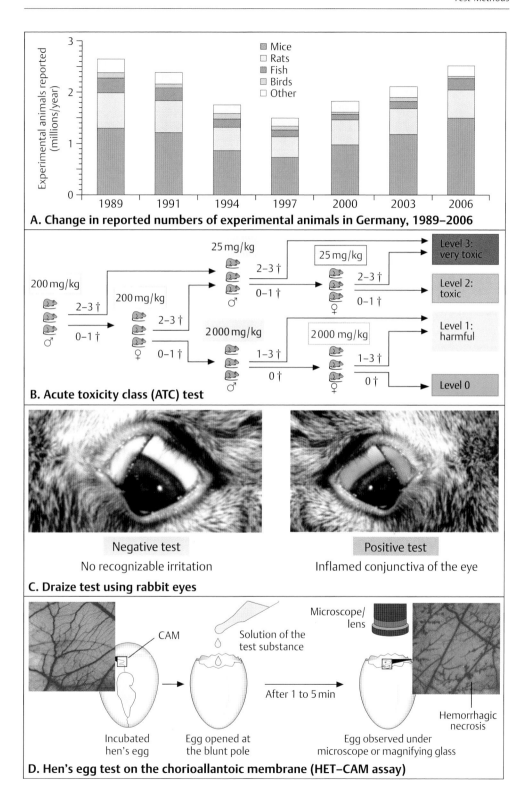

A. Change in reported numbers of experimental animals in Germany, 1989–2006

B. Acute toxicity class (ATC) test

Negative test
No recognizable irritation

Positive test
Inflamed conjunctiva of the eye

C. Draize test using rabbit eyes

D. Hen's egg test on the chorioallantoic membrane (HET–CAM assay)

■ In-Vitro Methods

These include tests for cytotoxicity, mutagenicity, and, teratogenicity.

Dye Tests

Dye tests are used for detecting *cytotoxicity*. Certain dyes, such as *neutral red*, are taken up by live cells only. The amount of dye taken up is then measured.

Other dyes are only formed after precursors have been taken up by the cell and then activated by cellular enzymes. In the presence of the test substance and *XTT* (a tetrazole salt), the formation of *formazan* by the action of cellular dehydrogenases occurs in living cells only; the amount of this dye is determined by photometry (**A**).

Still other dyes, such as *trypan blue*, do not penetrate the membrane of intact cells; they end up in damaged cells only, and the stained cells are counted under the microscope.

Ames Test

The Ames test is used for detecting *mutagenicity* in bacteria. Specifically altered strains of *Salmonella* or *E. coli* contain an abnormal gene and grow only on special culture media, whereas the wild-type strains also grow on normal agar (**B**). After exposure to a mutagen, some of the altered bacteria regain the ability of the wild type to grow on normal agar as a result of back-mutation (reversion). The colonies formed by such *revertants* can be easily counted. Many mutagens have an effect only after metabolic activation; hence, an *activator* (S9 mix, a microsomal fraction of rat liver) is added during the incubation phase.

HGPRT Test

The HGPRT test is used for predicting *carcinogenicity* in mammalian cells. The cells used in this test (e.g., V79 Chinese hamster fibroblasts) carry a mutation in the hypoxanthine guanine phosphoribosyltransferase (*HGPRT*) gene, which makes them resistant to thioguanine (TG).

When TG-resistant cells are incubated together with wild-type cells in the presence of TG, the resistant cells die as well because of metabolic cooperation by cell-to-cell communi-

cation. Tumor promoters (e.g., phenobarbital, DDT) suppress this communication, and the resistant cells survive (**C**).

Limulus Test

This test is used to detect *pyrogens*. It uses an aqueous extract of blood cells (amoebocytes) from the horseshoe crab *Limulus polyphemus*. In contrast to the rabbit test, which measures a rise in temperature after parenteral application of pyrogens, only pyrogens of Gram-negative bacteria (endotoxins) react. The end point is the formation of a gel in the test tube (positive test) (**D**).

Sister Chromatid Exchange Assay

This test is used for detecting *clastogenic effects*. Sister chromatid exchange (SCE) occurs spontaneously during cell division, but it occurs more frequently in the presence of agents causing chromosome breaks (clastogens). The SCE assay uses actively dividing mammalian cells. Newly formed DNA strands are labeled with 5-bromodeoxyuridine (BrdUrd) during the first mitosis. After the second mitosis, the label should appear only on one of the sister chromatids. Abnormal distribution of the label is observed if the test substance causes SCE (**E**).

Limb Bud or Whole Embryo Culture Assay

This test is used for detecting *teratogenicity* in rat or mouse embryos. After explantation from the uterus, whole embryos or isolated limb buds are exposed to the test substance for up to 4 days. End points include vitality, growth, and morphological abnormalities.

Micronucleus Test

This test is used for detecting *genotoxicity*, and it requires cultured cells or biopsy material. Micronuclei are formed when abnormal chromosomes lag behind during cell division or when acentric chromosome fragments are not included in the reconstituted nucleus of a daughter cell. Clastogenic agents promote the formation of micronuclei. Test samples are scored for the presence of extranuclear DNA-containing bodies (**F**).

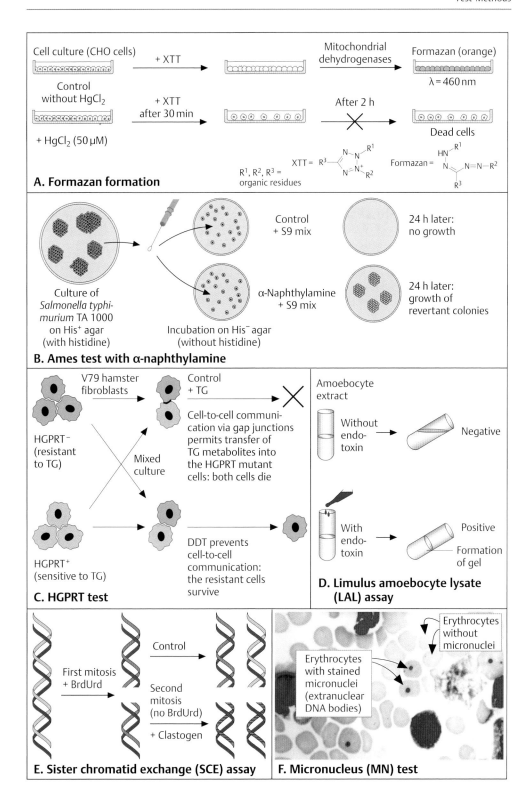

A. Formazan formation

Cell culture (CHO cells) + XTT → Mitochondrial dehydrogenases → Formazan (orange) λ = 460 nm

Control without HgCl₂ + XTT after 30 min → After 2 h ✗ → Dead cells

+ HgCl₂ (50 µM)

XTT = R³, R¹, R², R³ = organic residues

Formazan =

B. Ames test with α-naphthylamine

Culture of *Salmonella typhimurium* TA 1000 on His⁺ agar (with histidine)

Incubation on His⁻ agar (without histidine)

Control + S9 mix → 24 h later: no growth

α-Naphthylamine + S9 mix → 24 h later: growth of revertant colonies

C. HGPRT test

V79 hamster fibroblasts

HGPRT⁻ (resistant to TG)

HGPRT⁺ (sensitive to TG)

Mixed culture

Control + TG ✗

Cell-to-cell communication via gap junctions permits transfer of TG metabolites into the HGPRT mutant cells: both cells die

DDT prevents cell-to-cell communication: the resistant cells survive

D. Limulus amoebocyte lysate (LAL) assay

Amoebocyte extract

Without endotoxin → Negative

With endotoxin → Positive — Formation of gel

E. Sister chromatid exchange (SCE) assay

First mitosis + BrdUrd

Control

Second mitosis (no BrdUrd)

+ Clastogen

F. Micronucleus (MN) test

Erythrocytes without micronuclei

Erythrocytes with stained micronuclei (extranuclear DNA bodies)

■ Basics

The range of methods used in toxicology has been expanded by the introduction of the new **"omics" technologies** (e.g., genomics, proteomics, and metabolomics) developed in molecular biology (**A**). With these methods, changes in entire families of cellular molecules (e.g., DNA/ RNA, proteins, and intermediary metabolites) can be studied simultaneously. After cells or organisms are exposed to foreign substances (xenobiotics), changes in the complex patterns of cell activity (*fingerprints*) are analyzed to uncover their mechanisms of action. The highly complex activity profiles are collected in data banks and evaluated. In the United States, the *National Institute of Environmental Health Sciences (NIEHS)* has established a major new extramural program, the *Toxicogenomics Research Consortium (TRC)* (www.niehs.nih.gov/research/ supported/centers/trc).

Toxicogenomics

This subdiscipline of genomics studies the changes in gene expression at the mRNA level that occur after exposure of organisms to xenobiotics, environmental stressors, or pathological dysfunctions. The altered gene activities are analyzed using **microarray** technology in which defined DNA sequences (cDNA or oligonucleotides) are immobilized on a solid support, such as a microscopic glass slide, silicon chip, or nylon membrane (DNA chips).

Messenger RNA (mRNA) transcribed from active genes is isolated from exposed and unexposed tissues or cells, labeled with marker molecules for later identification, and then incubated with DNA chips. Comparative analysis of the hybridization patterns of mRNA bound to the DNA chips provides information about changes in the activity of specific genes following the exposure to xenobiotics (**B**).

A single **DNA chip** can carry the sequences of as many as 10 000 genes or gene fragments. Evaluation of the hybridization patterns includes comparison with information stored in data banks (bioinformatics). DNA chips may carry specific genes that are active in human organs (e.g., liver, kidneys, skin) or involved in phase I and phase II metabolism. The use of microarray technology in toxicology has con-firmed the mechanism of action of many xenobiotics that leads to specific changes in the activity of genes for enzymes or receptor proteins. Toxic substances with similar mechanisms of action induce similar transcription patterns, as demonstrated by a study in which the effects of 15 hepatotoxic compounds were tested in rat hepatocytes using DNA microarrays.

It should be pointed out, however, that changes in gene activity are not necessarily reflected by similar changes in protein synthesis or degradation. Essential information for unraveling the molecular basis of toxic effects is therefore also provided by the study of protein metabolism (proteomics).

Proteomics

Proteomics is the study of the full set of proteins (proteome) encoded by the genome. There are many more proteins than genes in an organism. One reason is the existence of protein isoforms, which appear in different compositions in different cells depending on their stage of differentiation. Proteome analysis is therefore not geared to the entire proteome of an organism but only to the proteins present in a certain cell type or tissue at a specific point in time. In toxicology, proteome analysis is used to identify and characterize changes in protein patterns after exposure to xenobiotics or environmental stressors.

Proteome analysis is usually done by two-dimensional gel electrophoresis. Automated image analysis software and evaluation (bioinformatics) makes it possible to identify up to 10 000 protein spots.

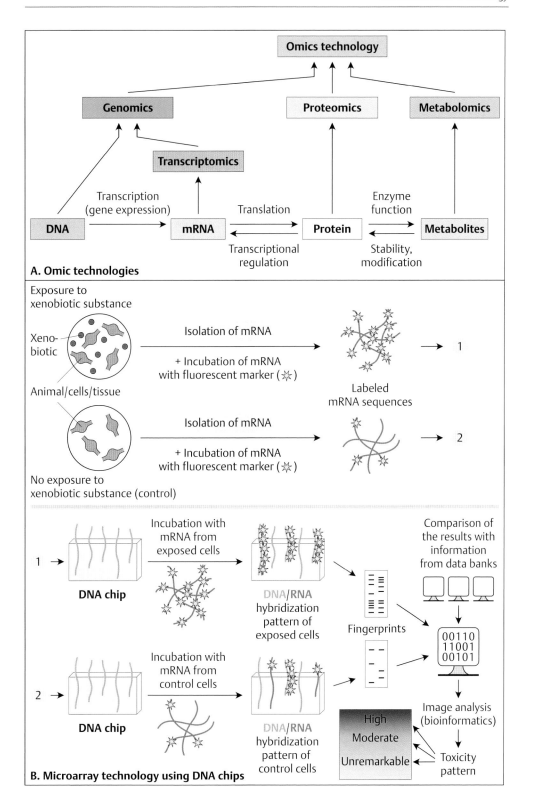

A. Omic technologies

B. Microarray technology using DNA chips

Proteomics (continued)

Protein chip technology involves capturing individual proteins from complex mixtures by means of protein-binding microarrays and subsequently identifying these proteins by mass spectrometry. The chips are coated with specific target molecules (peptide aptamers) or other molecules reacting specifically with proteins (e.g., antibodies) and thus capture only a specific fraction of cellular proteins. Toxicologically interesting proteins are then located in cells or tissues using green fluorescent protein (GFP) as a protein fusion tag. Formerly unknown proteins have thus been identified in the liver of experimental animals after exposure to hepatotoxic substances, and the same proteins were shown to be produced in liver cell cultures after exposure. In the development of new drugs, these methods can be used to reveal their mode of action, thereby saving valuable time in drug toxicology studies.

Metabolomics

The systematic study of all metabolites in an organism (metabolome) is concerned with uncovering the changes in cellular metabolism after exposure to xenobiotics or stressors. Metabolomics therefore applies to all intermediary metabolites and biomolecules, such as lipids and carbohydrates (but not nucleic acids and proteins). These substances are quantified by MRI and mass spectroscopy.

■ Other Methods

Transgenic Model Systems

The **knockout method** uses targeted inactivation of a specific gene during embryogenesis and subsequent screening for changes in the developing organism. The inactivation of a gene may have positive or negative effects. For example, when the gene for a growth factor in mice is knocked out, the transgenic mice are smaller than normal and are not viable, although they are only missing a few whiskers (**A**). Transgenic mouse models have been successfully used in pharmaceutical research (e.g.,

transgenic mice endowed with specific enzymes essential for the regulation of blood pressure). Transgenic animal models for carcinogenicity testing of chemicals are currently still unsatisfactory because every transgenic model is only useful for studying the toxic effects on one particular gene involved in the multistep process of chemical carcinogenesis.

RNA interference is a promising method that permits inhibition of the expression of individual genes. This type of gene regulation always involves RNA as the target-recognizing molecule. Recent research has demonstrated that RNA interference may be used at the chromatin level, the post-transcriptional level, and the translational level.

Cloning (from the Greek: *klon*, young shoot or twig) is a biological process that generates identical copies of a DNA sequence, cell, or organism. This does not necessarily mean that the resulting clones always have identical properties. For example, a litter of cloned cats had different coat colors (**B**), and "Dolly," the first cloned sheep (**C**), had a shortened lifespan.

Adult and Embryonic Stem Cells

Embryos and adult tissues contain undifferentiated stem cells that have the potential to develop into organ-specific tissues, both in vivo and in vitro. The experimental or therapeutic use of embryonic stem (ES) cells of human origin has not been uniformly accepted worldwide. The fluorescent embryonic stem cell test (FEST) uses mouse ES cells as a developmental system and green fluorescent protein (GFP) as a marker for gene expression (**D**). This highly accurate test is a suitable screening method for embryotoxic chemicals and takes less than 14 days. For example, ES stem cells are transfected with a cardiac tissue-specific reporter gene construct (*gfp* fusion gene). Expression of the reporter gene after development of ES cell aggregates into embryoid bodies and differentiation of various cell types (**E**) leads to fluorescence in cardiomyocytes only. Fluorometric analysis of reporter gene expression after exposure of embryoid bodies to a xenobiotic substance versus incubation in control medium establishes the degree of embryotoxicity of the test substance.

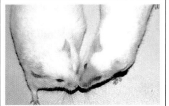

The large mouse carries an active gene for growth factor production	The small mouse carries a knockout gene for growth factor production

A. Transgenic knockout mice

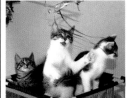

Cloned cats with identical genetic material but different coat colors

B. Cloned cats

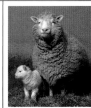

"Dolly" and her first-born lamb "Bonnie"

The first cloned sheep was born in Edinburgh, Scotland, on July 5, 1996, and was named after the country singer Dolly Parton. It lived only 6.5 years; the normal lifespan of a sheep is 12 years.

C. Cloned sheep

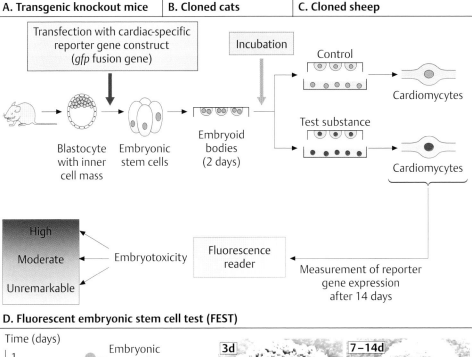

Transfection with cardiac-specific reporter gene construct (*gfp* fusion gene)

Incubation

Control

Cardiomycetes

Test substance

Cardiomycetes

Blastocyte with inner cell mass

Embryonic stem cells

Embryoid bodies (2 days)

High

Moderate

Unremarkable

Embryotoxicity

Fluorescence reader

Measurement of reporter gene expression after 14 days

D. Fluorescent embryonic stem cell test (FEST)

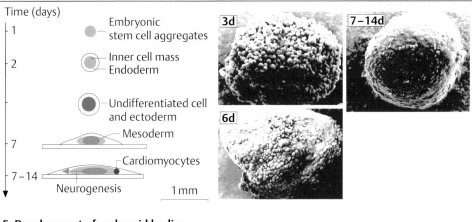

Time (days)

Embryonic stem cell aggregates

Inner cell mass Endoderm

Undifferentiated cell and ectoderm

Mesoderm

Cardiomyocytes

Neurogenesis

1 mm

3d

7–14d

6d

E. Development of embryoid bodies

27

▨ Threshold Values

Basics

Setting threshold values in toxicology has always been controversial. For example, one important question is whether or not a carcinogen has a no-effect threshold (NET). Great efforts must be made to minimize the exposure to carcinogens if there is no threshold. However, the question of whether or not such a threshold exists is difficult to answer experimentally, since possible effects at very low doses may be obscured by background incidence and, in the case of animal studies, by small group sizes that constrain the power of the assay. Furthermore, the question cannot be answered theoretically, since the multistep model of chemical carcinogenesis (see Glossary) is complex and does not allow us to make easy-to-check predictions.

Carcinogens

It is currently assumed that most genotoxic carcinogens do *not* have a threshold dose, although tumor promoters do. Examples of nonthreshold genotoxic carcinogens with a clear dose–effect relationship are aflatoxin B1 (p. 210), diethylnitrosamine (p. 128), and the tobacco-specific 4-(N-methyl-N-nitrosamino)-1-(3-pyridyl)-1-butanone (p. 126). Furthermore, no threshold has been detected for the hepatocarcinogen 2-acetylaminofluorene (**A**) after exposure at low doses (**B**), despite the use of large numbers of test animals (24 000 mice).

However, these results do not necessarily apply to all genotoxic carcinogens. In case of the carcinogen vinyl acetate, the existence of a NET has been clearly demonstrated in mice and rats at doses of less than 500 mg/kg per day (**C**).

Tumor Promoters

These substances act by promoting tumor development (epigenetic effect) rather than by binding to DNA. Some of them induce gene damage that leads to cell proliferation. Others stimulate cell division by binding to receptors and activating them. However, activation of a signaling pathway requires a certain amount of activated receptor to trigger a specific effect. This may explain the existence of a threshold.

Possible Mechanisms of No-Effect Threshold

Theoretically, the existence of a NET may be explained by the following mechanisms (**D**):

1. Carcinogen activation: Xenobiotic-metabolizing enzymes (e.g., cytochrome P450 monooxygenases) activate compounds, thus inducing genotoxic effects. No such activation occurs in organisms lacking these enzymes. The long-tailed macaque (*Macaca fascicularis*) (**E**) does not express the key enzyme cytochrome P450 1A2, required for the activation of carcinogenic heterocyclic aromatic amines; it is therefore resistant to these substances.

2. Carcinogen detoxification: After exposure to styrene oxide, a threshold dose is observed in the presence of human microsomal epoxide hydrolases. However, it is well known that detoxifying enzymes sometimes fail to deactivate a few carcinogen molecules, which then cause DNA damage.

3. DNA repair mechanisms: These are considered as possible causes of a NET. Certain prereplicative DNA repair mechanisms are thought to be error-free, for example, the repair of premutagenic lesions of O^6-alkylguanine by alkyltransferase. However, there are usually several enzymes involved in these repair reactions, and overexpression of one enzyme may result in unbalanced repair and hypermutable reactions without a NET.

4. Apoptosis: This mechanism eliminates mutated cells. However, only severely damaged cells are eliminated from the population by means of DNA damage sensor proteins.

5. Immune system: This effectively eliminates tumor cells. Presumably, it can even recognize and eliminate initiated cells that do not yet show phenotypic changes. This could mean that there is a threshold dose below which the immune system reacts optimally and above which it is saturated.

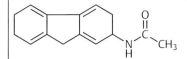

2-Acetylaminofluorene is a synthetic product originally developed as a pesticide. It was later abandoned as such because of its carcinogenic effect. It is now used as a model carcinogen in scientific research.

A. 2-Acetylaminofluorene causes tumors of the liver, bladder, and kidneys

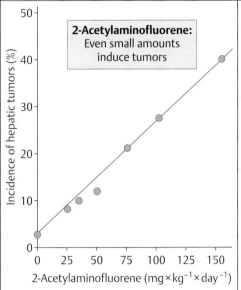

2-Acetylaminofluorene: Even small amounts induce tumors

Incidence of hepatic tumors (%)

2-Acetylaminofluorene (mg×kg^{-1}×day^{-1})

B. No-threshold carcinogen

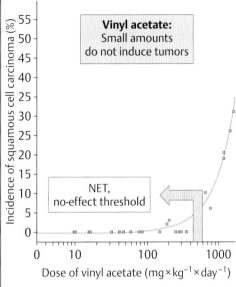

Vinyl acetate: Small amounts do not induce tumors

Incidence of squamous cell carcinoma (%)

NET, no-effect threshold

Dose of vinyl acetate (mg×kg^{-1}×day^{-1})

C. Threshold carcinogen

Multi-step model of carcinogenesis	Possible influence on threshold dose
Procarcinogen ←	Metabolic activation
Genotoxic ultimate carcinogen ⟶	Metabolic inactivation
DNA damage	Pre-replicative DNA repair
↓ Replication ⟶	Replicative damage repair ("error-prone DNA polymerases")
Fixation (mismatches) ⟶	Post-replicative DNA repair
↓ Mutation ⟶	Apoptosis
↓ Proliferation ⟶	Immune system
Expansion	
↓ Proliferation ←	Exogenous tumor promoters, cytokines
Tumor	

Explanation of arrows: ← exogenous factors   ⟶ effects

D. Mechanisms explaining no-effect threshold (NET)

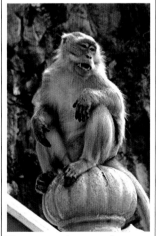

The cynomolgus monkey *(Macaca fascicularis)* is resistant to carcinogenic heterocyclic aromatic amines.

E. Long-tailed macaque

First Aid for Poisoning (Lay Responders)

First aid treatment for poisoning by lay people is normally not recommended. If the poison has been swallowed, vomiting should not be induced by a lay person, except in very rare cases. Inducing vomiting is only useful within the first hour after uptake and should remain restricted to poisons such as paraquat, arsenic, alkyl phosphates, and amatoxin. It is paramount that the local poison control center is contacted (see p. 64) as it can provide information on first aid. Inducing vomiting is more dangerous than helpful, especially with children because they normally ingest only small amounts; this also applies particularly to swallowing cigarettes. Spontaneous vomiting occurs with many types of poisoning. The patient should therefore be placed in a lateral position with the head lying low (**A**), thus preventing aspiration of the vomit. This is especially important if the patient is unconscious or disoriented. If poisonous or corrosive substances come into contact with the skin, immediate rinsing with ample amounts of water is essential. This should be followed by washing with soap to decontaminate the affected skin areas. It may be necessary to undress the patient completely to prevent further contamination from clothes. If acid or an alkaline solution has got into the eyes, the eyes should be rinsed under running tap water or by squeezing water from a soaked tissue directly into the palpebral fold (**B**). These measures can be performed by lay persons while waiting for the emergency physician. In case of accidental swallowing of corrosive substances, the patient should be encouraged to drink plenty of water to dilute the poison.

Primary Care by a Physician

When providing primary care to a poisoned person, the physician or a paramedic will observe the **five-finger rule** (**C**). This calls for *elementary aid, removal of the poison, antidote therapy* (insofar as the antidote is known), *transport* to a suitable clinic, and *securing of evidence.*

Basic First Aid (D)

Basic first aid follows the **ABC rule**: *A* stands for *airways*; keep them open and remove anything remaining in the mouth. *B* is for *breathing*; provide ventilation, if needed. *C* is for *circulation*; stabilize circulation by increasing the volume and/or administering catecholamines. In a worst-case scenario, cardiopulmonary resuscitation is applied. Resuscitation follows the **DEF rule**. *D* is for *drugs*; administer drugs to assist or restore circulation. *E* is for *ECG*; use it for diagnosis of asystole or ventricular fibrillation. *F* stands for *fibrillation*; treat by defibrillation.

In most cases of poisoning, the vital functions can be secured by endotracheal intubation to keep the airways free and, if necessary, by using a respirator. Foreign bodies in the upper airways of small children can be removed by having the child hang loosely upside down and simultaneously compressing the thorax from the front and back. In case of circulatory collapse, cardiac massage at a ratio of 5:1 is indicated, i.e., 60 heart massages and 12 resuscitation attempts per minute (provided two assistants are present, which is normally the case). For resuscitation the following drugs are used: epinephrine, sodium hydrogen carbonate, atropine, and—after successful defibrillation—lidocaine as an antiarrhythmic agent. Dopamine is used for stabilizing the blood pressure.

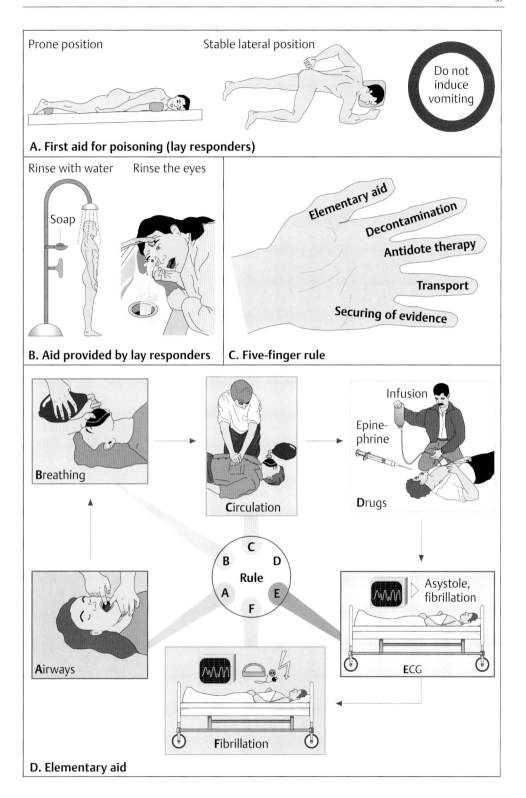

A. First aid for poisoning (lay responders)

Prone position   Stable lateral position   Do not induce vomiting

B. Aid provided by lay responders

Rinse with water   Rinse the eyes   Soap

C. Five-finger rule

Elementary aid
Decontamination
Antidote therapy
Transport
Securing of evidence

D. Elementary aid

Breathing
Circulation
Drugs — Infusion, Epine-phrine
Airways
ECG — Asystole, fibrillation
Fibrillation

Rule
B C D
A F E

31

Detoxification (A)

If a poison has been swallowed, it can be removed from the stomach by inducing vomiting or by gastric lavage. As noted previously, in the case of a pharmaceutical drug, this only makes sense within the first hour. Vomiting should only be induced by administering ipecac syrup (derived from the plant *Cephaelis ipecacuanha*) and only in patients who are fully conscious; it must not be used after the swallowing of foaming agents, solvents, acids, or alkaline solutions. Gastric lavage is performed in conscious patients after placing them in the prone position. Disoriented or unconscious patients can undergo gastric lavage in supine position after intubation of the trachea and subsequent sealing by a tracheal cuff. Tap water at body temperature is used for adults, and the rinsing is done with 10–20 L of water in 0.5-L portions. For children, isotonic sodium chloride solution is used. Gastric lavage is followed by instillation of activated charcoal (1 g/kg BW) by means of a gastric tube or probe to bind the poison remaining in the gastrointestinal tract. Charcoal is usually administered together with a laxative; this accelerates intestinal passage and thus the forced excretion of poison bound to the charcoal. Normally, sodium sulfate at a dose of 0.4 g/kg BW for adults and 0.5 g/kg BW for children is used for this purgative measure. Once absorption has taken place, the following procedures are available as secondary detoxification measures: forced diuresis, hemodialysis, hemoperfusion, and plasmapheresis. The range of indications for all these procedures is very limited. Before such a procedure is performed, the local poison control should always be contacted.

Antidote Therapy (B)

Antidotes. These are substances which specifically interfere with the poison's mechanism of action and therefore alleviate or abolish its action, or contribute to its accelerated elimination. For example, dimethylaminophenol (DMAP) is a life-saving antidote that leads to detoxification of cyanide by forming methemoglobin. It must always be available in the emergency kit (Tox Box). Charcoal binds the poison in the gastrointestinal tract and thus prevents its absorption. Chelating agents lead to the forced renal elimi-

nation of heavy metals in the case of heavy metal poisoning. There should always be a sufficient supply of antidotes in intensive care units and emergency vehicles.

Transport

In addition to immediate therapeutic measures, logistics (e.g., transport) often play an important role in the outcome of acute exogenous intoxication. Transporting the patient is only possible once the circulation has been stabilized and the airways cleared, i.e., when the patient is conscious and in the prone or lateral position, or after intubation if unconscious.

Securing Evidence

It is very important to collect and preserve various samples that may be critical in the diagnosis of poisoning. Samples that can always be obtained are urine, blood in EDTA tubes, and native blood to obtain serum. In certain circumstances, stool samples (in case of food poisoning or fungal poisoning) or exhaled air collected in a respiratory balloon (in the case of gas poisoning) must be obtained. The samples must be identified by accurate labeling (e.g., personal data, sample type, time of collection; see also biomonitoring, p. 38). Blood and urine samples should be secured before any antidote is administered, because the antidote may interfere with the method of determination, e.g., by binding the poison.

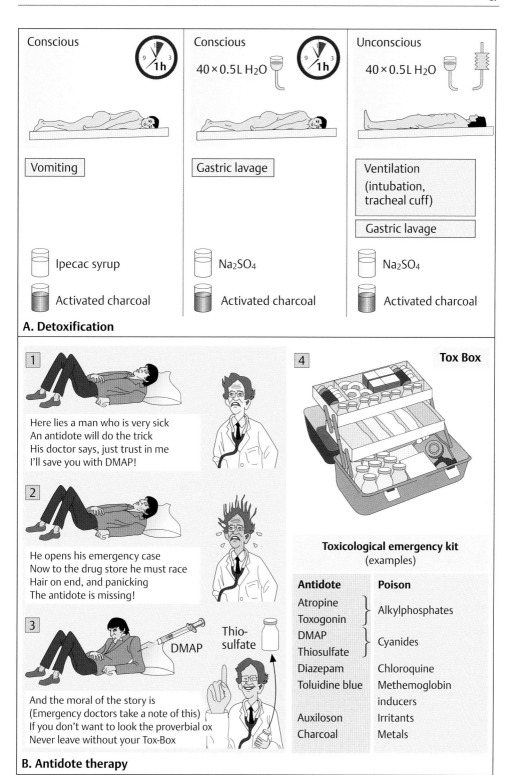

Conscious	Conscious	Unconscious
1h	40 × 0.5L H_2O 1h	40 × 0.5L H_2O
Vomiting	Gastric lavage	Ventilation (intubation, tracheal cuff)
		Gastric lavage
Ipecac syrup	Na$_2$SO$_4$	Na$_2$SO$_4$
Activated charcoal	Activated charcoal	Activated charcoal

A. Detoxification

1

Here lies a man who is very sick
An antidote will do the trick
His doctor says, just trust in me
I'll save you with DMAP!

2

He opens his emergency case
Now to the drug store he must race
Hair on end, and panicking
The antidote is missing!

3

DMAP Thio-sulfate

And the moral of the story is
(Emergency doctors take a note of this)
If you don't want to look the proverbial ox
Never leave without your Tox-Box

4 **Tox Box**

Toxicological emergency kit
(examples)

Antidote	Poison
Atropine	} Alkylphosphates
Toxogonin	
DMAP	} Cyanides
Thiosulfate	
Diazepam	Chloroquine
Toluidine blue	Methemoglobin inducers
Auxiloson	Irritants
Charcoal	Metals

B. Antidote therapy

33

▓ Basics

Definition

Environmental medicine. This is an interdisciplinary field of medicine. It deals with the effects of environmental factors (toxic substances, noise, and radiation) on human health.

Disciplines of Environmental Medicine (A)

We distinguish between *preventive disciplines*, such as environmental hygiene and environmental toxicology, which deal with the detection of toxic substances in our natural surroundings, and *disciplines in which physicians attend patients*, such as clinical toxicology, dermatology (allergology), otorhinolaryngology, internal medicine (pulmonology or respiratory medicine), and pediatrics. In addition to these two main groups, there are occupational (or industrial) medicine and the public health services. These also deal with problems of environmental medicine: occupational medicine because it has acquired extensive experience with toxic substances that affect industrial workers, and the public health services because they function as the protectors of public health. Physicians working in occupational medicine have compiled information on occupational diseases caused by exposure to chemicals, and have advocated appropriate preventive measures as well as the elimination of toxic workplace chemicals.

Alternative Disciplines

With the growth of the ecological movement, many practitioners interested in alternative health care have also become involved in environmental medicine. The spectrum ranges from physicians practicing homeopathy to those who offer fringe methods for the diagnosis of environmental poisoning and for detoxification (e.g., bioresonance, electroacupuncture) which may not always be founded on commonly accepted scientific principles. These practitioners have formed their own associations, some of which are politically active.

Human Exposure to Environmental Factors

Environmental media. Air, water, and soil may be polluted with toxic substances. Plants grown in such an environment and used as food may therefore be contaminated as well. In particular, residues of herbicides and pesticides, in excess of approved national legal limits for these chemicals, may be present on or in fruits and vegetables. Animal-derived foods may be polluted if the animals raised for meat production have been fed with contaminated plants or treated unlawfully or in a manner contrary to national regulations, for example, with growth-promoting drugs.

Sources of emission. Pollution can also derive from sources of emission. Depending on its distribution, expansion, and dilution, any emission can find its way into the air, water, and soil. *Motor vehicles and combustion engines of all kinds* are powerful emitters, as are the *waste air* and *waste water* of industrial plants. There is mass transfer between the environmental media, for example, through deposition, precipitation, leaching, or outgassing. Toxic substances get into the human body as gases or bound to dust via the respiratory tract; as food and ingested dust particles via the gastrointestinal tract; or by direct contact with chemicals or textiles via the skin.

Other forms of pollution (B). The emission of sound waves (noise); electromagnetic fields, for example, from power lines or cell phones or radar units (e.g., measuring equipment); radioactive radiation (α-, β-, γ-rays); and ultraviolet irradiation (UV-A, -B, -C rays; e.g., sunlight, tanning parlors) represent an additional burden for the human body. For details, see under Noise, p. 302, and Radiation, p. 294.

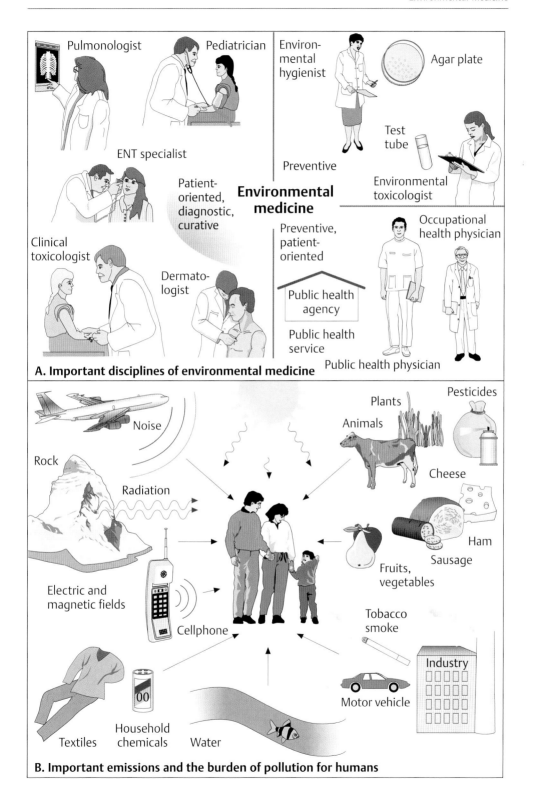

A. Important disciplines of environmental medicine

Pulmonologist

Pediatrician

Environmental hygienist

Agar plate

ENT specialist

Test tube

Preventive

Environmental toxicologist

Patient-oriented, diagnostic, curative

Environmental medicine

Clinical toxicologist

Dermatologist

Preventive, patient-oriented

Occupational health physician

Public health agency

Public health service

Public health physician

B. Important emissions and the burden of pollution for humans

Noise

Plants

Animals

Pesticides

Rock

Cheese

Radiation

Ham

Electric and magnetic fields

Sausage

Fruits, vegetables

Cellphone

Tobacco smoke

Industry

Motor vehicle

Textiles

Household chemicals

Water

Invasion and Elimination

Toxic substances may be eliminated in the urine, feces, sweat, breast milk, hair, and skin, or metabolized in the body (largely in the liver). When the elimination mechanisms are overwhelmed, or when the substances have a strong affinity to certain structures—such as heavy metals to enzymes, or lipophilic substances to fatty tissue—toxic substances concentrate in tissues (*accumulation*). The mere presence of foreign materials in the body does not mean that they always have a damaging effect. Certain substances taken up from the environment may even be important for physiological processes, for example, trace elements such as copper, iron, and zinc, and iodine. The science of toxicology is primarily involved when toxic substances lead to temporary or persistent adverse effects of normal physiological processes. As a rule, toxic substances may damage enzymes, membrane components, or the genome, unless they are rapidly excreted and thus prevented from having an effect. Continuous action of a substance may lead to an overload of the system and thus cause damage after a latency period.

The probability of damaging effects increases with the concentration of the substance in the body (dose–response relationship). The only known exceptions to this rule so far are carcinogens. Most dose–response relationships have a threshold dose below which there is no observed effect (no observed effect level, NOEL) (**A**). Most toxic substances show a specific poisonous effect above a certain dose (lowest observed effect level, LOEL) (**A**). There is little convincing scientific evidence that nonspecific feelings of ill-health, unaccompanied by measurable organ manifestations, can be induced by toxic substances in the low-dose range.

Continuing Medical Education

Most medical associations in the United States and European countries award the advanced qualification of "specialist in environmental medicine" or a similar title on physicians who have completed a course of specialization and have been active for several years in a specialty concerned with environmental medicine. The topics for continuing education include (**B**):

1. Basics and methods of environmental medicine: Information on institutions dealing with environmental medicine, procurement of information, environmental analysis, toxicology, epidemiology, biomonitoring, risk assessment, and setting guidance values.

2. Groups of pollutants relevant to environmental medicine: Outdoor and indoor air pollution, iatrogenic pollution, pollution from consumer goods, foods, drinking-water and bath water, wastewater renovation or disposal, toxic substances in soil and water, waste management, noise and radiation pollution, environmental factors affecting the sensory organs, meteorology and climatology, and ecological balance.

3. Clinical aspects of environmental medicine: Medical history of the patient, diagnostic procedures, differential diagnosis, therapeutic options, alternative methods, consultations, risk groups in environmental medicine, environmental psychology including psychotherapy and counseling, and prevention.

4. Environmental legislation: The following types of laws, regulations, etc. concern the environment: environmental law and health law; laws on pollution control, lead in gasoline, chemicals, environmental compatibility testing, and health care services; regulations on hazardous material, poison information, agriculture, and occupational diseases; and technical instructions on prevention of air pollution.

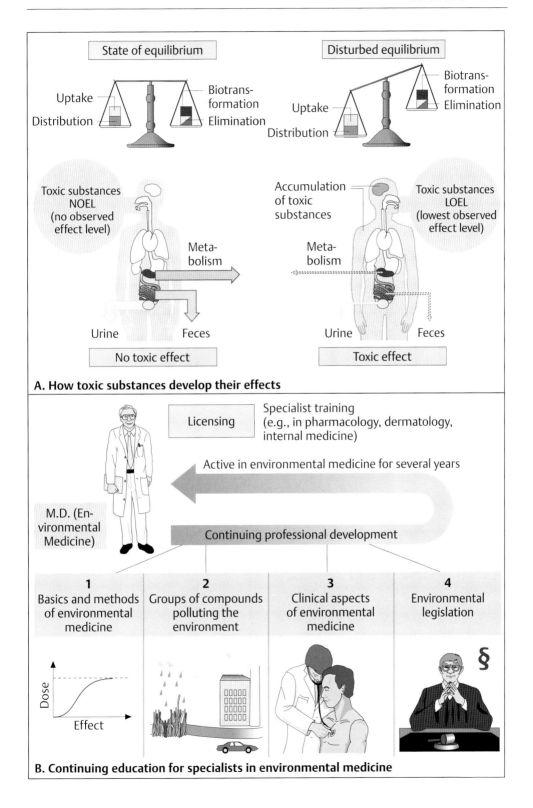

State of equilibrium

Uptake
Distribution

Biotrans-
formation
Elimination

Toxic substances
NOEL
(no observed
effect level)

Meta-
bolism

Urine   Feces

No toxic effect

Disturbed equilibrium

Uptake
Distribution

Biotrans-
formation
Elimination

Accumulation
of toxic
substances

Toxic substances
LOEL
(lowest observed
effect level)

Meta-
bolism

Urine   Feces

Toxic effect

A. How toxic substances develop their effects

Licensing

Specialist training
(e.g., in pharmacology, dermatology,
internal medicine)

Active in environmental medicine for several years

M.D. (En-
vironmental
Medicine)

Continuing professional development

1
Basics and methods
of environmental
medicine

2
Groups of compounds
polluting the
environment

3
Clinical aspects
of environmental
medicine

4
Environmental
legislation

Dose

Effect

§

B. Continuing education for specialists in environmental medicine

■ Biomonitoring

Basics

Biomonitoring involves measuring the concentration of toxic substances and/or their metabolites in biological samples. When these are human samples, it is called *human biomonitoring*. Materials that can be examined include blood, serum, feces, urine, breath, breast milk, hair, teeth, and semen. The purpose of human biomonitoring is to assess the exposure to toxic substances in specific groups of the population at a specific time. In this way, substances are detected that have been transferred from the environment into the human body where they are normally not present. Therefore, only reference values rather than normal values are given. They are determined by means of studies on toxic substances in unexposed individuals within a specific geographic region. They reflect the basic exposure to pollutants (**A**). When test results exceed the reference values, this does not necessarily mean they are "toxic" or "dangerous." For proper interpretation of the results, information on the place and time of uptake of the toxic substance and knowledge of its absorption, distribution, metabolism and excretion (ADME), as well as its toxicological characteristics, are required.

Environmental Media

Toxic substances may be taken up by *inhalation, ingestion,* or *percutaneous absorption* (**B**). They originate from the environment (*water, soil, air*); from *food* containing residues of toxic substances; or from *consumer goods* and *commodities,* such as furniture or clothes. Concentrations in the blood or serum are typically more indicative of a recent acute exposure, but the urine may contain substances that have remained in the body for a moderate period of time and are possibly excreted as a result of the testing, for example, through mobilization with chelating agents. Exposure to toxic substances that occurred a long time previously is best detected by the analysis of hair and teeth or, in rare cases, by the analysis of tissues. Detection of concentrations in breast milk is important for substances that accumulate preferentially in fatty tissues (bioaccumulation). It is very important in assessing the exposure in neonates and young children (**C**).

Securing Evidence

When obtaining samples for biomonitoring, proper sample collection is essential. Blood should be drawn using disposable needles, and it should be collected in vials coated with potassium EDTA (K-EDTA) as an anticoagulant and free of toxic substances. When collecting blood for the detection of solvents and halogenated hydrocarbons, glass vessels with Teflon-coated caps must be used. These blood samples should be shaken immediately after collection so that microcoagulation does not take place. Urine is collected in polyethylene vials. For specific tasks, for example, analysis for heavy metals, the vials must be pretreated with acid and rinsed with water. A 24-h urine specimen is more representative than a random spot sample. Variations in the volume of urine are taken into account by reference to the excretion of creatinine. Hair can sometimes be used to determine the time at which an exposure has taken place. The hair must be washed, in order to distinguish between incorporated poisons and those applied externally. All biological samples must be properly labeled (**D**). The time of sampling is important, particularly with volatile substances (e.g., solvents). The questions most frequently asked by patients in environmental outpatient clinics relate to mercury from amalgam fillings, or poisoning by indoor wood preservatives (e.g., pentachlorophenol, hexachlorocyclohexane) or formaldehyde.

Toxic substance	Biological sample	Mean values		Upper limit
Lead	Blood	50 – 70	µg/L	150 µg/L
γ-HCH (lindane)	Blood	0.2 – 0.5	µg/L	1.0 µg/L
PCB	Blood	0.01 – 2.0	µg/L	3.0 µg/L
PCDD/PCDF (dioxins)	Blood	1 – 500	pg/g blood lipids	900 pg/g blood lipids
PCP	Urine	2 – 5	µg/g creatinine	12 µg/g creatinine
Hg (no amalgam fillings)	Urine	0.1 – 0.3	µg/L	1 µg/L
Hg (with 8 amalgam fillings)	Urine	0.3 – 1.0	µg/L	5 µg/L

A. Reference values for some environmental pollutants in human biological samples

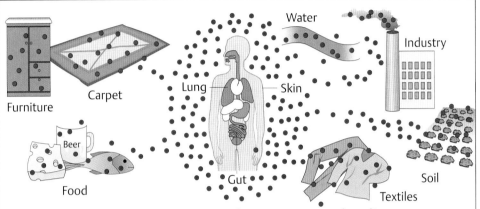

B. Pathways of uptake of toxic substances from environmental media

Recent exposure

Exposure some time ago

Exposure a long time ago

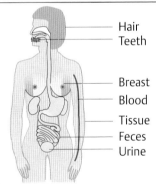

Hair
Teeth

Breast
Blood
Tissue
Feces
Urine

C. Securing body materials for the determination of toxic substances

Test sample

Identification number
Name of patient
Type of saved material
Date and time of collection
Suspected toxic substance
Assumed time of uptake of toxic substance

D. Recommended labeling of the biological test sample

Environmental Poisons and Psychiatric Disorders

"Doctor Hopping"

Some people increasingly blame nonspecific symptoms on environmental factors. Suggested threats to human health from the domestic environment or from amalgam fillings have been widely discussed in the mass media, thus creating unease and a feeling of apprehension in the population at large. The result is that anxious people suddenly blame environmental poisons whenever they do not feel well. Individuals who have suffered from ill-health for a long time are often relieved to have found an explanation for their symptoms.

Fear of environmental poisoning can certainly make one sick, and may contribute to psychiatric or psychosomatic illnesses. Unfortunately, the fixation on environmental poisons is encouraged by some well-meaning physicians, which may result in some patients not receiving the appropriate psychotherapeutic treatment. Instead, they visit many different specialists ("doctor hopping"), and may be offered very different diagnoses, which range from being physically completely healthy to chronically poisoned beyond recovery, or from being a malingerer to being a psychopath (**A**).

Biomonitoring studies for various environmental exposures often reveal exposures within the normal range or slightly above. High levels such as those found with acute poisoning, or when exceeding safe limits established by national or international regulatory authorities, are found only very infrequently. The significance of these findings may differ—depending on the physician, the findings may be interpreted either as chronic poisoning or as harmless background exposure. Some physicians no longer accept a dose–response relationship (which is the norm in pharmacology and toxicology) or the paradigm of Paracelsus ("only the dose makes the poison"). It is interesting that patients frequently report nonspecific symptoms, regardless of the putative poison to which they claim they have been exposed. The symptoms often resemble the "symptom complex" that psychiatrists have described as somatization disorder (**B**).

Another argument for the possibility that "environmental poisoning" could represent a psychiatric disorder is that these symptoms had already been described long before certain substances (e.g., pentachlorophenol) were present in the environment. In earlier times, they were interpreted as spinal irritation (in the 19th century), neurasthenia (at the beginning of the 20th century), or chronic brucellosis (in the 1930s).

Five Stages of Manifestation in "Environmental Victims"

In terms of phenomenology, we distinguish five stages of manifestation in "environmentally poisoned" individuals, with the strongest manifestation being *multiple chemical sensitivity* (MCS) or *idiopathic environmental intolerance* (IEI) (**C**):

1. **Flexible individuals looking for information.** These are patients who feel ill and are looking for an external cause of their disease.

2. **Fixed individuals looking for information.** They are already sure that an external noxious agent is to blame, but they are still open to accepting other causes, such as allergies or infections, in addition to poisoning.

3. **Poisoned individuals looking for information.** They are sure that poisoning has taken place and are now searching only for the poison that is to blame for their condition.

4. **Poisoned optimists.** They believe they can be cured by measures such as detoxification or sanitation of their home and/or workplace.

5. **Poisoned victims.** They feel chronically ill and have lost any hope of cure. They adapt their entire life to the disease.

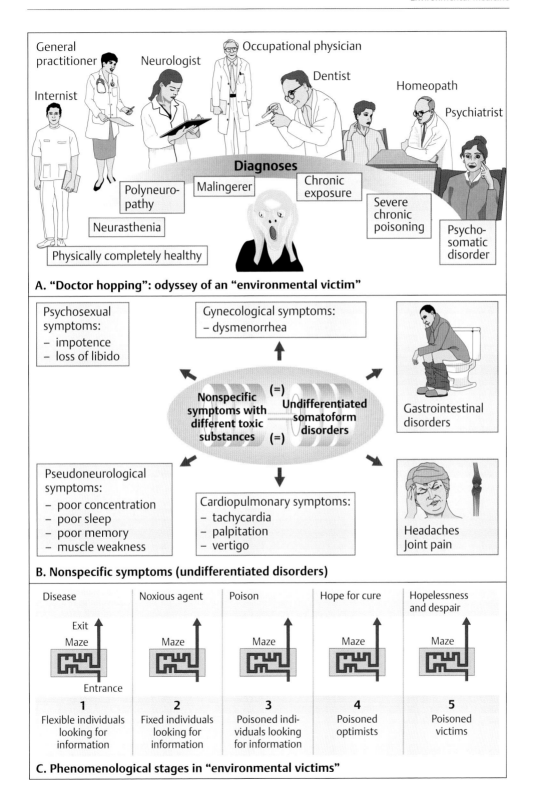

A. "Doctor hopping": odyssey of an "environmental victim"

General practitioner

Neurologist

Occupational physician

Dentist

Homeopath

Psychiatrist

Internist

Diagnoses

Polyneuro-pathy

Malingerer

Chronic exposure

Neurasthenia

Severe chronic poisoning

Psycho-somatic disorder

Physically completely healthy

Psychosexual symptoms:
– impotence
– loss of libido

Gynecological symptoms:
– dysmenorrhea

Nonspecific symptoms with different toxic substances (=) Undifferentiated somatoform disorders (=)

Gastrointestinal disorders

Pseudoneurological symptoms:
– poor concentration
– poor sleep
– poor memory
– muscle weakness

Cardiopulmonary symptoms:
– tachycardia
– palpitation
– vertigo

Headaches
Joint pain

B. Nonspecific symptoms (undifferentiated disorders)

Disease	Noxious agent	Poison	Hope for cure	Hopelessness and despair
Exit ↑ Maze Entrance	Maze	Maze	Maze	Maze
1 Flexible individuals looking for information	**2** Fixed individuals looking for information	**3** Poisoned individuals looking for information	**4** Poisoned optimists	**5** Poisoned victims

C. Phenomenological stages in "environmental victims"

41

Psychosocial Consequences for the "Environmentally Poisoned"

As "environmentally poisoned" individuals are convinced that they are continuously threatened by pollutants, they develop behavioral disorders with psychosocial consequences (**A**). Psychiatric disorders caused by environmental pollutants do not all have the same origin. According to modern diagnostic criteria for psychiatric disorders, they include affective disorders, anxiety disorders, somatoform disorders, and—in rare cases—psychotic disorders. If the poisons themselves actually cause psychiatric disorders, these should be classified as organically caused psychiatric disorders. Within the group of people with affective disorders, "environmentally poisoned" individuals are usually those suffering from adjustment disorder with a depressive emotional response (formerly known as neurotic depression).

Exteriorization of Problems

A psychiatric disorder can be triggered by "environmental poisoning." The underlying cause may be a subconscious, repressed conflict that should be resolved. However, if it cannot be resolved, the person is looking for causes in the environment. An "environmental poison" is particularly suitable for this purpose: one exteriorizes the problem and invests all one's energy into fighting this "environmental poison." This may temporarily suppress the depressive mood (**B**).

Toxicophobia, Somatotropic Disorders, and Hypochondriasis

Toxicophobia. This anxiety disorder is characterized by a fear of being poisoned, although this is not in fact the case. It may be chronic, or occur suddenly in the form of panic attacks, for example, triggered by odors (**C**).

Somatotropic disorder. The clinical symptoms of this disorder are bodily complaints or an irrational fear of disease.

Hypochondriasis. When the fear is particularly incomprehensible and the patient always interprets all bodily sensations as severe illness, the condition is called hypochondriasis (**D**).

Somatoform Disorders

Somatization disorder is suspected when there have been multiple physical symptoms over a period of at least 6 months and the patient is less than 30 years old. When the first manifestation occurs in patients older than 30 years, it is called undifferentiated somatoform disorder. Patients with these somatoform disorders make up the largest portion of "environmental victims." For those patients who ascribe their complaints to pollutants (*attribution*), the cause of their disease is already absolutely clear (*fixed disease concept*). The main symptoms of somatization disorders are in the gastrointestinal tract, while other symptoms are only secondary (see environmental poisons, p. 40).

According to depth psychology, somatization disorders may have their origins in early childhood:

1. The mother behaves toward the child in a very *possessive* and *overbearing* way, and the child (who, indeed, had been in the mother's possession during pregnancy) has no chance to separate and realize its own body (*lack of identity*).

2. Another relationship pattern exists that could be called *lack of relationship*: the child is not noticed, but is ignored or even despised. The conflicts thus created in the child are so prominent that they need to be vigorously suppressed.

It is therefore very difficult to persuade patients with somatization disorder to enter therapy. In most cases, it is better for these patients to let them hold on to their fixed disease concept, rather to confront them with psychogenic causes of their disease.

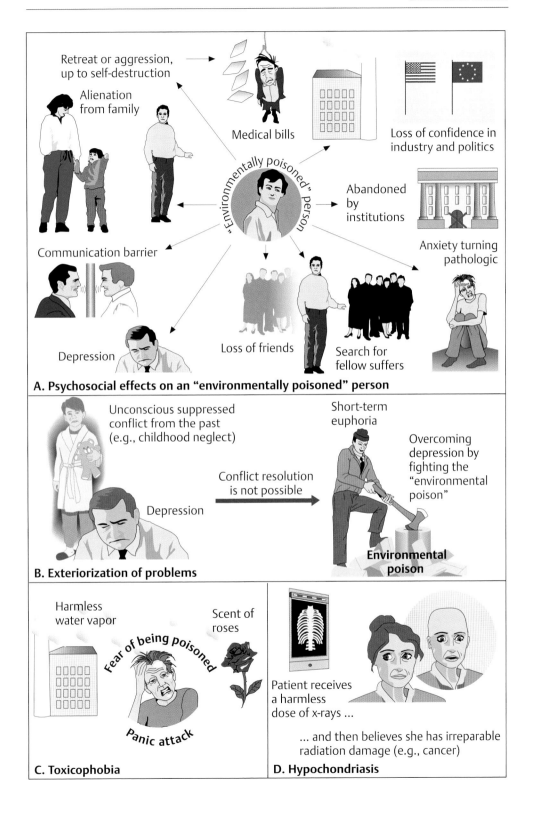

A. Psychosocial effects on an "environmentally poisoned" person

Retreat or aggression, up to self-destruction

Alienation from family

Medical bills

Loss of confidence in industry and politics

"Environmentally poisoned" person

Abandoned by institutions

Anxiety turning pathologic

Communication barrier

Depression

Loss of friends

Search for fellow suffers

B. Exteriorization of problems

Unconscious suppressed conflict from the past (e.g., childhood neglect)

Depression

Conflict resolution is not possible

Short-term euphoria

Overcoming depression by fighting the "environmental poison"

Environmental poison

C. Toxicophobia

Harmless water vapor

Scent of roses

Fear of being poisoned

Panic attack

D. Hypochondriasis

Patient receives a harmless dose of x-rays ...

... and then believes she has irreparable radiation damage (e.g., cancer)

Environmental Poisons as Causes of Disease

Patients with a psychosomatic illness adjust their symptoms to the trends of the time. They strive to present symptoms that are commonly enough observed in conventional medicine to make them plausible (see nonspecific symptoms, p. 40). It is thus possible that, time after time, these patients find a physician who confirms the somatic cause of their illness. Environmental poisons are particularly suited to being regarded as a cause of disease because it is possible to measure low doses in body media (see biomonitoring, p. 38). The patients then perceive any test results as confirmation, even when they indicate extremely low levels that would not be expected to be associated with adverse health outcomes.

Environmental Delusion

Psychotic disorders. These are defined as gross impairment in reality testing, as evidenced by delusion and hallucinations. These disorders are rare, but they are usually easy to confirm by differential diagnosis. In most cases, the diseased person suspects in an incoherent way that a certain institution or person wants to poison them. How the poison is administered is unclear and often even physically impossible. These patients are often elderly, and the delusion is singular, i.e., not associated with other psychotic disorders or disorganized behavior (**A**).

Sometimes it is difficult to distinguish psychotic disorders from somatoform disorders in individuals who are not yet delusional and who claim to have somatic reactions to the suspected administration of poison (see nonspecific symptoms, p. 40).

Organic Psychoses

Organic psychiatric disorders. These occur in individuals with genuine chronic poisoning (**B**). There are usually distinct changes in personality, such as emotional instability, aggression, tantrums, apathy, indifference, or suspicion. Furthermore, there may be disturbances of short-term and long-term memory, delirium, dementia, delusion, hallucinosis, and affective disorders. However, these disorders usually occur only after severe intoxication or during alcohol or drug withdrawal, as well as after hypoxemia or hypoglycemia. They are of a temporary nature and very distinct and pronounced. The noxious agent is usually known.

Many "environmentally poisoned" individuals claim to have such disturbances, and they are even supported by some neurologists and psychiatrists. Although there is as yet no evidence for the theory that environmental noxious agents lead to organic mental disorders, many patients find an excellent explanation for their disorders, which are often characterized as psychogenic: one is certainly mentally ill, but it is not one's own fault because one has been poisoned. A cure is impossible because one cannot avoid the noxious agent. Even if the noxious agent has actually been eliminated, the damage done is too severe and can no longer be repaired. This may take the burden off the patient. However, this interpretation may also prevent a cure by psychotherapeutic means.

Such "environmentally poisoned" patients frequently form self-help groups and become active lobbyists. They go to court and may even win their case (**C**). This does great harm to the general public, but it is the price our modern society has to pay for the increasing "chemicalization" and "energization" of our lives.

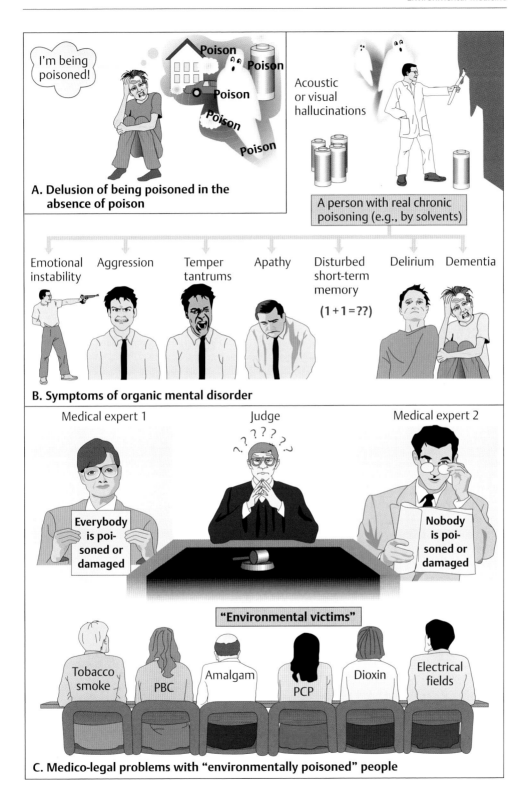

A. Delusion of being poisoned in the absence of poison

I'm being poisoned!

Poison Poison Poison Poison Poison

Acoustic or visual hallucinations

A person with real chronic poisoning (e.g., by solvents)

Emotional instability · Aggression · Temper tantrums · Apathy · Disturbed short-term memory $(1+1=??)$ · Delirium · Dementia

B. Symptoms of organic mental disorder

Medical expert 1 — Judge — Medical expert 2

Everybody is poisoned or damaged

Nobody is poisoned or damaged

"Environmental victims"

Tobacco smoke · PBC · Amalgam · PCP · Dioxin · Electrical fields

C. Medico-legal problems with "environmentally poisoned" people

■ Toxicological Evaluation

Humans are frequently exposed to environmental stresses caused by a mixture of pollutants, the toxicological evaluation of which is difficult (**A**). The specific exposure conditions leading to contact with environmental media (air, water, and soil) by means of exposure pathways (inhalation, food ingestion, skin contact) differ from case to case, which complicates the toxicological evaluation further. However, only the amount of material that has actually been taken up by an individual is of medical importance.

In recent years, numerous methods have been developed that make it possible to quantify the average risk to human health and to assess the greatest risks that may be posed by pollutants (*risk assessment*). For this purpose, toxicologically based limits, or guidance values, are used which take into account any scientific knowledge available on the mode of action and dose–response relationship of the substance in question. To prevent human exposures, such guidance values are now established for the concentration of substances, e.g., in drinking-water, in food, or in the air at the workplace (**B**). For certain substances, additional limits are established for the maximum amount that is not expected to be associated with an adverse health impact when taken up by humans, even with daily exposure over a lifetime: the *tolerable daily intake (TDI)* and the *acceptable daily intake (ADI)* are the most common terms used internationally to express these thresholds. These are based on the highest dose of the substance at which no effect is detectable in animal experiments (*no observed [adverse] effect level, NO[A]EL*). Depending on the biological significance of the substance, the uncertainty in the database on which the value is based, and on our current knowledge, certain *safety factors* are included in the limits. The better the agreement between dose–response relationship, mode of action, and toxicokinetic behavior in animals and humans, the smaller the safety factor between NO(A)EL values and ADI derived from it. Under conditions where data are derived from human exposures, a safety factor as small as 10-fold may be used. If the assessment is based on laboratory studies in animals, a safety factor of at least 100 is applied. This includes a safety factor of 10-fold to account for the possibility that humans may be more sensitive to the substance than the animal species used for testing, and an additional 10-fold safety factor because sensitivity may vary by a factor of 10 even within the human population. Exceeding guidance values, such as the ADI or TDI, is not necessarily considered dangerous to human health because of the safety factors that have been incorporated.

Epidemiology and Risk Assessment

Toxicological experiments cannot be performed in humans. Hence, both evaluation and risk assessment have to rely on experience in the workplace and on cases of poisoning. In addition to reports on individual cases about symptoms and the course of poisoning, epidemiological studies involving exposed groups versus control groups can help to uncover the toxic effects of substances. The connection between tobacco smoke and lung cancer was discovered in this way.

A quantitative risk assessment for humans based on a bioassay should include all available data, such as epidemiology, mutagenicity studies, toxicokinetics, metabolism, mode of action, and structural relationships.

Combined Action

When different substances act in the same way at their sites of action and therefore influence physiological factors in the same way, their effects may be enhanced (additively or synergistically). Inhibition of the normal elimination of one substance by another may lead to its accumulation and thus to an increased or prolonged action, e.g., inhibition of enzyme systems, or hindrance of transport processes by cell membranes (**C**).

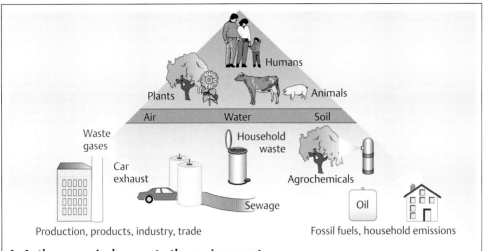

A. Anthropogenic damage to the environment

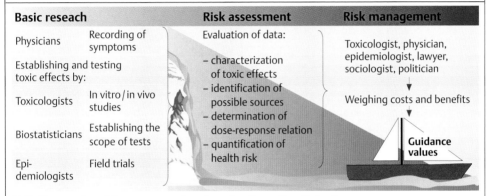

Basic reseach		Risk assessment	Risk management
Physicians	Recording of symptoms	Evaluation of data:	Toxicologist, physician, epidemiologist, lawyer, sociologist, politician
Establishing and testing toxic effects by:		– characterization of toxic effects	
Toxicologists	In vitro / in vivo studies	– identification of possible sources	Weighing costs and benefits
Biostatisticians	Establishing the scope of tests	– determination of dose-response relation	
Epi-demiologists	Field trials	– quantification of health risk	Guidance values

B. Pathways for risk assessment and evaluation of pollutants

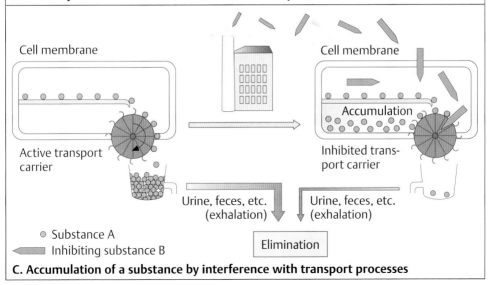

Cell membrane

Cell membrane

Accumulation

Active transport carrier

Inhibited transport carrier

Urine, feces, etc. (exhalation)

Urine, feces, etc. (exhalation)

Elimination

○ Substance A

◁▭ Inhibiting substance B

C. Accumulation of a substance by interference with transport processes

■ Air

Basics. Among the different environmental media, the air and its pollutants have been studied most intensively. Like other living organisms, humans are exposed to air right from their first breath and throughout their lifetime. Constituents of air—such as the gases naturally present (**A**) as well as particles and anthropogenic emissions—have a *direct* effect on the bronchopulmonary system. Furthermore, depending on an individual's level of physical activity, different amounts of (toxic) material may be taken up through increased breathing volumes, even if the concentration in the air remains unchanged. The pollutants may lead to functional and morphological changes in the organism, which are either acute or occur after long-term, chronic, exposure. For environmental monitoring and clean air maintenance, air pollutants are measured according to regulations and air quality standards mostly at a national level, e.g., the US National Ambient Air Quality Standards, the Clean Air Act in the United Kingdom, or the Federal Immission Control Act in Germany. Measuring stations are maintained by government agencies or authorized institutions according to established procedures described in the different national regulations and clean air legislation.

Emissions and mass transport. Airborne emissions are distributed and diluted by vertical and horizontal movements in the air. The vertical dispersion of pollutants can be prevented by transport barriers, such as inversion layers (air of uniform density and temperature). Hence, meteorological conditions with little air movement may lead to the formation of smog in the layer near the ground. The increased amounts of sulfur dioxide, nitrogen oxides, dust particles, and organic trace elements from industrial waste gas are deposited either locally or far away from the source once the flue gases have risen to higher altitudes by convection. The more persistent compounds eventually become distributed globally (e.g., tetrachloromethane). Various photochemical reactions in the atmosphere, however, degrade gaseous and particle-bound organic compounds. Reactions in the gaseous phase and at surfaces determine the chemical lifespan of a substance; a rough estimate is possible, based on the reaction mechanisms (**B**). A substance with a lifespan of more than a year is likely to become distributed globally.

Components of air pollution. Anthropogenic mass pollutants primarily include sulfur dioxide, nitrogen oxides, hydrogen chloride and hydrogen fluoride, and small dust particles. Next come organic compounds from industry and from combustion generated by domestic heating, motor vehicle traffic, power stations, and waste disposal procedures (see p. 54). Humans living in different areas are affected by very different concentrations of pollutants (**C**). Naturally occurring aerosols, pollen, and fungal spores are also a form of air pollution and facilitate airborne infections. Indoor air may be far more polluted than outdoor air as a result of various emissions that lead to disturbances in individuals' well-being and occasionally also to health problems.

Guidance values. National regulations and clean air acts such as the Federal Immission Control Act in Germany or the U.S. National Ambient Air Quality Standards have set limits for the emission and absorption of certain substances. Depending on the toxicity of a substance, different guidance values apply for short-term and long-term pollution. If a limit is exceeded temporarily, this does not necessarily mean acute danger to health. Special regulations apply to limits for certain pollutants and emitters (e.g., heavy metals, dioxins, and furans). Because of the special action mechanisms of certain substances, the aim is to minimize these substances (e.g., during production).

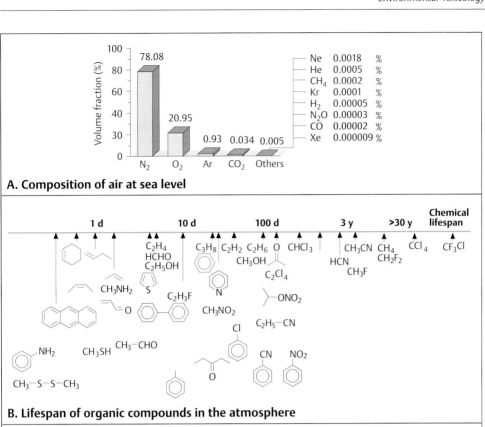

A. Composition of air at sea level

B. Lifespan of organic compounds in the atmosphere

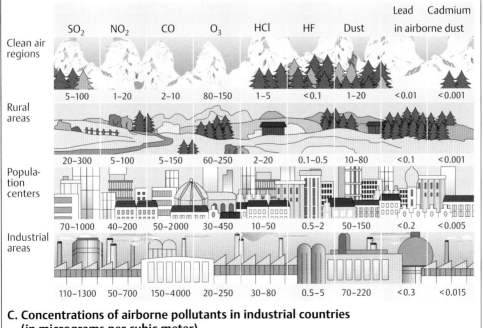

C. Concentrations of airborne pollutants in industrial countries (in micrograms per cubic meter)

Toxicology. Gaseous and particulate emissions may pose a health risk; pre-existing diseases (e.g., asthma) may intensify the symptoms. Inhaled pollutants initially affect the lungs, but other target organs and organ functions may also be affected once the uptake of foreign substances and their metabolic transformation (e.g., in the liver) have taken place (**A**).

Experimental studies have provided some ideas about threshold concentrations of certain pollutants. For example, healthy individuals showed increased flow resistance in the airways only after exposure to very high levels of SO_2 (> 14 mg/m^3 for 5 min). Asthmatic individuals were more sensitive to acute exposure, but they tolerated high SO_2 concentrations without pathological reactions when the exposure was gradual. Below 1.35 mg SO_2/m^3 (~ 0.5 ppm), no reactions were observed. In patients with a particularly sensitive response, symptoms were also observed after light physical work, cold air, cigarette smoke, and diesel exhaust. There was no evidence for synergistic or potentiating effects of different substances.

Epidemiology. Individual observations and studies on the relationship between air pollutants and diseases of the respiratory tract in industrial areas go back several decades. In most cases, concentrations of pollutants have been recorded only incompletely with respect to place and time. Furthermore, conflicting or less informative results were obtained when interfering factors were ignored in the epidemiological analyses, for example, during the causal allocation of air pollutants in retrospective studies. Influencing factors should be controlled; for example, differences in age and social situation, smoking habits, or additional exposure routes. If the study is to yield reliable results, these must be known and should be uniformly distributed over both test group and control group. Differences in the length of stay in a polluted area, or specific exposures in the workplace, distort the results. Studies have shown that the impairment of an individual's well-being cannot be correlated with specific contaminants in the outdoor air because, more often than not, the same people are also exposed to considerable indoor pollution (active and passive smoking, open fires, gas stoves, domestic heating). It has been unambiguously es-

tablished that smokers have a several-fold higher risk of dying of chronic bronchitis and asthma. Other components of indoor air, such as solvents present in paints and glues, also contribute to health problems.

Preventive measures. To limit the emission of pollutants, elaborate measures are required for clean-up of exhaust gases from motor vehicle traffic and industry, especially old plants, which represent significant local sources of emission (**B**). Highly concentrated residues must be treated separately. Indoor sources of pollutants (e.g., open fireplaces) should be eliminated, and smoking should not be permitted in public places.

Clean air control in industrialized countries. Except for oxides of nitrogen, all important pollutants (and small dust particles, in particular) have been significantly reduced in recent years (**C**). Episodes of smog, like those regularly observed in the past whenever meteorological conditions created inversion layers over population centers, have become rare in recent years (see p. 122).

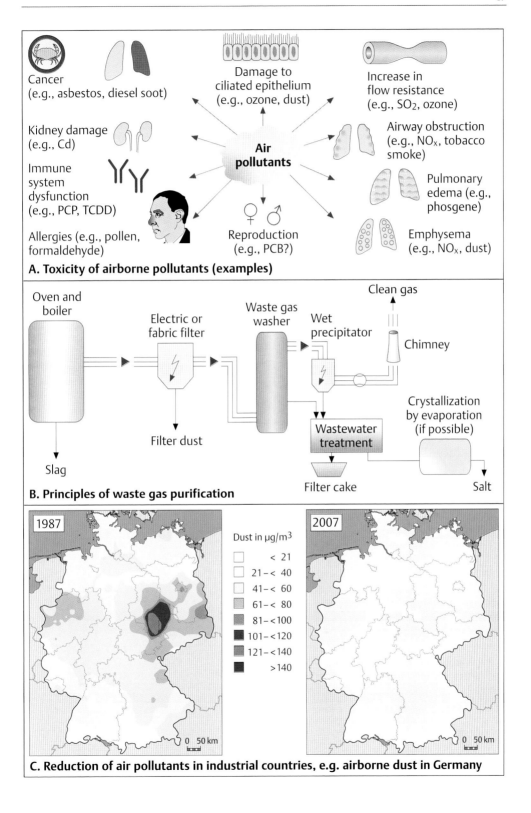

A. Toxicity of airborne pollutants (examples)

Cancer
(e.g., asbestos, diesel soot)

Kidney damage
(e.g., Cd)

Immune
system
dysfunction
(e.g., PCP, TCDD)

Allergies (e.g., pollen,
formaldehyde)

Damage to
ciliated epithelium
(e.g., ozone, dust)

**Air
pollutants**

Reproduction
(e.g., PCB?)

Increase in
flow resistance
(e.g., SO_2, ozone)

Airway obstruction
(e.g., NO_x, tobacco
smoke)

Pulmonary
edema (e.g.,
phosgene)

Emphysema
(e.g., NO_x, dust)

B. Principles of waste gas purification

Oven and
boiler

Electric or
fabric filter

Waste gas
washer

Wet
precipitator

Clean gas

Chimney

Crystallization
by evaporation
(if possible)

Wastewater
treatment

Filter dust

Slag

Filter cake

Salt

C. Reduction of air pollutants in industrial countries, e.g. airborne dust in Germany

1987

2007

Dust in $\mu g/m^3$

< 21
21 – < 40
41 – < 60
61 – < 80
81 – <100
101 – <120
121 – <140
>140

0 50 km

0 50 km

Water and Soil

Basics. Water and soil, like the air, may contain anthropogenic contaminants and thus contribute to the chemical load on humans when taken up through the skin or by mouth. Ingestion of foreign material from the soil is only possible through direct contact (or direct uptake by small children), or indirectly as a result of transfer of pollutants into foods. As an essential dietary component, drinking-water can directly contribute to acute health problems. In order to secure good water quality, governments therefore set guidance values that are usually guided by analytical detection limits for substances contained in the water. They do not necessarily represent threshold values for toxic effects.

Emission sources and pollutant pathways. Modern analytical methods have only recently uncovered many sources of water and soil pollution by foreign material. Among important sources of pollution are disused industrial sites from which harmful substances have contaminated the environment directly or by means of waste water. The closed production systems currently in use largely prevent pollution by toxic substances. Intensive agriculture is potentially dangerous because it contributes to the pollution of water and soil by using fertilizers, insecticides, and other crop protection agents. Waste disposal also contributes to pollution by generating dangerous deposits and by the inappropriate disposal of waste waters and other residues (see p. 54). Today, these residues and other legacy hazardous materials that may be hazardous to health still exist in many countries, for example, at sites formerly used as tanneries, metal refining facilities or gasoline stations. Here, health hazards may still exist when rising vapors lead to indoor pollution in residential areas due to the seepage of chemicals into the groundwater, or the presence of volatile substances in the soil. Furthermore, any air pollution contributes to increased entry of pollutants into the water and soil because dust particles and aerosols precipitate with the rain (**A**).

Constituents and their effects. The extent of any pollution with foreign material is different for groundwater and surface water. Since both of these are increasingly used as sources of drinking-water, their quality has become an important health issue. A considerable problem is the nitrate content in drinking-water, as it directly affects the health of infants. Other contaminants in the water and in the soil (mainly heavy metals, organic compounds like aromatic hydrocarbons [p. 96] and halogenated compounds) can accumulate in the human body and thus lead to chronic effects.

Preventive measures. Whenever there is a possibility that residues from agricultural food production pose a health hazard, restrictions on the use of water and soil are in order. The use of an area as a playground may also have to be restricted because of elevated levels of dangerous substances (e.g., if the soil is contaminated with heavy metals or PCDD/PCDF) (**B**). One criterion for usability may be the specification of toxicity equivalency factors (TEF) (see Glossary; and also p. 116).

Legislative measures aim at avoiding future contamination of water and soil. Currently, water treatment plants can adequately remove most foreign matter, although this diverts toxic substances into the sewage sludge (and thus often into the soil). Biological, physico-chemical, and thermal procedures for soil sanitation are expensive, but they may sometimes have to be used when there are increased concentrations of toxic substances (e.g., on old hazardous sites) which cannot be effectively removed by other means (**C**).

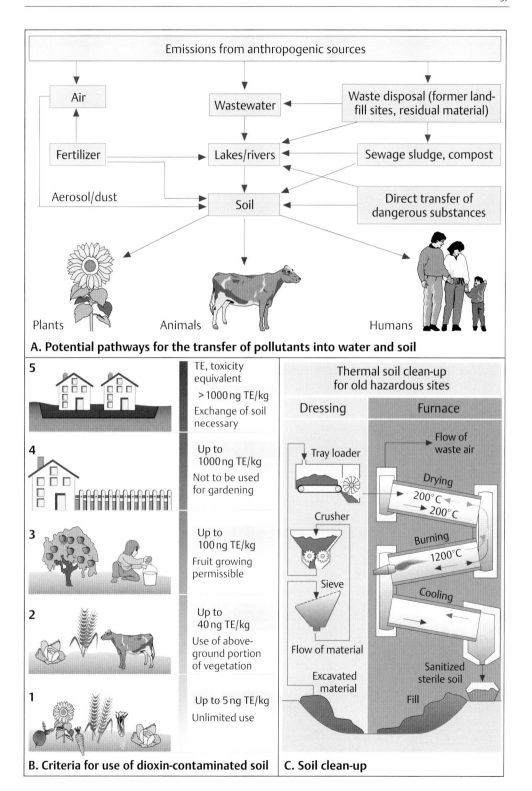

A. Potential pathways for the transfer of pollutants into water and soil

Emissions from anthropogenic sources

Air

Wastewater

Waste disposal (former land-fill sites, residual material)

Fertilizer

Lakes/rivers

Sewage sludge, compost

Aerosol/dust

Soil

Direct transfer of dangerous substances

Plants

Animals

Humans

B. Criteria for use of dioxin-contaminated soil

TE, toxicity equivalent

5 — > 1000 ng TE/kg — Exchange of soil necessary

4 — Up to 1000 ng TE/kg — Not to be used for gardening

3 — Up to 100 ng TE/kg — Fruit growing permissible

2 — Up to 40 ng TE/kg — Use of above-ground portion of vegetation

1 — Up to 5 ng TE/kg — Unlimited use

C. Soil clean-up

Thermal soil clean-up for old hazardous sites

Dressing — Furnace

Tray loader

Crusher

Sieve

Flow of material

Excavated material

Flow of waste air

Drying — 200°C — 200°C

Burning — 1200°C

Cooling

Sanitized sterile soil

Fill

◼ Waste

Basics

Ever since toxic substances like dioxins and furans (see p. 116) were detected in the flue ash of waste incineration plants, people have been equating waste disposal with health hazards caused by similar emissions. Indeed, many toxicologically important compounds find their way into municipal waste, for example, mercury from batteries and fluorescent tubes, cadmium from accumulators, and polychlorinated compounds from waste oil. The amount of municipal waste per inhabitant is about 500–700 kg per year in industrialized countries (**A**). The disposal methods themselves are also toxicologically important. This applies not only to the disposal of exhaust gas, slag, and residues from flue-gas purification (from incinerators) but also to the disposal of seepage water (from landfills).

Emissions from waste disposal (B). Although much waste can be avoided by reuse and recycling, emissions from the residual waste can only be minimized by appropriate disposal methods. Depending on the composition of the waste, foreign matter gets into the environment by emission of gas and particles or by seepage of water. To avoid any health hazards caused by waste disposal, in the future only extensively mineralized waste will be deposited in landfills. These specifications require pretreatment; so far, they can only be met by thermal procedures. Because old landfills are not sealed, many substances (including carcinogenic ones) are still being emitted even today. Future landfills must be equipped with several safety barriers. Landfill gas and seepage water must undergo treatment, and any waste that needs to be controlled, such as PCBs, hospital waste, or sewage sludge, must be collected separately. Procedures for biological–mechanical pretreatment, such as composting, are used for degrading organic components; however, since some pollutants remain in the compost unchanged, they will tend to accumulate in the soil.

Emissions from landfills and waste incineration plants contain not only carbon monoxide (like any other emission from incomplete combustion processes) but also inorganic and organic compounds as reaction products (e.g., PAK, PCB, PCDD/PCDF) (**B**). Toxicologically significant components can be determined directly in the waste gas. Carbon monoxide is used as an indicator of incomplete combustion. The dust particle content may serve as an approximate measure of the amount of unknown compounds in the waste gas, as long as these substances are nonvolatile and particle-bound.

Exposure and toxicology. The immediate surroundings of waste disposal plants may pose a human health hazard because of pollution of the air, soil, and water. The ubiquitously distributed air pollutants contribute to the contamination of food because they accumulate in plants, animal feed, and foods with high fat content, such as meat, butter, eggs, and milk (**C**). With the exception of old hazardous sites, it is assumed that modern waste disposal management ensures that the air we breath and the food we eat will not pose a health hazard. This means that in areas surrounding waste disposal plants, the concentrations of organic compounds or heavy metals in breast milk do not differ from the concentrations present elsewhere. In individual cases, it may be necessary to monitor additive effects because of other exposure pathways (e.g., ingestion of soil by children) (**C**).

Preventive measures for health protection. These include emission limits for waste disposal plants; safe storage and treatment of residues and filter dust.

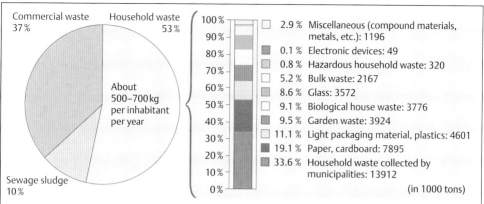

Commercial waste 37%

Household waste 53%

About 500–700 kg per inhabitant per year

Sewage sludge 10%

2.9%	Miscellaneous (compound materials, metals, etc.): 1196
0.1%	Electronic devices: 49
0.8%	Hazardous household waste: 320
5.2%	Bulk waste: 2167
8.6%	Glass: 3572
9.1%	Biological house waste: 3776
9.5%	Garden waste: 3924
11.1%	Light packaging material, plastics: 4601
19.1%	Paper, cardboard: 7895
33.6%	Household waste collected by municipalities: 13912

(in 1000 tons)

A. Composition of municipal waste in industrial countries, e.g. Germany in 2006

Landfill and sealing components

Gas flaring

CH_4 CO CO_2 NO_x

Surface sealing

Base sealing   Waste

Base sealing

Groundwater

Composting

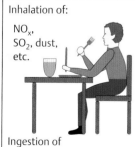

H_2S CH_4 CO_2

Modern waste incineration plant

Purified flue gas

SO_2 HF NO_x HCl

CO/CO_2 Dust particles and organic components

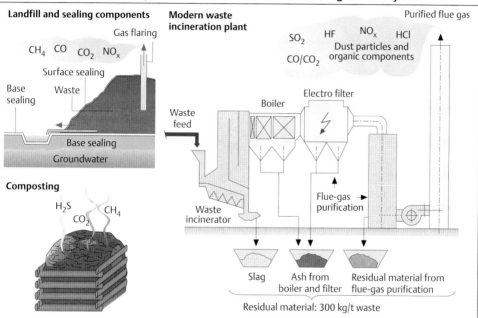

Electro filter

Boiler

Waste feed

Flue-gas purification

Waste incinerator

Slag   Ash from boiler and filter   Residual material from flue-gas purification

Residual material: 300 kg/t waste

B. Disposal processes and important emissions

Inhalation of:

NO_x, SO_2, dust, etc.

Hand-to-mouth contacts in small children

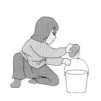

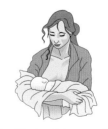

Ingestion of contaminated food (e.g., PCB)

Ingestion of contaminated soil particles up to 10 g/d (e.g., heavy metals, organic compounds)

Uptake of toxic substances with mother's milk (e.g., dioxins, furans, PCB, halogenated benzene derivatives)

C. Potential health hazards through inappropriate waste disposal

Consumer Goods

Consumer goods often contain substances that may pose a health risk. As a result of frequent contact with them, damage to human health cannot be excluded. Sources of toxic substances include building materials, furniture, floor coverings, cleaning agents, disinfectants, sealants, electronics, ceramics (e.g., aluminum compounds), jewelry (e.g., nickel), cosmetics, and smoking.

The following pollutants may be found in consumer goods (**A**):

Asbestos. This was formerly used for the reinforcement of plastics, for insulation against noise and heat, and also as a building material. Inhalation of asbestos fibers causes lung cancer or asbestosis.

Formaldehyde. This is found in particle board, wood adhesives, paints, and tobacco smoke. Frequent contact leads to mucosal irritation, headaches, and allergic reactions.

Isocyanates. These compounds are found in floor coverings and polyurethane foams. Isocyanates are considered to be allergens. Prolonged inhalation causes eye irritation, damage to the pulmonary alveoli, and isocyanate-induced asthma.

Solvents (e.g., hydrocarbons). These are used for producing adhesives, textiles, paints, and imitation leather; frequent contact leads to various health problems.

Ozone. This is produced by laser printers, for example, and causes eye irritation.

Phenols. These compounds are found in synthetic resins (e.g., on wooden toys); frequent contact induces damage to the liver and kidneys.

Polycyclic aromatic hydrocarbons. These compounds are carcinogenic and are found in tobacco smoke and combustion gas.

Polychlorinated biphenyls. They are found in PVC floor coverings and sealants; frequent contact results in damage to the liver.

Radon. This radioactive noble gas is released by certain rocks (e.g., building materials, ground under buildings). Low doses of radon are used for treating rheumatism, gout, etc. High doses, however, may induce gastrointestinal disorders and may be important in the induction of bronchial carcinoma.

To minimize the concentration of pollutants, it is important to ventilate rooms regularly. Airborne dust is a carrier of pollutants and is best removed by wet wiping; vacuum cleaning only stirs up fine dust particles.

Pollutants can also get into the body by contact of textiles with the skin. The compatibility of fabrics with skin is determined by both the fiber material and the substances used to treat the fibers (**B**). Heavy sweating or tight-fitting clothes may increase the risk of health problems due to foreign substances in textiles (e.g., contact allergies to azo dyes). **Azo dyes** are used as disperse dyes; they are suspected of giving off carcinogenic aromatic amines (e.g., benzidine). To prevent mold spots or moth damage during long-term storage, textiles are often treated with **salicylic acid, formaldehyde, inorganic salts,** or **sulfonamides.** Textiles infested by insects can be treated without chemicals by simply placing them in a domestic freezer for a day. The cold will kill the eggs and larvae. Sensitive people (e.g., allergic individuals) can avoid health problems by not wearing dyed undergarments, by washing clothes before wearing them for the first time, or by buying only clothes that are color fast. Leather garments may have been treated with **chromium salts** and **azo dyes** during tanning, or with **PCP** for preservation, although the EU does not permit such treatments. **Paraffin** emulsions render textiles waterproof, but may cause skin irritation after long-term contact.

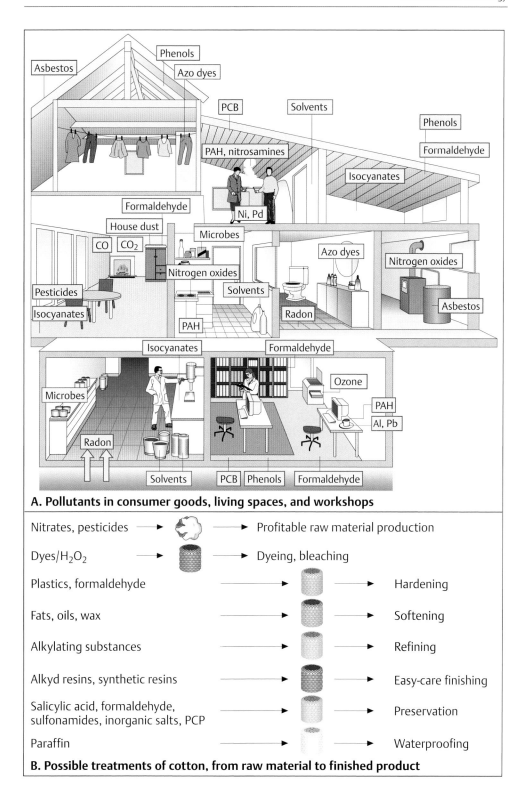

A. Pollutants in consumer goods, living spaces, and workshops

Nitrates, pesticides ⟶ ⟶ Profitable raw material production

Dyes/H_2O_2 ⟶ ⟶ Dyeing, bleaching

Plastics, formaldehyde ⟶ ⟶ Hardening

Fats, oils, wax ⟶ ⟶ Softening

Alkylating substances ⟶ ⟶ Refining

Alkyd resins, synthetic resins ⟶ ⟶ Easy-care finishing

Salicylic acid, formaldehyde, sulfonamides, inorganic salts, PCP ⟶ ⟶ Preservation

Paraffin ⟶ ⟶ Waterproofing

B. Possible treatments of cotton, from raw material to finished product

■ Risk and Epidemiology

Risk. *Absolute risk* for a group of individuals with similar exposure is the ratio of the number of disease cases to the total number of individuals in that group. *Relative risk* is the ratio of the absolute risk of the exposed group to that of the unexposed group. *Risk assessment* is the quantitative determination of possible health hazards caused by chemicals or radiation depending on activity, dose, and exposure time. *Risk evaluation* is the rating of a risk according to aspects of social acceptability and health care policies.

The insurance industry defines risk as the product of probability of occurrence and amount of damage; the calculation of insurance premiums is based on this. Whether a small damage occurs frequently or a large one rarely, the risk remains the same. Calculation of a risk often suffers from a hidden error. Just like lay people, experts are subject to "cognitive dissonance"; in other words, they do not recognize important information that interferes with established habits. For example, in 1985 NASA published a risk study for the space shuttle, according to which the probability of a crash was 1 : 100 000. Studies performed by other committees, however, assumed a risk of 1 : 270 to 1 : 57. The space shuttle actually crashed on its 25th flight.

According to recent studies, it is approximately 650 times less likely to be killed by lightning, and almost 10 times more likely to die from smoking cigarettes than it is to die from the effects of alcohol (**A**). The risk of being killed by a meteorite is greater than that of being killed in a plane crash. The probability of the earth being hit by an asteroid is extremely small, but millions of people would die; hence, the risk is enhanced.

Various risks contribute to the reduction in life expectancy: for example, in cigarette-smoking men the reduction is almost 7 years on average (**B**). Risk acceptance in the population is a complex and incalculable phenomenon:

1. Rare dangers (e.g., snake bites) are overrated, whereas common threats (e.g., death by myocardial infarction due to overweight and lack of exercise) are underestimated.

2. Probabilities are incorrectly assessed (e.g., some people are frightened of flying but never

of driving a car, although driving is more dangerous than flying).

3. People overestimate their own capabilities (e.g., they believe they are immune to disease, or will live a long live).

4. Habits that are believed to be controllable are ignored despite their obvious risks (e.g., smoking, or drinking alcohol).

5. Matters that are believed to be beyond one's own control cause anxiety (e.g., special landfill sites, or toxic substances in foods).

Epidemiology. This investigates the frequency of diseases, the physiological variables and social consequences of disease in human populations, and also the factors influencing these frequencies.

A minimum number of pathological cases is required in order to establish statistically significant risks (**C**). When the spontaneous rate of individual malformations in the population is 0.05%, an 80-fold increase in risk becomes recognizable with 4 pathological cases out of 100 children exposed in the womb; with 400 exposed children, only a 20-fold increase in risk is required for the same number of cases. By contrast, with a malformation rate of 0.8% (e.g., heart defects), a 9-fold increase in risk becomes apparent, with 7 pathological cases out of 100 exposed children, and a 3-fold increase in risk implies 13 pathological cases out of 400 exposed children.

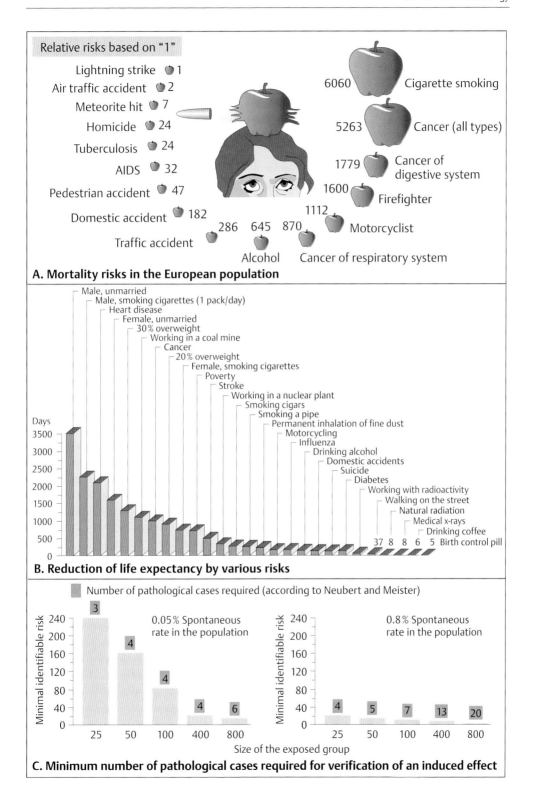

Relative risks based on "1"

Lightning strike 1
Air traffic accident 2
Meteorite hit 7
Homicide 24
Tuberculosis 24
AIDS 32
Pedestrian accident 47
Domestic accident 182
Traffic accident 286 645 870

6060 Cigarette smoking
5263 Cancer (all types)
1779 Cancer of digestive system
1600 Firefighter
1112 Motorcyclist
Alcohol Cancer of respiratory system

A. Mortality risks in the European population

Male, unmarried
Male, smoking cigarettes (1 pack/day)
Heart disease
Female, unmarried
30 % overweight
Working in a coal mine
Cancer
20 % overweight
Female, smoking cigarettes
Poverty
Stroke
Working in a nuclear plant
Smoking cigars
Smoking a pipe
Permanent inhalation of fine dust
Motorcycling
Influenza
Drinking alcohol
Domestic accidents
Suicide
Diabetes
Working with radioactivity
Walking on the street
Natural radiation
Medical x-rays
Drinking coffee
37 8 8 6 5 Birth control pill

Days
3500
3000
2500
2000
1500
1000
500
0

B. Reduction of life expectancy by various risks

Number of pathological cases required (according to Neubert and Meister)

Minimal identifiable risk
240
200
160
120
80
40
0

3
4
4
4
6

0.05 % Spontaneous rate in the population

25 50 100 400 800

Minimal identifiable risk
240
200
160
120
80
40
0

4
5
7
13
20

0.8 % Spontaneous rate in the population

25 50 100 400 800

Size of the exposed group

C. Minimum number of pathological cases required for verification of an induced effect

Ecotoxicology

Ecotoxicology is the science concerned with predicting the actions and interactions of environmental chemicals in existing ecosystems. In toxicology, human health has top priority, but ecotoxicology focuses on protecting the structure and function of ecosystems and on protecting endangered species.

Although many chemical substances are known to cause specific damage to human health, in many cases rigid criteria have not yet been established for assessing their effect on the environment. Problems still exist regarding the following issues (**A**): How significant are the effects observed in single organisms for the total population? Do laboratory results apply for conditions in the field? Do results obtained for certain animal species apply for other species?

The most important characteristics for evaluating the harmfulness of a substance (*environmental hazard potential*) include:
- knowledge of its distribution in air and water, or in water and soil/sediment
- mobility
- accumulation
- biological availability
- metabolism
- dose–response relationship.

Ecotoxicological tests are performed both in vitro and in vivo, to estimate the hazard potential of a chemical on the environment or on ecosystems; e.g., controlled tests at the cellular and subcellular levels (e.g., enzyme tests), tests on single species (e.g., altered swimming behavior in fish, or reduced reproduction of daphnia and algae), and controlled multispecies tests, including observations on the environment (**B**). In-vitro procedures offer several advantages: they are easy to reproduce, they are standardized, and they are highly effective in terms of objective and costs. For evaluating the risks of environmental hazards, however, in-vivo experiments are essential.

For estimating the *no observed effect concentration* (NOEC), the activity of enzymes (e.g., ATPase) is studied, e.g., in fish after acute and chronic exposure to environmental chemicals (e.g., PCBs).

Organisms used to predict the hazard potential of chemicals in environmental media include midges (*Chironomus riparius*) for sediments, springtails (*Collembola*) for the forest floor, and earthworms (*Lumbricus*) for agricultural land.

To estimate the effect of environmental chemicals, extrapolation factors are used (**C**); e.g., the hazardous concentration (HC; ecologically acceptable concentration) and the level of concern (LOC; concentration of a chemical at which damage to the population in the field is expected). Extrapolation is done on the basis of NOEC data from field ecosystems and from single-species tests. When there are at least three chronic NOEC values, the lowest NOEC is divided by a safety factor of 10. When there are only data on lethal or effective concentrations (LC_{50}/EC_{50}) for fish, invertebrates, and algae, or only one value of the acute test (LD_{50}/ED_{50}) in only one species, a safety factor of 100 or 1000 must be used. The aim of the procedure is absolute protection of the organisms at a specific concentration in the environment.

Ecoterrorism

Ecoterrorism is the deliberate targeting and damaging of ecosystems. For example, the calculated flaring of petroleum causes severe soot formation in the atmosphere and therefore damages the micro- and macroflora and -fauna (e.g., during the 1991 Iraq War). Deliberate discharge of oil, chemicals, or radioactivity into the sea destroys aquatic and terrestrial ecosystems (**D**).

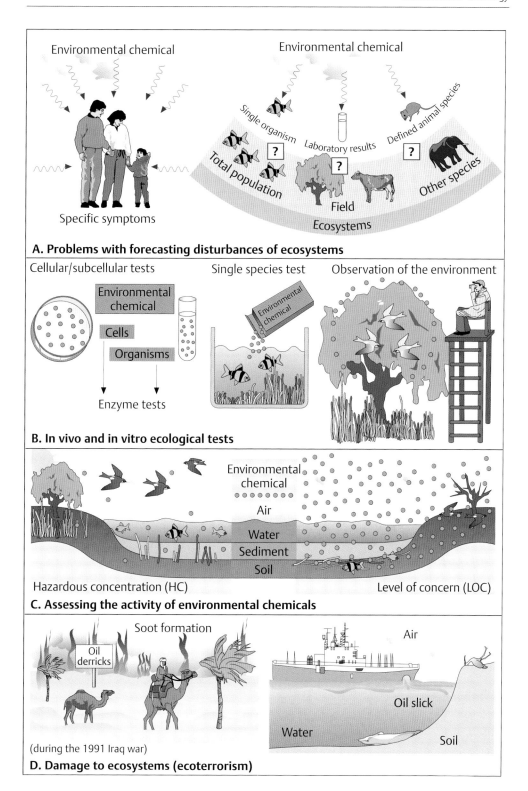

A. Problems with forecasting disturbances of ecosystems

Environmental chemical

Environmental chemical

Specific symptoms

Single organism

Laboratory results

Defined animal species

Total population

Field

Other species

Ecosystems

B. In vivo and in vitro ecological tests

Cellular/subcellular tests

Single species test

Observation of the environment

Environmental chemical

Cells

Organisms

Enzyme tests

Environmental chemical

C. Assessing the activity of environmental chemicals

Environmental chemical

Air

Water

Sediment

Soil

Hazardous concentration (HC)

Level of concern (LOC)

D. Damage to ecosystems (ecoterrorism)

Soot formation

Oil derricks

Air

Oil slick

Water

Soil

(during the 1991 Iraq war)

Toxic Substances in Foods

Native Toxins

These include all naturally occurring constituents of plants and animals that may be harmful to human health when ingested. Based on experience over thousands of years, humans have selected from the rich offerings of nature the foods most suitable for their nutrition. Food for adults therefore usually contains harmless amounts of native toxins. However, toxic effects may be observed in children, or in elderly, sick, or very sensitive individuals. Native toxins are found in food derived from plants (**A**) as well as animals (**B**).

Native toxins in plants. These include hemagglutinins in beans and cereals, saponins in red beets and asparagus, and oxalic acid in rhubarb and spinach. Bitter almonds contain the cyanogenic glycoside amygdalin, green potatoes contain solanin, and liquorice (made from the glycyrrhiza plant) contains glycyrrhetic acid (**A**). Many of these toxins are degraded by traditional methods of preparation, such as washing, soaking, cooking, etc. Phytic acid (in wheat) is degraded by prolonged fermentation of the dough when baking bread (a method rarely used today) (**C**). The essential vitamins A and D may also act as native toxins when larger amounts are consumed (hypervitaminosis).

Native toxins in animals. Depending on what the animals normally eat, native toxins occur in almost all bivalve mollusks (saxitoxin), some shrimp (anatoxin A), and fish from the Pacific Ocean, e.g., ocean perch (maitotoxin complex) (**B**). Most of these substances are produced by microorganisms (mainly dinoflagellates) that live in or on the host organism. Anatoxin originates from the cyanobacterium *Anabaena flosaquae*. In case of doubt, the only protection is not to eat these foods.

Anthropogenic Toxic Substances

These substances may get into food by spoiling or through unsuitable preparation methods (**D**). Incorrect storage is responsible for the presence of the following toxins in food: mold metabolites (aflatoxins) from some *Aspergillus* species, bacterial toxins from salmonellae, and the very poisonous botulinum toxin from *Clostridium botulinum*. Anthropogenic toxic substances, such as benzopyrene (in smoked and barbecued food), heated and oxidized fats, and heavy metals released from unsuitable cooking pots or water pipes, may finally be taken up by humans (bioaccumulation) (**D**). Food additives, such as food coloring agents (tartrazine), preservatives (nitrite pickling salt, sulfur), acidifying agents (phosphates), flavoring agents, emulsifiers, antioxidants, thickening and gelatinizing agents, are added to food for technological and cosmetic reasons.

Anthropogenic toxic substances in foods also include residues from fertilizers (nitrates), pharmaceuticals (antibiotics), and plant protection agents (pesticides) from agriculture and forestry, and also constituents of waste gas, municipal wastes, and waste water from private households, traffic, and industry (**D**).

No harmful effects on human health from genetically modified (GM) foods, such as tomatoes, potatoes, baker's yeast, and products manufactured from these (novel foods) (see p. 214), have been documented. The same holds true for food irradiation. Irradiation of food is prohibited in Germany but in some EU countries it is used for seven groups of food, including dried herbs and spices, cereal flakes, legumes, dried fruit and vegetables, shrimp, poultry meat, and gum arabic. The permissible concentrations of most anthropogenic toxic substances in food are subject to legislation in many countries. By contrast, in many other jurisdictions guidance values exist only for many heavy metals, and often even these are not legally binding.

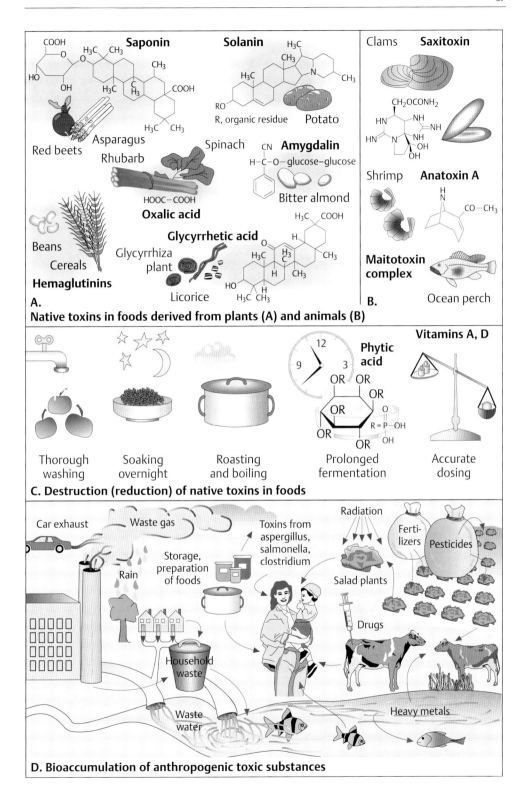

Saponin

COOH

HO

OH

Red beets

Asparagus

Rhubarb

Beans

Cereals

Hemaglutinins

A.

Solanin

R, organic residue

Spinach

Amygdalin

H—C—O—glucose–glucose

Bitter almond

Oxalic acid

HOOC—COOH

Glycyrrhetic acid

Glycyrrhiza plant

Licorice

Potato

Clams   Saxitoxin

CH₂OCONH₂

Shrimp   Anatoxin A

Maitotoxin complex

B.   Ocean perch

Native toxins in foods derived from plants (A) and animals (B)

Thorough washing

Soaking overnight

Roasting and boiling

Phytic acid

OR

OR

OR

OR

OR

OR

R = P—OH

Prolonged fermentation

Vitamins A, D

Accurate dosing

C. Destruction (reduction) of native toxins in foods

Car exhaust

Waste gas

Storage, preparation of foods

Rain

Household waste

Waste water

Toxins from aspergillus, salmonella, clostridium

Radiation

Ferti-lizers

Pesticides

Salad plants

Drugs

Heavy metals

D. Bioaccumulation of anthropogenic toxic substances

▨ Basics

The advent of the personal computer and access to the Internet has made important toxicology information easily accessible to everyone.

Poison Control Centers

These centers offer help with toxicological problems at the workplace and in the home, including those caused by food and consumer goods, environmental factors, and pharmaceutical products. Poison control centers can usually be reached by telephone 24 hours a day (**A**). The following link provides access to the "WHO world directory of poisons centers (Yellow Tox)" of the International Program on Chemical Safety (IPCS): www.who.int/ipcs/poisons/centre/directory/en/. Clicking on the country in question takes you to a list of all poison centers, with full address and contact details.

For nonacute problems, information on the toxicity of chemical compounds, their action, and the necessary first aid and poison control measures can be found in extensive databases. They are available in printed form, on electronic media (CD-ROM), or online. Some of these databases are listed below.

Databases in Printed Form

Many sources of information are available internationally on the toxicology of a wide range of substances. These sources include, for example, databases compiled by the European Union (e. g., ECDIN, European Chemicals Data and Information Network); by the US federal government, including the Environmental Protection Agency (EPA) or the National Institute of Occupational Safety and Health (NIOSH) (e.g., RTECS, Registry of Toxic Effects of Chemical Substances); or by worldwide organizations, such as the World Health Organization (WHO) (e.g., publications of the International Agency for Research on Cancer, IARC) or the United Nations (e.g., IRPTC, the International Register of Potentially Toxic Chemicals). These databases are available in printed form or on electronic media.

Online Databases

These provide up-to-date information that is often not available in printed form. Examples of these online services are:

- for toxicology, environmental health, and chemical database, www.toxnet.nlm.nih.gov
- for health and human services, www.healthfinder.gov
- for chemical safety information from an intergovernmental organization, www.inchem.org
- for information from the Canadian Centre for Occupational Health and Safety, www.ccohs.ca
- for information from the European Medicines Agency (EMEA), www.emea.europa.eu
- for information from Health Technology Assessment International, www.htai.org
- for general health information, www.who.int

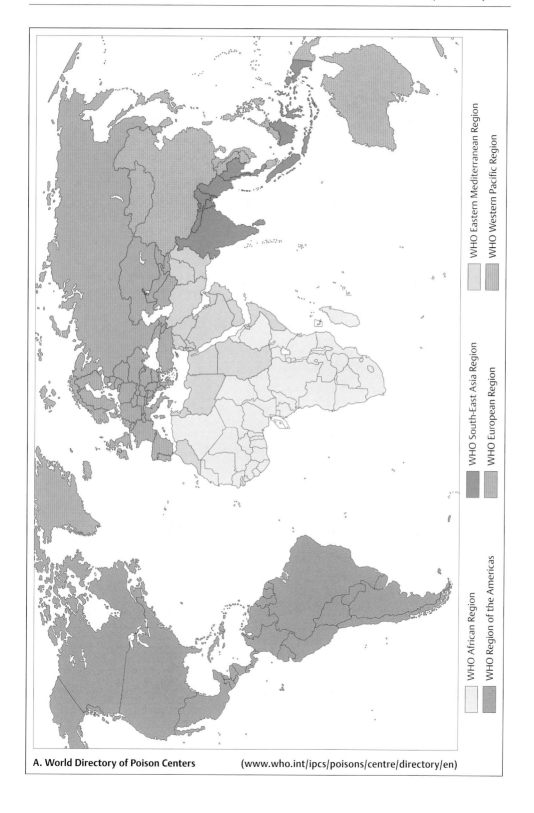

A. World Directory of Poison Centers   (www.who.int/ipcs/poisons/centre/directory/en)

WHO Eastern Mediterranean Region

WHO Western Pacific Region

WHO South-East Asia Region

WHO European Region

WHO African Region

WHO Region of the Americas

Applied Toxicology

▪ Alkaloids

Atropine

The tertiary nitrogen compound atropine (**A**) is a pharmaceutical drug used as an antidote for poisoning with parathion (E605). It is also used as an anticholinergic, bronchodilator, antispasmodic, antiparkinsonian, and mydriatic.

Atropine is potentially deadly. Eating as few as 3–5 berries of the deadly nightshade *Atropa belladonna* (**A**) can kill a child, and 10–20 berries are lethal for adults. Especially in children, intoxication is frequently caused when medication is confused with eye drops containing atropine. Nevertheless, lethal incidents are rare despite the dramatic symptoms, thanks to the characteristic symptoms of poisoning, the wide therapeutic window (or index), and the excellent treatment options.

The alkaloid hyoscyamine (see p. 268) undergoes racemization into atropine, and this explains why the two compounds lead to similar symptoms of poisoning. Hyoscyamine is found in several species of the nightshade family (see p. 268).

Signs of intoxication. Typical symptoms of poisoning (**B**) include parasympatholytic (anticholinergic) peripheral and central effects, depending on the dose of atropine administered. A dose of 0.5–1.0 mg causes mild bradycardia, dry mouth and skin, and minor dilatation of the pupils. Doses of 2.0 mg and more result in tachycardia, accelerated pulse, intense thirst, mydriasis, and impaired accommodation. With doses of 5.0 mg and more, the above symptoms are more pronounced, and the inhibition of glandular secretion results in hoarseness, difficulty in swallowing, and impaired speech; restlessness and headache are also observed, and body temperature may rise (hyperthermia) as the result of impaired sweat secretion. Because of disturbed regulation, the skin appears dry, hot, and bright red, especially in the face. Effects on the intestinal muscles manifest themselves as reduced intestinal peristalsis (obstipation) and lack of tonus, and/or effect on the genitourinary tract as voiding difficulties leading to urinary retention. Doses of 10 mg and more have additional effects on the central nervous system, such as restlessness, clonic spasms,

frenzy, confusion, delirium, and hallucination. This phase of excitement may turn into a state of exhaustion associated with deep unconsciousness. Death occurs as the result of central respiratory paralysis.

Above a dose of 1.5 mg/kg BW, atropine is life-threatening to adults. A dose of 10–20 mg/kg BW is definitely fatal; the lethal dose for children is 1–10 mg/kg BW.

Therapy. The initial treatment of atropine poisoning (**C**) consists of general measures, such as gastric lavage and administration of activated charcoal to prevent further absorption of the poison. In addition, the vital functions of respiration, body temperature, and micturition must be maintained by artificial respiration, thermolytic physical measures (e.g., a cold bath), and forced diuresis by means of a bladder catheter. Oral and ocular mucosae need to be moistened. Small IV doses of benzodiazepines (diazepam) or short-acting barbiturates are administered for sedation. The indirect parasympathomimetic physostigmine salicylate is considered the most effective antidote. This cholinesterase inhibitor can abolish the peripheral symptoms and, unlike pyridostigmine and neostigmine, also the central symptoms. It is administered by means of IM injection or slow IV infusion at a dose of 0.5–2.0 mg/kg BW for adults and 0.02 mg/kg BW for children. Since the antagonist is rapidly metabolized, one repeat administration of 1 mg/20 min (preferably as a brief infusion) is indicated if there is prolonged decrease in vigilance.

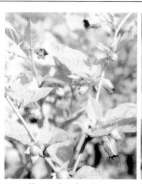

Deadly nightshade
(*Atropa belladonna*)

Ripe berry

Tropine

Tropic acid

Atropine
(alkaloid)

A. Occurrence of atropine

Peripheral symptoms

Dry mouth, thirst, difficulty swallowing, hoarseness (inhibition of glandular secretion)

Tachycardia (initially often mild bradycardia)

Hyperthermia

Dry, red, hot skin

Obstipation

Urinary retention

Central symptoms

– Restlessness, frenzy, confusion, hallucination
– Clonic spasms
– Coma
– Respiratory depression
– Death by respiratory paralysis

Mydriasis and impaired accommodation

Normal eye

B. Acute toxicity of atropine

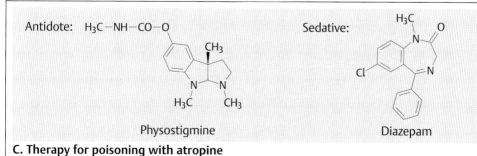

Antidote: H₃C—NH—CO—O

Physostigmine

Sedative:

Diazepam

C. Therapy for poisoning with atropine

Colchicine

The alkaloid of the meadow saffron *Colchicum autumnale* (**A**) is a mitotic poison. It is also the drug of choice for treating acute attacks of gout. Most cases of poisoning are therefore not caused by accidental ingestion of seeds and leaves but by therapeutic overdosage.

The lethal dose is 20 mg colchicine (5 g of seeds) for adults and 5 mg (1.25 g of seeds) for children.

Signs of intoxication. The symptom-free latency period lasts for up to 6 hours after ingestion. It is followed by acute symptoms of poisoning (**B**), such as gastrointestinal problems (bloody diarrhea, colicky abdominal pain, nausea, and vomiting). Cholera-like diarrhea with vomiting is accompanied by symptoms that manifest themselves first in the mouth and throat as a scratchy feeling, burning, and difficulty in swallowing, and then as a choking feeling and cyanosis (**C**). Later in the course of poisoning, the symptoms include bone marrow depression, blood clotting disorders, kidney damage, hepatonecrosis, dehydration, electrolyte imbalances, generalized spasms, and ascending paralysis. Death occurs after 2 or 3 days due to cardiac arrest, respiratory failure, or sepsis.

Therapy. Emergency procedures include detoxification by induction of vomiting, administration of activated charcoal, and gastric lavage. To interrupt enterohepatic cycling, an indwelling duodenal catheter is used for continuous aspiration of the duodenal juice. Plasma volume expanders are administered for shock treatment.

Morphine and Opioids

These drugs (**D**) have a central stimulant action and are potent analgesics. Because of the potential risk of causing addiction, they are subject to national drug regulations, e.g., the Controlled Substances Act in the United States.

Signs of intoxication. The cardinal symptoms of acute poisoning (**E**) include extreme miosis, somnolence or coma, and respiratory depression (2–4 breaths/min). The central respiratory paralysis (hypoxia) usually observed after 7–12 h is often preceded by Cheyne–Stokes respiration and cyanosis. Furthermore, there are symptoms of circulatory collapse, hypotension, bradycardia, hypothermia, loss of tone, areflexia, flush, and pulmonary edema. Plasma concentrations of 0.1 mg/L and higher are toxic, and concentrations above 0.5 mg/L are dangerous. The lethal dose of morphine in adults is >0.1 g after parenteral application and 0.3–1.5 g after oral application (maximum daily dose 200 mg). Infants are much more sensitive (lethal dose 30 mg).

Chronic morphine poisoning (**E**) is called *morphinism*, a state of physical and emotional dependence. Opioid addicts suffer from spastic obstipation and disturbed micturition, and they have constricted ("pinpoint") pupils. Characteristic changes also include weight loss, impotence, all kinds of infections, and physical and mental deterioration.

Therapy. In acute cases of poisoning with morphine or its derivatives (as well as synthetic opioid analogs such as pethidine, methadone, and pentazocine), emergency procedures include artificial ventilation with oxygen and shock treatment. Administration of the specific antidote naloxone hydrochloride (0.4 mg/mL) (**D**) is used to counteract oxygen deprivation as quickly as possible. Intravenous application of this short-acting opioid antagonist abolishes the central depressant and peripheral effects of opioids within minutes. The initial dose is 0.4 mg IV or IM (for children 10 µg/kg BW) every 2–3 min until the respiratory depression ceases and a maximum dose of 2–4 mg in total is reached. Since morphine antagonists trigger life-threatening withdrawal symptoms in morphine addicts (ventricular fibrillation, collapse), the dose of the antagonist in such cases should be reduced and the dosage interval shortened. Stimulation of central α_2-receptors by clonidine (17 µg/kg BW per day) diminishes the norepinephrine-mediated withdrawal symptoms.

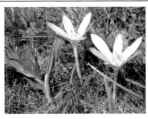

Meadow saffron
(Colchicum autumnale)

Colchicine (alkaloid)

A. Occurrence of colchicine

Burning, scratching, difficulty swallowing

Hepatonecrosis, hepatic failure

Kidney damage

Colic, hemorrhagic enteritis, diarrhea resembling cholera (dehydration, loss of electrolytes)

Death
Cardiac arrest, respiratory failure, sepsis, respiratory paralysis

Granulocytopenia, thrombocytopenia

Blood-clotting disorders (intravascular coagulation)

Shock (cardiovascular disorder, coma)

Spasms, ascending paralysis, myopathy, cardiac insufficiency, dyspnea (cyanosis)

In persons surviving the poisoning: hair falling out after 10–14 days

B. Acute toxicity of colchicine

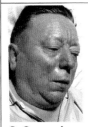

C. Cyanosis

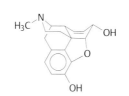

D.   Morphine

Antidote:

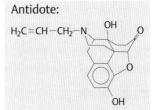

Naloxone

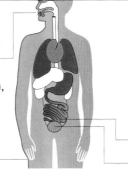

Acute toxicity

Somnolence ⟶ coma

Extreme miosis

Respiratory depression

Cyanosis ⟶ hypoxia ⟶ respiratory arrest

Shock ⟶ hypotension, bradycardia, pulmonary edema

Loss of tone of skeletal muscles, areflexia

Hypothermia

Chronic toxicity

Narrow pupils (miosis)

Normal eye   Miosis

Infections, impotence, weight loss, physical and mental deterioration

Spastic obstipation

Disturbed micturition

E. Toxicity of morphine

71

Ergot Alkaloids

These mycotoxins occur in the sclerotium (**A**) of the ergot fungus *Claviceps purpurea*, which grows as a parasite in the ears of cereal plants, especially rye (*Secale cereale*). The isolated alkaloids are used as pharmaceuticals for treating circulatory disorders, headaches, and migraine, and for stopping postpartum hemorrhages.

In medieval times, epidemic mass poisonings with ergot-contaminated rye frequently caused *ergotism*, associated with gangrene and central nervous system disorders. Peripheral vasoconstriction caused hands and feet to die off, with dry gangrene accompanied by burning pain.

Signs of intoxication. The most potent of these vasoconstrictive alkaloids is ergotamine (**B**), a derivative of lysergic acid (see p. 92). Acute poisoning by ingestion is characterized by nausea, vomiting, abdominal pain, diarrhea, paresthesia (tingling in fingers and toes), coldness and numbness in the extremities, and central nervous system symptoms, such as headache, vertigo, anxiety, spasms, dyspnea, and mydriasis (**C**). Exceeding the *maximum daily dose* of ergotamine (> 10 mg) results in circulatory collapse and unconsciousness. Respiratory paralysis and cardiac arrest may then lead to death. As a result of long-term use at high dosage (*chronic poisoning*), irreversible vascular damage occurs, thus leading to gangrenous tissue (**C**). However, this occurs only after extensive vasospasms, ischemia, necrosis, and endothelial damage associated with thrombus formation.

Therapy. Treatment of acute poisoning after ingestion consists of eliminating the poison by administration of activated charcoal, gastric lavage with sodium sulfate, and hemostatic measures, such as dextran infusion and heparin administration. Arterial vasospasms associated with ergotism are treated with organic nitrites (e.g., amyl nitrite), nitroglycerine (0.4 mg sublingually), or papaverine (30–60 mg IM or IV). In case of spasms, diazepam (5–10 mg IV) is used as an effective anticonvulsive. Respiratory paralysis should be counterbalanced by artificial respiration.

Physostigmine (Eserine)

Calabar beans (**D**), the seeds of the West African legume *Physostigma venenosum*, contain 0.1 % of this alkaloid (**E**). As an indirect parasympathomimetic, this carbamate is used in ophthalmology as a topical solution (0.25–1 %) for treating glaucoma, and also for treating atonic intestine and bladder, and myasthenia gravis. Its salicylate derivative is used in toxicology as a systemic antidote for atropine poisoning (see p. 68), and also as an antagonist to antidepressants, tricyclic antihistamines, and curare. Its acute toxicity in humans is high, and poisoning frequently occurs from cholinesterase inhibitors used as insecticides and also as a result of antidote overdosage. The lethal dose is 6–10 mg after ingestion, but less following parenteral application.

Signs of intoxication. By inhibiting cholinesterase, the availability of neurotransmitters at cholinergic nerve endings, ganglia, and motor endplates is increased. The resulting symptoms of muscarinic and nicotinic receptor activation manifest themselves in salivation, nausea, vomiting, and diarrhea due to intestinal irritation and inhibition of cardiac function. Characteristic symptoms include fascicular and fibrillar muscle twitches (**F**), which persist long after the poisoning. Physostigmine is a tertiary amine that can penetrate into the central nervous system where it has a cholinomimetic effect. Overdosage therefore results also in central symptoms, such as spasms, delirium, coma, and cyanosis; death finally occurs due to respiratory failure, triggered by severe bronchial secretion and constriction and, ultimately, central respiratory paralysis.

Therapy. Treatment primarily consists of eliminating the poison by means of gastric lavage and activated charcoal. Parenteral application of the antidote atropine sulfate (1–2 mg IM, using a 10 mg/mL solution) (see p. 69) is effective against the peripheral muscarine-like symptoms, and diazepam is effective in controlling spasms. Artificial respiration is used when respiratory paralysis sets in.

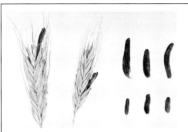

A. Ergot *(Secale cereale)*

Ergot alkaloids:
Synonyms:
– secale alkaloids
– indole alkaloids

Basic structure
and cyclic
peptide portion

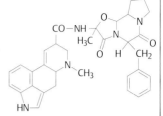

B. Ergotamine

| Acute toxicity |

Headache, vertigo, nausea,
vomiting, tonic-clonic seizures,
anxiety, confusion, paresthesia,
dyspnea, paralysis,
unconsciousness, respiratory
paralysis

Mydriasis

Cardiac arrest

Abdominal pain,
diarrhea

Vasoconstriction,
coldness or numbness in limbs,
endothelial damage (→ thrombus)

C. Toxicity of Ergotamine

| Chronic toxicity |

Convulsions
(convulsive ergotism)

Vascular spasms, ischemia,
necrosis

Gangrene in limbs,
later also in brain and coronaries
(gangrenous ergotism)

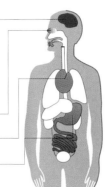

Gangrene
of the nose
and right
auricle

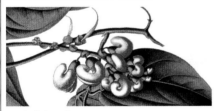

D. Calabar beans

$H_3C-NH-CO-O$

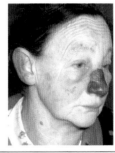

E. Physostigmine

Peripheral symptoms

Salivation,
nausea,
vomiting,
diarrhea,
muscle twitching
(fibrillar, fascicular)

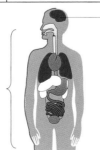

Central symptoms

Delirium,
spasms,
coma,
cyanosis,
respiratory paralysis

F. Acute toxicity of physostigmine

▓ Barbiturates

These drugs are frequently abused because they are potentially addictive and may also be used as a means of committing suicide. Barbiturate-containing hypnotics and sedatives with a limited therapeutic window have therefore been largely replaced by benzodiazepines (**A**). In the context of intoxication with sleeping pills, this has resulted in a decline in both the severity and frequency of poisonings with this group of drugs.

Signs of intoxication. The typical symptoms of acute poisoning include confusion and unconsciousness (isoelectric EEG, **B**), areflexia, dilated and unresponsive pupils, tissue hypoxia due to central respiratory depression, acidosis, a drop in blood pressure, hypothermia, and renal insufficiency. Death may occur by central respiratory paralysis or, after 2–4 days, as the result of secondary disorders (failure of heart, circulation, or kidney), bronchopneumonia, or shock lung (**C**). Toxic plasma concentrations are reached at 5–20 mg/L, and concentrations of 50–100 mg/L are lethal; more than 5–10 g is a lethal dose.

Therapy. Initial treatment of the symptoms of severe poisoning consists of artificial respiration and treatment of shock. Rapid excretion of barbiturates is facilitated by forced diuresis and simultaneous alkalization of the urine through sodium bicarbonate infusion, and also by hemodialysis or hemoperfusion. After endotracheal intubation, gastric lavage may be performed within 24 h after ingestion to remove nonabsorbed poison. Subsequent instillation of 30 g activated charcoal followed by saline laxative (15 g sodium sulfate) will promote further detoxification.

Barbiturate addiction is *chronic intoxication*; it occurs when normal doses are exceeded by a factor of 15. Abrupt withdrawal may lead to seizures and psychosis; the dose should therefore be slowly reduced in hospital.

▓ Benzodiazepines

Therapeutic doses may lead to physical and emotional dependence after 10–14 days (*low dose dependence*). These tranquilizers are therefore subject to drug regulations. Some authorities have argued that the increase in human suicidal poisonings from 13% to 16% in the 1990s was due to the introduction of benzodiazepine analogues.

Signs of intoxication. Acute poisoning manifests itself in symptoms that are characterized by dizziness, ataxia, confusion, and coma (**D**).

Symptoms of *chronic intoxication* include indolence (indifference, lack of interest). The patient may be in a bad mood, irritable, and have a tendency to aggressive outbursts. Agitation, confusion, anxiety, and insomnia are some of the *paradoxical* consequences of continuous use (**D**).

The toxic dose is 1–3 mg/kg BW. Fatal poisoning due to ingestion of up to 1 g of benzodiazepines has not been described in the literature because of the wide therapeutic window of these drugs. However, synergistic interactions with other central depressive pharmaceuticals and alcohol have been described. The main danger of such severe polydependencies lies in central respiratory depression, unconsciousness, and areflexia accompanied by toxic shock syndrome.

Therapy. Emergency measures: stabilization of vital signs by artificial respiration and circulatory support, and monitoring of pulse rate and blood pressure. In hospital, the central depressive action of benzodiazepines is counteracted by administering the specific antagonist flumazenil. The initial dose is 0.2 mg IV within 15 s. This is followed by further injection of single doses of 0.1 mg at intervals of 60 s. If needed, this is repeated up to a maximum dose of 1 mg flumazenil. The usual dose is in the range of 0.3–0.6 mg. It is important to note that the half-life of the antagonist is less than 1 h, thus making follow-up injections necessary when treating intoxication with long-acting benzodiazepines. Gastric lavage and activated charcoal may suffice in less life-threatening situations.

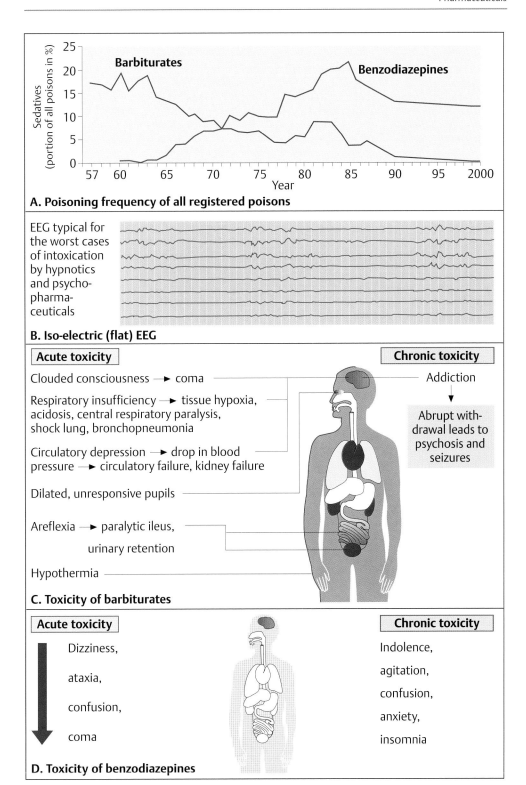

A. Poisoning frequency of all registered poisons

EEG typical for the worst cases of intoxication by hypnotics and psycho-pharmaceuticals

B. Iso-electric (flat) EEG

Acute toxicity

Chronic toxicity

Clouded consciousness ➞ coma

Addiction

Respiratory insufficiency ➞ tissue hypoxia, acidosis, central respiratory paralysis, shock lung, bronchopneumonia

Abrupt withdrawal leads to psychosis and seizures

Circulatory depression ➞ drop in blood pressure ➞ circulatory failure, kidney failure

Dilated, unresponsive pupils

Areflexia ➞ paralytic ileus,

urinary retention

Hypothermia

C. Toxicity of barbiturates

Acute toxicity

Chronic toxicity

Dizziness,

Indolence,

ataxia,

agitation,

confusion,

confusion,

coma

anxiety,

insomnia

D. Toxicity of benzodiazepines

■ Iron

Iron compounds are used for oral and parenteral treatment of iron deficiency with hemoglobin values of less than 12 g Hb/dL blood.

Excessive doses may lead to acute or chronic iron poisoning. Acute poisoning occurs occasionally in adults after attempted suicide and in children after accidental ingestion.

Signs of intoxication. The symptoms of poisoning after acute over dosage take the following clinical course (**A**): Vomiting, diarrhea, hemorrhagic gastroenteritis, cardiovascular collapse, or shock may lead to death within the first 6 h (stage 1). If the patient survives this phase, there will be a short recovery phase (stage 2). Poisoning due to very high doses and delay of treatment cause additional symptoms (stage 3), such as fever, leukocytosis, metabolic acidosis, disturbed blood clotting (prolonged prothrombin, thrombin, and thromboplastin times), central and peripheral paralysis, spasms, coma, toxic hepatitis and renal tubular necrosis, and persistent damage to liver, kidneys, and the central nervous system. The re-convalescent stage of poisoning (stage 4) is characterized by sclerotic adhesions in the gastrointestinal tract which are associated with ileus-like symptoms (stenosis of pylorus and antrum).

In children, 1 g ferrous sulfate taken by mouth has a caustic effect topically and is toxic systemically. The lethal dose for children is around 2 g; for adults it is 10–50 g.

Therapy. Iron intoxication is associated with a depletion in the capacity to bind iron, thus causing an increase of free iron in the blood. Therefore, treatment of acute poisoning consists of the inhibition of iron absorption on the one hand, and facilitation of renal iron elimination on the other. In addition, symptoms of shock have also to be treated. Depending on the state of consciousness, the first measure may be the induction of vomiting to empty the stomach. Gastric lavage with 1% $NaHCO_3$ lowers the proton concentration and results in the formation of poorly soluble ferrous carbonate. Administration of milk or raw eggs results in the formation of iron–protein complexes; however, they bind iron only temporarily and may therefore further increase its bioavailability. The chelating agent deferoxamine (**B**) is used as an antidote, since it has a high affinity to iron. It binds iron only from ferritin, transferrin, and hemosiderin and eliminates it via the kidneys.

Deferoxamine (1 g binds ~85 mg iron) should be administered when serum iron levels are ≥ 350 µg/dL (**C**). The initial dose is 0.5–1 g IM, or 15 mg/kg BW/hour IV as a 5% glucose solution (maximum daily dose 80 mg/kg BW), and the maximum dose for adults is 1–2 g/day. The daily dose of deferoxamine should not be exceeded, as the antidote may itself have a toxic effect. Tachycardia and a drop in blood pressure have been observed when the infusion was too rapid. Prolonged use of the antidote may lead to opacity of the lens, hypotension, a tendency to collapse, kidney damage, and neurotoxic effects. Renal insufficiency is considered a contraindication for the deferoxamine.

Chronic iron poisoning. This includes *hemosiderosis* and *hemochromatosis* (**A**), which may be caused by parenteral iron overload and deposition of iron in the reticuloendothelial system (RES), or by a genetic defect. In *acquired hemochromatosis*, iron is flushed out with deferoxamine; for *genetic hemochromatosis* blood-letting is a useful therapy.

Acute toxicity

Stage 1 (1–6 h after ingestion)
Vomiting, diarrhea, abdominal
pain, hemorrhagic gastroenteritis,
coma, cardiovascular collapse
(vasodilatation) or shock

Stage 2 (10–14 h after ingestion)
Short recovery phase
with apparent improvement

Stage 3 (12–48 h after ingestion)
Fever, leukocytosis, metabolic
acidosis, disturbed blood-clotting,
spasms and paralysis, coma,
inverted T wave in ECG, toxic
hepatitis, liver damage (GPT ↑),
renal tubular necrosis, renal damage

Stage (2–5 weeks later)
Sclerotic adhesions in the GIT,
stenosis of pylorus and antrum,
intestinal obstruction, liver
cirrhosis, CNS damage

Chronic toxicity

Hemosiderosis
Deposition of up to 40 g
iron in the RES

Hemochromatosis
Concurrent tissue damage,
like liver cirrhosis,
diabetes mellitus

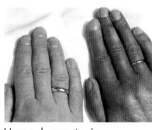

Hemochromatosis
of the right hand

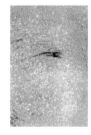

Hemo-
chromatosis
of the body
(bronze
diabetes)

A. Toxicity of iron

B. Deferoxamine

$$H_2N-(CH_2)_5-\underset{HO}{\overset{}{N}}-\underset{O}{\overset{}{C}}-(CH_2)_2-\underset{O}{\overset{}{C}}-\underset{H}{\overset{}{N}}-(CH_2)_5-\underset{HO}{\overset{}{N}}-\underset{O}{\overset{}{C}}-(CH_2)_2-\underset{O}{\overset{}{C}}-\underset{H}{\overset{}{N}}-(CH_2)_5-\underset{HO}{\overset{}{N}}-\underset{O}{\overset{}{C}}-CH_3$$

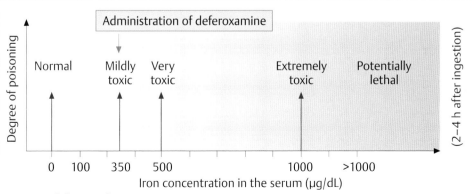

Administration of deferoxamine

Degree of poisoning

Normal   Mildly   Very   Extremely   Potentially
          toxic   toxic   toxic   lethal

0   100   350   500   1000   >1000

Iron concentration in the serum (µg/dL)

(2–4 h after ingestion)

C. Start of therapy for iron poisoning

Cardiac Glycosides

Digitoxin, Digoxin

The pharmacological effects of glycosides originating from the foxglove plants *Digitalis purpurea* and *D. lanata* (**A**) are positively inotropic, negatively chronotropic, negatively dromotropic, and positively bathmotropic. These glycosides are therefore used for treating cardiac insufficiency. The two main compounds, digitoxin and digoxin, affect the dynamics and rhythm of the heart; however, like all cardioactive steroids, they have a narrow therapeutic window. The primary glycosides are cardenolides (**A**), which have a terminal glucose attached to the digitoxose of their oligosaccharide side chain. Cleavage of the glucose produces the secondary glycosides (e.g., digitoxin, digoxin).

Signs of intoxication. Early signs of a toxic effect of these glycosides include gastrointestinal irritation, such as nausea, vomiting, and diarrhea, as well as central symptoms, such as headaches, fatigue, insomnia, vertigo, and confusion. Irregular respiration may lead to cyanosis (**B**). Other characteristic extracardiac effects of cardiac glycoside overdosage include neurological symptoms, such as tinnitus, impaired vision (halo or scotoma, xanthopsia) as well as delirium and hallucination. Life-threatening signs of intoxication are arrhythmias; depending on the original condition of the poisoned person (i. e., whether or not they have heart disease), these signs manifest themselves in various forms of *bradycardia* (sinus bradycardia, AV block, death due to asystole) or *tachycardia* (ventricular tachyarrhythmia, atrial extrasystoles, death due to ventricular fibrillation) (**B**).

In contrast to acute suicidal or accidental poisonings, chronic poisoning may occur when a change in the pathological condition (renal insufficiency or drug interaction) causes a therapeutic dose to become toxic. The optimal plasma concentration is 0.8–1.4 ng/mL of digoxin or 10–30 ng/mL digitoxin. When the therapeutic dose is exceeded by a factor of 1.5–3, toxic effects are to be expected. A plasma level of more than 2.0 ng/mL digoxin (30–40 ng/mL digitoxin) borders on the toxic range. A level of 6.3 ng/mL digoxin causes ventricular fibrillation (**B**).

Therapy. Treatment of acute intoxication after ingestion consists of gastric lavage and inhibition of intestinal absorption by the administration of activated charcoal (20 g) or colestyramine (8 g) (**C**). In cases of bradycardia, atropine (0.5 mg IV) is indicated. A temporary pacemaker is considered the treatment of choice. In case of tachycardia and normokalemia or hypokalemia, infusions of potassium ions are given while monitoring electrolytes and ECG (10 mmol/h = 0.75 g KCl, up to 40–60 mmol/d). The contraindications are hyperkalemia, atrioventricular block, renal insufficiency, and treatment failure. In such cases, class I antiarrhythmic agents, such as phenytoin (5 mg/kg IV) or lidocaine (initially 50–100 mg IV, then as an infusion up to 1 g/day), may be administered. If there is ventricular tachycardia, IV administration of antiarrhythmic agents (such as phenytoin or lidocaine) may lead to cardiac arrest due to an increase in serum potassium (> 5 mmol/L). Treatment of severe arrhythmias is therefore preferentially performed with specific digoxin- and digitoxin-binding antibody Fab fragments obtained from the serum of immunized sheep (digitalis antidote BM, Digibind). The immunological binding of free cardiac glycoside molecules in the blood and in the interstitial space result in inactivation of the poison and subsequent renal elimination due to the low molecular weight of the Fab–glycoside complex. One vial (80 mg) of the antidote will bind 1 mg of the glycoside in the body; frequently, up to six vials (480 mg in total) need to be injected.

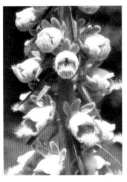
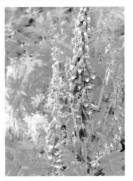

Cardenolides
(steroids with a five-membered unsaturated lactone in position 17)

R, residue	
R = H:	**digitoxin**
R = OH:	**digoxin**

Aglycon: digitoxigenin

Sugar component: digitoxose

Woolly (or Grecian) fox-glove *(Digitalis lanata)* Purple (or common) fox-glove *(Digitalis purpurea)*

A. Plants of origin and formulas of digitoxin/digoxin

Extracardiac symptoms

Psychiatric

Confusion, fatigue, insomnia, hallucination, delirium, seizures

Visual

Impaired vision (halo or scotoma)

Impaired color vision (xanthopsia)

Respiratory

Dyspnea, cyanosis, increased ventilation

Gastrointestinal

Abdominal pain, diarrhea

Extracardiac symptoms

Central nervous system

Nausea, vomiting, headache, vertigo, loss of appetite, dizziness, neuralgia, paresthesia, muscle weakness

Cardiac symptoms

Arrhythmias

– Bradycardia:
  sinus bradycardia
  AV block of 2nd and 3rd degrees

– Tachycardia:
  atrial tachycardia
  atrial extrasystoles
  AV tachycardia
  ventricular extrasystoles (bi/trigeminy)
  ventricular tachycardia
  ventricular fibrillation

B. Acute toxicity of digitoxin and digoxin

Specific treatment:

– administration of K^+ (IV)

– atropine sulfate (IV)

– digitalis antidote BM

Symptomatic treatment:

e.g.

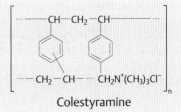

Colestyramine

C. Therapy for poisoning with digitalis and digoxin

Paracetamol (Acetaminophen)

This analgesic and antipyretic (**A**) is often used for suicide attempts. Ingestion of a single dose of more than 10 g is considered toxic for adults; subsequent liver damage is therefore to be expected. Ingestion of a single dose of more than 15 g is lethal. In a healthy adult, blood concentrations of paracetamol of more than 200 µg/mL are considered toxic. The lethal dose for children is assumed to be 2–8 g (≥ 40 mg/kg BW) depending on age, and for infants it is 0.5 g.

Signs of intoxication. The manifestations of poisoning are divided into four stages (**B**). Within the first 24 h after taking an overdose (stage 1), symptoms begin with minor gastrointestinal complaints, such as loss of appetite, nausea, vomiting, pallor, and upper abdominal pain. After 24 h (stage 2), signs of liver damage are indicated by an abnormal liver function test. Also observed are a steep increase in the transaminases GOT and GPT, indicating hepatonecrosis; a drop in clotting factors, resulting in increased prothrombin time; and an increase in serum bilirubin. Days 3 and 4 (stage 3) are characterized by the first signs of liver failure; icterus, metabolic acidosis, hypoglycemia, hemorrhagic diathesis, and hepatic encephalopathy may also occur. Hepatic functions either improve after day 5 (stage 4), or fulminating hepatonecrosis occurs and, in severe cases, also cramps, collapse, respiratory depression, and death in hepatic coma.

Therapy. Primary treatment of acute poisoning within the first 6 h consists of the induction of vomiting, gastric lavage, and SC injection of apomorphine (0.07 mg/kg BW). This should be followed by administration of activated charcoal (1 g/kg BW). Specific treatment with SH-group donors is indicated when, 4 h after ingestion of an overdose, the plasma concentration of paracetamol is 150 µg/mL (1000 µmol/L) (Rumack–Matthew nomogram). Infusion of the antidote *N*-acetylcysteine (NAC) (**C**) should be started within the first 10 h so that liver damage is minimized by binding of the cytotoxic paracetamol metabolites. The duration of treatment with the currently available 20% injection solution depends on the clinical picture. Termination of treatment is necessary only if there are first signs of an anaphylactic reaction. Dosage instructions for NAC use are as follows: the initial dose is 150 mg/kg BW in 200 mL of 5% glucose by IV application over 15 min; this is followed by infusion of 50 mg/kg BW in 500 mL over 4 h, and by another infusion of 100 mg/kg BW in 1000 mL (up to a total dose of 300 mg/kg BW) applied over a total treatment time of up to 20 h and 15 min. A useful additional measure for very severe poisoning, particularly in cases of renal insufficiency, is hemoperfusion using synthetic resin. Forced diuresis is not recommended.

The mechanism of acute intoxication is based on the formation of various reactive paracetamol metabolites (**A**) by the cytochrome P450 system of the liver. When the glutathione (GSH) reserves of this system are exhausted, the metabolites can no longer be detoxified and thus lead to liver damage, and finally hepatonecrosis, by binding to liver proteins. In-vivo studies in hamsters have confirmed that the irreversible binding of metabolites to macromolecules correlates with the extent of cell death. The binding of paracetamol to proteins increased when the GSH level dropped to less than 30% of the normal value (**D**).

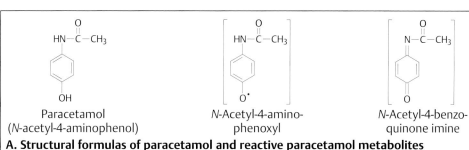

Paracetamol
(*N*-acetyl-4-aminophenol)

N-Acetyl-4-amino-
phenoxyl

N-Acetyl-4-benzo-
quinone imine

A. Structural formulas of paracetamol and reactive paracetamol metabolites

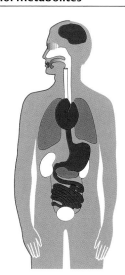

Stage 1 (up to 24 h)
GIT symptoms (nausea, loss of appetite, vomiting, pallor, upper abdominal pain)

Stage 2 (after 24 h)
Liver damage (GOT and GPT ↑), blood-clotting factors ↓, bilirubin ↑

Stage 3 (days 3 and 4)
Liver failure, jaundice, metabolic acidosis, hypoglycemia, hemorrhagic diathesis, hepatic encephalopathy

Stage 4 (after 5 days)
Liver necrosis, spasms, collapse, respiratory depression, hepatic coma

B. Acute toxicity of paracetamol

Antidote: $HS-CH_2-CH-COOH$
$\qquad\qquad\quad HN-C-CH_3$
$\qquad\qquad\qquad\; \| $
$\qquad\qquad\qquad\; O$

N-Acetylcysteine (NAC)

C. Therapy for poisoning with paracetamol

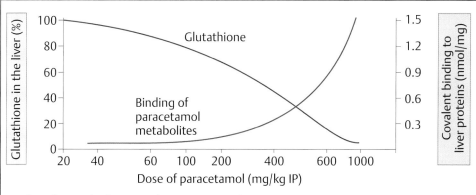

D. Glutathione depletion and increased binding of paracetamol metabolites to proteins

■ Addictive Substances

Definition. Addictive substances include natural or synthetic compounds. Their repeated use may lead to dependency in some individuals. Dependency is characterized by the habit of taking an addictive substance because of the irresistible urge either to achieve a sensation of well-being or to eliminate uncomfortable feelings or pain. The World Health Organization (WHO) has defined seven groups of substances that may lead to dependency (**A**).

■ Morphines

Heroin

Basics. Heroin is considered to be the addictive substance with the highest potential for developing dependency. Dihydrocodeine (DHC) is a heroin substitute available on the black market, whereas methadone is used under strictly supervised conditions for the medical treatment of opiate addicts. Heroin, or diacetylmorphine, was originally designed (in the 1890s) as an antitussive. The acetylation of morphine promotes rapid penetration into the central nervous system.

Absorption, distribution, metabolism, and elimination. Heroin is quickly distributed in the brain, kidney, liver, and lung, where it is rapidly metabolized to 6-monoacetylmorphine and then to morphine (**B**). Morphine binds predominantly to μ-receptors, which are distributed throughout the entire central nervous system. Their density is particularly high in the area postrema, nucleus accumbens, nucleus locus ceruleus, and limbic cortex (**C**). This explains the strong effect of morphine not only as a respiratory depressant but also as a euphorigenic agent. Heroin is taken up by addicts primarily by inhalation of the vapor over a heated foil, or else injected intravenously (*heroin fix*). It is also effective when ingested, which makes it particularly dangerous for *body packers* who conceal heroin packages in their gastrointestinal tract (**D**). The half-life of heroin in the serum is less than 20 min; that of 6-monoacetylmorphine is slightly longer. The detection of this metabolite is used to prove heroin poisoning.

Effects. The half-life of morphine is about 3 h (**B**). Severely addicted individuals must therefore use heroin several times a day to obtain a sufficiently euphorigenic effect or to avoid undesired withdrawal symptoms.

Toxicity. Heroin poisoning is recognized by the combination of miosis, respiratory depression, cyanosis, drop in blood pressure, and bradycardia (**E**). When such a patient is examined, the arms usually reveal thrombosed venous cords (track marks) corresponding to multiple sites of venipuncture (**F**). Among the known dangerous, undesired effects, which are nevertheless accepted by heroin users, are neurological disorders with epileptic seizures, posthypoxic brain damage, pulmonary edema, rhabdomyolysis, abscesses, endocarditis, and nephritis (**E**). Associated diseases due to needle sharing include severe infectious diseases, such as hepatitis B and C as well as HIV infection.

Therapy. Treatment of acute heroin poisoning consists of intubation and artificial respiration of the patient. Administration of volume substitutes and catecholamines may be necessary to stabilize the circulation. The opiate effect is abolished by administration of the antagonist naloxone (**G**). Care should be taken that the naloxone dose is titrated slowly (between 0.2 and 0.8 mg) to avoid unpleasant side effects, such as nausea, vomiting, and opiate withdrawal syndrome (e.g., circulatory collapse).

Group of compounds	Opioids	Alcohol	Cocaine	Amphetamine	Hallucinogens	Khatamines	Cannabis
Important representatives	Heroin DHC Methadone	Ethanol (beer, wine, liquor)	Freebase Crack	Amphetamine MDMA (ecstasy)	LSD Psilocybin Mescaline	Cathinone	Hashish Marihuana

A. Addictive substances

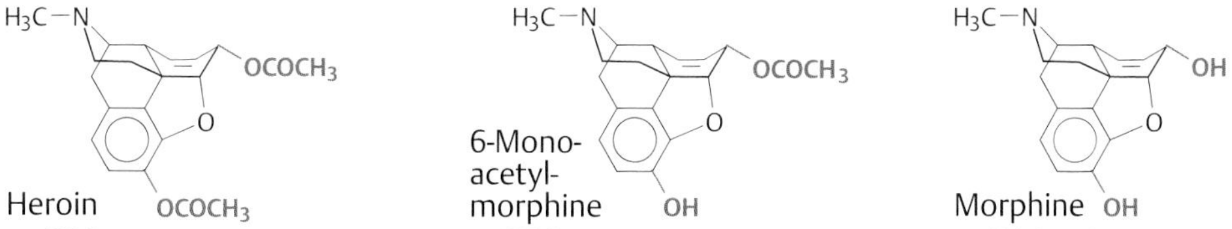
H3C—N
OCOCH3
O
OCOCH3
H3C—N
OCOCH3
O
OH
H3C—N
OH
O
OH

Heroin
Half-life 20 min

6-Monoacetylmorphine
Half-life 40 min

Morphine
Half-life 3 h

B. Structural formulas of heroin, 6-monoacetylmorphine, and morphine

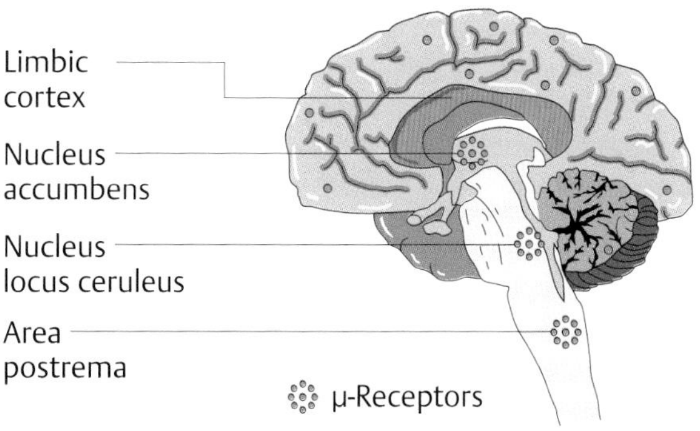
Limbic cortex
Nucleus accumbens
Nucleus locus ceruleus
Area postrema
μ-Receptors

C. Localization of μ-receptors

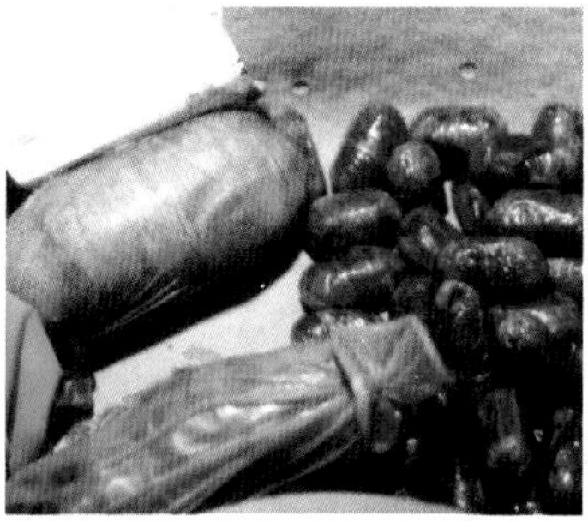

Heroin packed in condoms

D. Body packing

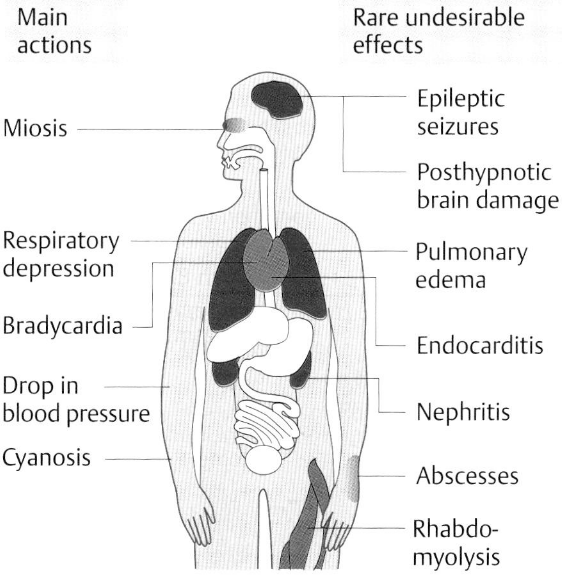
Main actions
Miosis
Respiratory depression
Bradycardia
Drop in blood pressure
Cyanosis
Rare undesirable effects
Epileptic seizures
Posthypnotic brain damage
Pulmonary edema
Endocarditis
Nephritis
Abscesses
Rhabdomyolysis

E. Acute toxicity of heroin

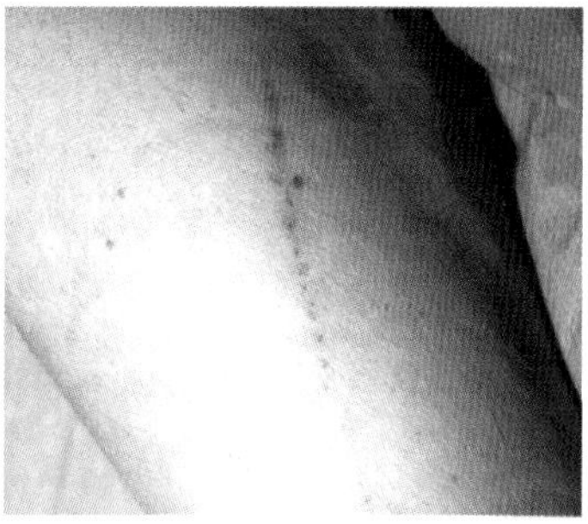

Track marks

F. Thrombosed venous cord

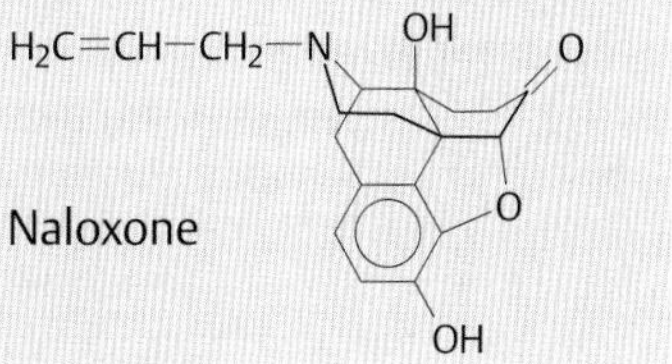
H2C=CH—CH2—N
OH
O
O
OH

Naloxone

G. Antidote

Alcohol

Basics. Alcohol (ethanol) is the most commonly used addictive substance in industrialized countries. It is largely consumed in the form of beer (50 g ethanol/L), wine (120 g/L), or hard liquor (400–600 g/L). Ethanol contributes to many human deaths. It plays a role in over 50% of all fatal car accidents, and 30% of people who commit suicide are under the influence of alcohol. There is a strong correlation between mortality from liver cirrhosis and alcohol consumption in the population. The incidence rate is around 30 deaths per year per 100 000 total population. Alcohol is considered the most important fetotoxic (teratogenic) substance in Western culture. In Germany, for example, around 2000 children are born every year with alcohol-related birth defects.

Absorption, distribution, and elimination. Ethanol is completely absorbed in the gastrointestinal tract (20% in the stomach, 80% in the small intestine). The speed of absorption depends on the stomach contents and the gastric emptying time (especially after rapid intake on an empty stomach). Ethanol is distributed to all tissues of the body, and this corresponds to the water content of individual tissues. Over 90% of the absorbed ethanol is metabolized in the body. The rest (10%) is largely eliminated in exhaled air and urine, and also in minute amounts with sweat (**A**).

Metabolism. Ethanol is degraded by means of two important metabolic pathways in the liver and in the gastrointestinal tract. In the cytoplasm, ethanol is degraded by alcohol dehydrogenase to acetaldehyde and then by acetaldehyde dehydrogenase to acetate (**B**). Both steps require NAD$^+$ as a cofactor. This system can be saturated. Therefore, ethanol degradation follows zero-order kinetics as long as alcohol levels are low. The second degradation system resides in the endoplasmic reticulum of liver cells and is called the *microsomal ethanol oxidizing system (MEOS)*. Ethanol is oxidized by the MEOS to acetaldehyde and then to acetate. The MEOS depends on NADPH and requires molecular oxygen. This system cannot be saturated, and its activity is increased by chronic alcohol consumption. The degradation of high alcohol levels therefore follows first-order kinetics (**B**).

Acute toxicity. The most important acute effect of ethanol manifests itself in the central nervous system. There is no specific receptor; rather, ethanol affects neuronal ion transport at the cell membrane and, therefore, transmembrane signal transmission. The cerebrum is particularly sensitive to the effects of ethanol, and the inhibitory neurons are initially more suppressed in their function than the stimulatory neurons. This results in disinhibition, excitement, and drunkenness, which is followed by disturbances in the occipital lobe (disturbed vision) and cerebellum (disturbed coordination, ataxia). Very high ethanol concentrations lead to depression of the reticular activating system (induction of sleep, coma) and, finally, to depression of the reticular formation (disturbed breathing) (**C**).

Therapy. The life-threatening phase of acute ethanol intoxication with coma and disturbed breathing is usually short, because ethanol intoxication mostly occurs with chronic alcoholics who have well-developed mechanisms of adaptation. This phase requires careful observation in an intensive care unit where respiration, oxygen saturation, blood pressure, and heart rate can be closely monitored. If the respiratory pathways have not been secured by intubation, the patient should be placed in lateral position to prevent aspiration of vomit (see also p. 86).

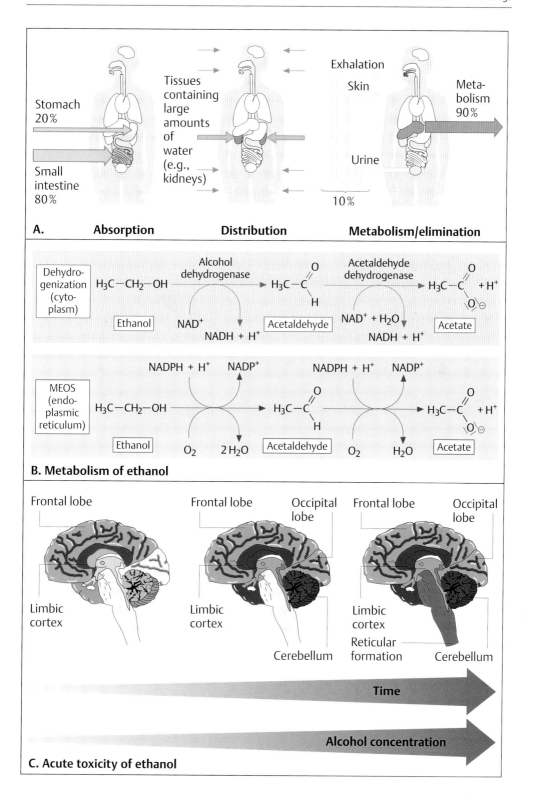

A. Absorption — Distribution — Metabolism/elimination

Stomach 20%
Small intestine 80%

Tissues containing large amounts of water (e.g., kidneys)

Exhalation
Skin
Urine
10%

Metabolism 90%

B. Metabolism of ethanol

Dehydrogenization (cytoplasm)

H_3C-CH_2-OH Ethanol — Alcohol dehydrogenase — NAD^+ → $NADH + H^+$ — $H_3C-C\overset{O}{\underset{H}{}}$ Acetaldehyde — Acetaldehyde dehydrogenase — $NAD^+ + H_2O$ → $NADH + H^+$ — $H_3C-C\overset{O}{\underset{O^{\ominus}}{}} + H^+$ Acetate

MEOS (endoplasmic reticulum)

H_3C-CH_2-OH Ethanol — $NADPH + H^+$ → $NADP^+$ — O_2 → $2H_2O$ — $H_3C-C\overset{O}{\underset{H}{}}$ Acetaldehyde — $NADPH + H^+$ → $NADP^+$ — O_2 → H_2O — $H_3C-C\overset{O}{\underset{O^{\ominus}}{}} + H^+$ Acetate

C. Acute toxicity of ethanol

Frontal lobe
Limbic cortex

Frontal lobe
Occipital lobe
Limbic cortex
Cerebellum

Frontal lobe
Occipital lobe
Limbic cortex
Reticular formation
Cerebellum

Time

Alcohol concentration

■ Chronic Alcoholism

Basics. Chronic alcoholism is a major problem for the health care system. The behavior of alcoholics leads to their social decline and calls for psychiatric and psychotherapeutic counseling. Secondary organic diseases are found in men who regularly consume about 80 g alcohol/day; this corresponds to around 1.5 L of beer or 0.6 L of wine. The limit in women is about 60 g alcohol/day. Secondary neurological diseases are especially severe (**A**).

Since alcoholics rarely admit their addiction and are often in a state of denial, biochemical test procedures can help the physician to recognize the condition. Tests for the liver enzymes glutamate pyruvate transaminase (GPT) and γ-glutamyl transpeptidase (γ-GT), mean corpuscular volume (MCV) of erythrocytes, and carbohydrate-deficient transferrin (CDT) are best suited for this purpose (**B**). Elevation of all these parameters unambiguously points to alcohol dependency. The increase in γ-GT alone is no proof in itself, but it raises suspicion.

Withdrawal symptoms. The withdrawal symptoms after voluntary or enforced abstinence from alcohol create a special problem (**C**). Discontinuation after long-term alcohol consumption may lead to alcohol withdrawal syndrome and, in the worst case, to delirium tremens, which still has a mortality of 1–4%.

There are three stages of alcohol withdrawal, and the symptoms may decline after the first or second stage, which usually takes 3–5 days. However, if delirium tremens sets in, it can last 10 days or more. Alcohol withdrawal syndrome is frequently preceded by epileptic seizures. The first symptoms are agitation and dysphoric mood. Autonomic symptoms include tremor of the hands, nausea, loss of appetite, and sweating. Pulse rate and blood pressure are increased. Predelirium is a state with violent autonomic signs, nervousness, and the beginnings of disorientation; the patient is still amenable to suggestion. The full state of delirium tremens is characterized by severe psychomotor unrest. Visual, tactile, and acoustic hallucinations occur. The patient often feels persecuted, sees small moving things, and suffers from panic attacks. The onset of delirium tremens is sudden; it occurs mostly in the evening and ends in postictal sleep (**C**).

Therapy. Treatment of alcohol withdrawal syndrome with drugs is not always necessary. As long as the patient shows only minor autonomic withdrawal symptoms, observation in a closed facility may suffice. However, if there are severe autonomic withdrawal symptoms and disorientation, pharmacotherapy is indicated. This may terminate the progression of symptoms and make the withdrawal symptoms disappear. The drugs of choice are clomethiazole in high doses (**D**) or benzodiazepines (see p. 74) in combination with neuroleptics (butyrophenone, chlorprothixene, **D**). Fully developed delirium tremens requires intensive care monitoring and IV administration of clomethiazole. Since this treatment is accompanied by severe sedation and pulmonary complications, high doses of IV clonidine in combination with benzodiazepines and neuroleptics may also be administered. Clonidine alleviates the autonomic symptoms, benzodiazepines sedate, and neuroleptics are effective against hallucinations.

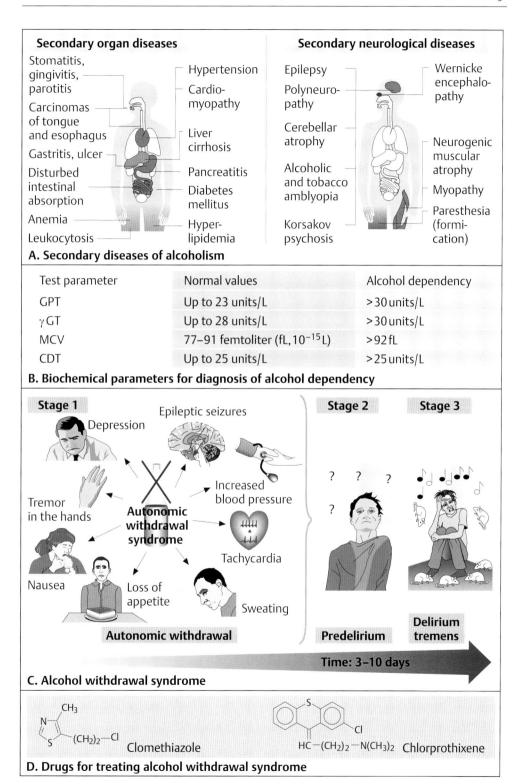

Secondary organ diseases

Stomatitis, gingivitis, parotitis

Carcinomas of tongue and esophagus

Gastritis, ulcer

Disturbed intestinal absorption

Anemia

Leukocytosis

Hypertension

Cardio-myopathy

Liver cirrhosis

Pancreatitis

Diabetes mellitus

Hyper-lipidemia

Secondary neurological diseases

Epilepsy

Polyneuro-pathy

Cerebellar atrophy

Alcoholic and tobacco amblyopia

Korsakov psychosis

Wernicke encephalo-pathy

Neurogenic muscular atrophy

Myopathy

Paresthesia (formi-cation)

A. Secondary diseases of alcoholism

Test parameter	Normal values	Alcohol dependency
GPT	Up to 23 units/L	>30 units/L
γGT	Up to 28 units/L	>30 units/L
MCV	77–91 femtoliter (fL, 10^{-15} L)	>92 fL
CDT	Up to 25 units/L	>25 units/L

B. Biochemical parameters for diagnosis of alcohol dependency

Stage 1

Depression

Epileptic seizures

Tremor in the hands

Autonomic withdrawal syndrome

Increased blood pressure

Tachycardia

Nausea

Loss of appetite

Sweating

Autonomic withdrawal

Stage 2

? ? ?

?

Stage 3

Predelirium

Delirium tremens

Time: 3–10 days

C. Alcohol withdrawal syndrome

Clomethiazole

Chlorprothixene

D. Drugs for treating alcohol withdrawal syndrome

▦ Cocaine

Basics. In 1859, Albert Niemann recognized that cocaine can be used as a local anesthetic. In 1884, Siegmund Freud recommended that depression be treated with cocaine. The author Arthur Conan Doyle made his hero Sherlock Holmes solve the most difficult crimes under the influence of cocaine. In 1886, John S. Pemberton developed a beverage containing cocaine and caffeine and sold it under the name Coca-Cola. It was only in 1906 that cocaine was removed from the formula.

Traditionally the drug of the rich and famous, cocaine is now a top street drug. The crystalline alkaloid, called benzoylmethylecgonine, is produced from the leaves of the coca plant *Erythroxylum coca* (**A**). On the market, it is available as cocaine hydrochloride in the form of crystals, small granules, or white powder. This form of cocaine is water-soluble and not volatile. Alkaline conversion and subsequent solvent extraction lead to the volatile free base of the drug (*freebase*), which is suitable for inhalation. *Crack* is the street name for the impure free base produced cheaply with baking soda and water (**A**).

Absorption, distribution, metabolism, and elimination. Cocaine hydrochloride is usually sniffed. The effect sets in within 20 min after sniffing, and lasts up to 3 h. By contrast, smoking the volatile free base (*freebasing*) leads to rapid absorption via the lungs and immediate onset of the euphoric effects; it is therefore highly addictive. Cocaine crosses the blood–brain barrier easily, and the highest tissue levels are found in the brain.

Cocaine is metabolized by the cholinesterases of the plasma and liver into a water-soluble metabolite, ecgonine methyl ester, and also by nonenzymatic hydrolysis into benzoylecgonine ester. Both metabolites appear in the urine (at 40% each); the remaining cocaine (20%) is excreted unchanged (**B**).

Mechanism of action. Cocaine blocks the reuptake of the neurotransmitters norepinephrine and dopamine in the neuronal synapses (**C**), thus causing excessive stimulation of their postsynaptic receptors. The desired effect of cocaine is intense euphoria. The drug has a stimulating effect, combats fatigue, facilitates social contacts, enhances the ability to concentrate, and produces mild and pleasant hallucinations.

Toxicity. The increase in sympathetic tone leads to mydriasis, tachycardia, tachypnea, and hypertension. Poisoning occurs after IV application of high doses or after frequent uninterrupted use (binges) over several days. The signs of intoxication appear in the form of cardiovascular, central nervous system, and pulmonary symptoms, leading to hypertonic crises, severe angina pectoris, arrhythmias, and myocardial infarction even in young people. In the central nervous system, poisoning manifests itself in the form of severe headaches, epileptic seizures, ischemic insults, and subarachnoidal or intracerebral hemorrhages. Bronchial constrictions and pulmonary infiltrations occur particularly after using crack cocaine. Necrosis of the nasal septum is always suggestive of chronic cocaine use (**D**).

Therapy. Treatment is symptomatic. The blood pressure must be lowered by α-blockade (labetalol). Other antihypertensive drugs that simultaneously protect the coronary arteries, such as nitroglycerine, may be used. Exclusive β-blockade has to be avoided because it leads to an increased α-adrenergic stimulus. Seizures are stopped by high doses of diazepam. Occasionally, relaxation by pancuronium may become necessary.

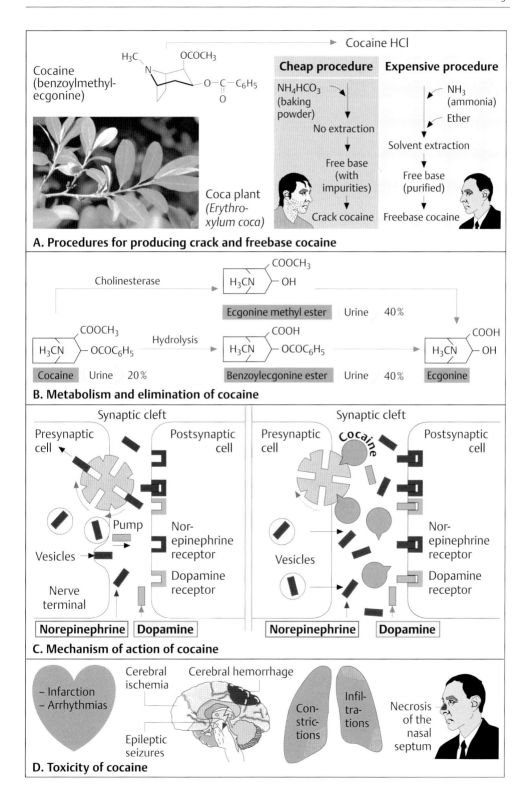

A. Procedures for producing crack and freebase cocaine

B. Metabolism and elimination of cocaine

C. Mechanism of action of cocaine

D. Toxicity of cocaine

■ Amphetamines

Basics. Amphetamines are substances that have primarily a stimulating effect on the central nervous system. In the past, they have been legally used as appetite suppressants (anorectics) and as strong stimulants to allow longer performance without sleep (performance-enhancing drugs). Methylphenidate (for treating children suffering from attention deficit hyperactivity disorder, ADHD) and fenfluramine (an appetite suppressant) are still legally available (**A**). Other amphetamines are potentially highly addictive and are therefore illegal. From these, *designer drugs* have been developed (all of them illegal) which have dose-related doping and hallucinogenic effects. The basic structure of amphetamine is β-phenylisopropylamine. Methylation of the amino group leads to methamphetamine, which is a stronger and longer-lasting stimulant than amphetamine. The most important designer drugs are produced by introducing methoxyl groups at the phenyl ring of the phenylisopropylamine molecule. Methylenedioxyamphetamine (MDA, *love pill*) and methylenedioxymethamphetamine (MDMA, *ecstasy*) are primarily stimulants, whereas 4-methyl-2,5-dimethoxyamphetamine (DOM, *peace pill*) and, even more so, 4-brome-2,5-dimethoxyamphetamine (DOB, *golden eagle*) are stimulants as well as hallucinogens (**A**).

Absorption, distribution, biotransformation, and elimination. Amphetamines are almost exclusively taken orally, although inhalation and IV injection are also possible. They are well absorbed by all mucosae; they are fat-soluble and easily cross the blood–brain barrier. In the liver, they are either deaminated at the side chain, or hydroxylated at the aromatic ring to produce *p*-hydroxyamphetamine which is then excreted in the urine. Upon acidification of the urine, up to 80% of the amphetamine is excreted unchanged (**B**).

Mechanism of action. The chemical structure of amphetamines is very similar to that of catecholamines. Amphetamines act as indirect sympathomimetics on the central and peripheral nervous systems. They increase the presynaptic release of catecholamines (dopamine, norepinephrine, epinephrine) and also act as monoamine oxidase inhibitors. At the same time, they stimulate serotonin receptors, and in animal experiments they lead to serotonin deprivation of neurons.

Desired effects. Because tolerance develops rapidly, amphetamines are abused only intermittently (usually at the weekends). Their effects include euphoria, increased self-confidence, decreased appetite, increased energy, enhanced physical performance, reduced sleep requirement, and dose- and substance-dependent hallucinations (**C**).

Toxicity. Mild intoxication is characterized by anxiety, restlessness, headache, palpitation, nausea, vomiting, and irritability. Signs of more pronounced intoxication include fever, confusion, stereotypy, hypertension, angina pectoris, and arrhythmias. Delirious states, malignant hyperthermia and hypertension, epileptic seizures, arrhythmias affecting the circulation, and focal neurological deficiencies indicate severe intoxication. Heat stroke with cerebral edema may occur, as can rhabdomyolysis with kidney failure, consumptive coagulopathy, and hepatotoxic effects up to fulminant liver failure (**C**).

Therapy. Treatment is symptomatic. Administration of a volume substitute is often required. High blood pressure should be lowered with β-blockers, nitroglycerine, or ACE inhibitors. In malignant hyperthermia, relaxation with dantrolene is required. Benzodiazepine or diazepam is often used for epileptic seizures (**D**).

Amphetamines

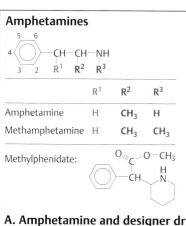

	R^1	R^2	R^3
Amphetamine	H	CH$_3$	H
Methamphetamine	H	CH$_3$	CH$_3$

Methylphenidate:

Designer drugs

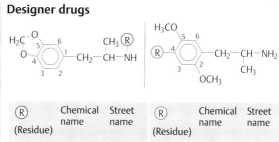

® (Residue)	Chemical name	Street name	® (Residue)	Chemical name	Street name
H	MDA	Love pill	CH$_3$	DOM	Peace pill
CH$_3$	MDMA	Ecstasy	Br	DOB	Golden eagle

A. Amphetamine and designer drugs

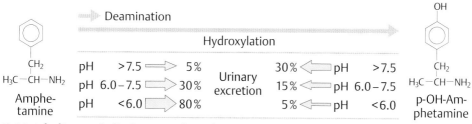

Deamination

Hydroxylation

Amphetamine		Urinary excretion		p-OH-Amphetamine
pH >7.5	5%		30%	pH >7.5
pH 6.0–7.5	30%		15%	pH 6.0–7.5
pH <6.0	80%		5%	pH <6.0

B. Metabolism and elimination of amphetamines

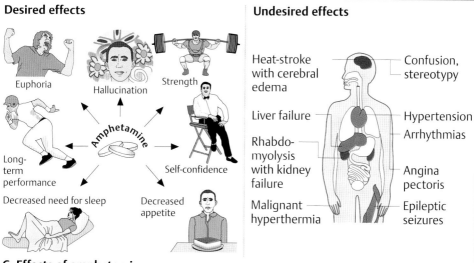

Desired effects

Euphoria

Hallucination

Strength

Long-term performance

Self-confidence

Decreased need for sleep

Decreased appetite

Amphetamine

Undesired effects

Heat-stroke with cerebral edema

Confusion, stereotypy

Liver failure

Hypertension

Arrhythmias

Rhabdomyolysis with kidney failure

Angina pectoris

Malignant hyperthermia

Epileptic seizures

C. Effects of amphetamines

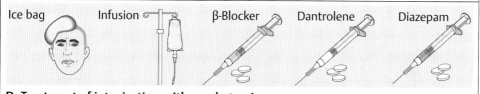

Ice bag   Infusion   β-Blocker   Dantrolene   Diazepam

D. Treatment of intoxication with amphetamines

91

■ Hallucinogens

These include substances like lysergic acid diethylamide (LSD), psilocybin (a mycotoxin, see p. 282), and mescaline (toxin of the peyote cactus). They cause misperception or alter sensory impression.

Lysergic acid diethylamide

LSD is a derivative of the secale alkaloid lysergic acid (**A**) (see p. 73). It is effective in the microgram range.

Adsorption, distribution, metabolism, and elimination. LSD is taken orally. It is well absorbed from the gastrointestinal tract. The serum half-life is 3 h. LSD is largely reduced, subsequently glucuronated, and then eliminated with the bile and in minor amounts in the urine (detection possible by radioimmunoassay, RIA) (**B**). LSD accumulates in the cortex, hippocampus, corpus striatum, and in small amounts in the cerebellum (**B**). It binds to postsynaptic serotonin receptors (5-HT$_2$). Symptoms that may occur up to 60 min after ingestion are tics, tachycardia, hypertension, hyperreflexia, redness of the face, and obligatory mydriasis.

Effects. At first, spatial perception changes; objects appear deformed; they move, vibrate, and become blurred. Noises are perceived louder than they really are, the sense of time is disturbed, colors change, and synesthesia may occur (colors are heard, and music is felt). Tolerance develops rapidly, and LSD is therefore not used continuously.

Toxicity. LSD does not cause severe poisoning. Mental disturbances lasting for 2–12 h manifest themselves in euphoria, and later in depression, depersonalization, and illusion. Particularly feared are *horror trips*, which are panic attacks. Other unpleasant effects are *flashbacks* (the experience of LSD effects long after the drug has worn off, up to half a year after the last ingestion) (**C**).

Therapy. Treatment is only necessary for horror trips. A calming talk is often all that is needed (*talking down*). Oral diazepam or haloperidol IM terminates this state of emergency immediately.

■ Khatamines

These sympathomimetic alkaloids are derived from *Catha edulis* (khat), a flowering shrub with evergreen leaves that has been cultivated in East Africa and the Arabian peninsula for centuries. Khat leaves are traditionally chewed for their euphoric properties, especially in Yemen where this is an integral part of social life. Khatamines are similar to amphetamines. The primary active constituent is (–)-*S*-cathinone. Its initial effects are euphoria, high blood pressure, and tachycardia. Negative effects that occur only later include anorexia, depression, insomnia, and emotional instability (**D**). Occasionally, there are persistent psychotic states; however, these can be easily treated with thioridazine.

■ Cannabis

Cannabis is derived from the hemp plant *Cannabis sativa* (**E**). Two preparations are used: marihuana (dried leaves and flowers) and hashish (dried resin, which has a higher cannabis content). The active constituent is tetrahydrocannabinol (THC) (**E**). Cannabis is the most often used illegal drug worldwide.

Adsorption, distribution, metabolism, and elimination. About 20% of the THC contained in the smoke is absorbed. Up to 99% of the THC is metabolized in the liver; only 1% appears unchanged in the urine.

Desired effects. Dose-related effects include comfort, euphoria, day-dreaming, pleasant relaxation, enhanced sensations (music becomes more pleasant), and altered sense of space and time.

Toxicity. Cannabis affects the short-term memory. High doses may lead to vertigo, anxiety, paranoia, and acute exogenous psychosis with hallucinations. The worst form is the amotivational syndrome (complete lack of motivation). The use of cannabis reduces fertility and leads to embryonic malformations. Cannabis is an entry drug (**E**): about 1–5% of cannabis smokers switch to harder drugs, and 99% of opiate addicts have smoked cannabis prior to their addiction. Flashbacks are also known to occur after cannabis use.

Therapy. Administration of benzodiazepines or neuroleptics.

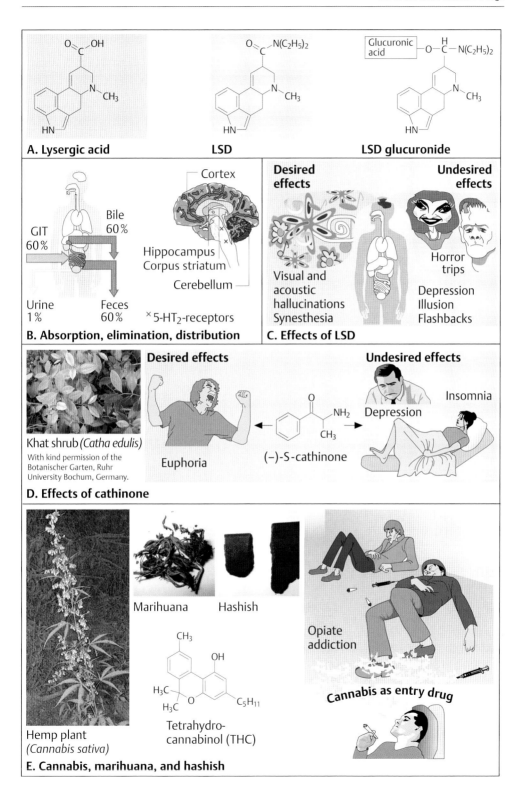

A. Lysergic acid **LSD** **LSD glucuronide**

B. Absorption, elimination, distribution

GIT 60%

Bile 60%

Urine 1% Feces 60%

Cortex

Hippocampus
Corpus striatum

Cerebellum

×5-HT$_2$-receptors

C. Effects of LSD

Desired effects

Visual and acoustic hallucinations
Synesthesia

Undesired effects

Horror trips

Depression
Illusion
Flashbacks

D. Effects of cathinone

Khat shrub *(Catha edulis)*
With kind permission of the Botanischer Garten, Ruhr University Bochum, Germany.

Desired effects

Euphoria

(−)-S-cathinone

Undesired effects

Depression

Insomnia

E. Cannabis, marihuana, and hashish

Marihuana Hashish

Tetrahydro-cannabinol (THC)

Hemp plant
(Cannabis sativa)

Opiate addiction

Cannabis as entry drug

Aliphatic and Alicyclic Hydrocarbons

Basics. Aliphatic hydrocarbons are organic compounds derived from open-chain hydrocarbons. Alicyclic hydrocarbons are organic compounds that contain one or more closed rings of carbon atoms, having only C–C single bonds or asymmetrically arranged double bonds in the carbocyclic ring structure. Examples include cyclopropane, cyclopentadiene, and cyclohexane. The gaseous alkanes (e.g., methane [marsh gas], ethane, propane, and butane) act primarily by displacing oxygen; high concentrations of these gases cause asphyxiation. Toxicologically more important are the solvents hexane and heptane; they are constituents of petroleum ether (benzine), in addition to octane.

Petroleum Ether (A)

Petroleum ether (also known as benzine, but not to be confused with benzene) is mainly used as a fuel (gasoline) and as a solvent. In chemical cleaning procedures (dry cleaning), it has increasingly replaced the more toxic chlorohydrocarbons (see p. 106). Acute poisoning with petroleum ether occurs by accidental inhalation of vapors or by inadvertent ingestion (the lethal dose is 7.5 mL/kg BW).

Toxicity. Petroleum ether has effects similar to diethyl ether, i. e., it acts as a sedative and narcotic (500–5000 mL/m^3 air), leading finally to respiratory paralysis. Although it is eliminated unchanged via the lungs, uptake by inhalation leads more quickly to dangerous concentrations than uptake by ingestion, and the effects set in more rapidly. Chronic exposure to *small* amounts (by ingestion or inhalation) has an euphoric effect and causes excitement and other central nervous symptoms. Respiratory arrest, cardiac arrest, and also severe polyneuropathy (with motor paralysis) have been observed in sniffing addicts after inhaling solvent vapors containing petroleum ether, and these symptoms may have been caused by the metabolite 2,5-hexanedione (less likely by heptanedione), which is excreted in the urine. Admixture of aromatic compounds (e.g., benzene) further increases toxicity.

Therapy. Administer activated charcoal and purgative.

Methanol (B) and Other Alcohols

Apart from ethanol (see p. 84), it is mainly methanol that is of special toxicological importance as a solvent; propanol, ethylene glycols (diethylene glycol is misused for sweetening wines), and propylene glycol compounds have a minor part to play. Exposure to methanol takes place by inhalation of vapor or by ingestion of denatured (methylated) alcohol and liquors; harmless amounts of methanol are found in fruits and tobacco smoke.

Toxicokinetics and toxicity. Some 30–60 % of methanol is exhaled unchanged; the rest is metabolized by enzymatic oxidation to formaldehyde (half-life 1 min) and formic acid. Its metabolism is slower per hour (25 mg/kg) than that of ethanol (175 mg/kg). Inhalation or ingestion leads to acute intoxication with nausea, vomiting, impaired vision (even blindness), respiratory paralysis, and gastrointestinal problems. Lethal methanol concentrations are 100–250 mg/100 mL blood. Chronic exposure causes mucosal irritation and nonspecific symptoms, such as vertigo, headache, and polyneuropathy.

Therapy. Treatment consists of primary detoxification and intensive care monitoring. Acute treatment with ethanol is required at methanol levels greater than 0.1 g/L, starting with 0.6 g ethanol/kg BW, and then 0.1 g ethanol/kg BW; hemodialysis may be required.

Formaldehyde (C)

This is used worldwide as a disinfectant and preservative (e.g., in medicine) and as a binding material and waterproofing agent in the lumber and textile industries. Formed during incomplete combustion, it can be detected in the air everywhere (0.1–1000 µg/m^3) (see p. 136).

Toxicokinetics and toxicity. After inhalation or ingestion, formaldehyde is rapidly absorbed and metabolized to formic acid (half-life 1 h). Acute and chronic inhalation leads to irritation of the mucosae, eyes, and airways, and causes skin lesions. The effective thresholds vary significantly between individuals.

Therapy. Treatment after ingestion consists of dilution by drinking plenty of water. Glucocorticoids are administered in case of inhalation.

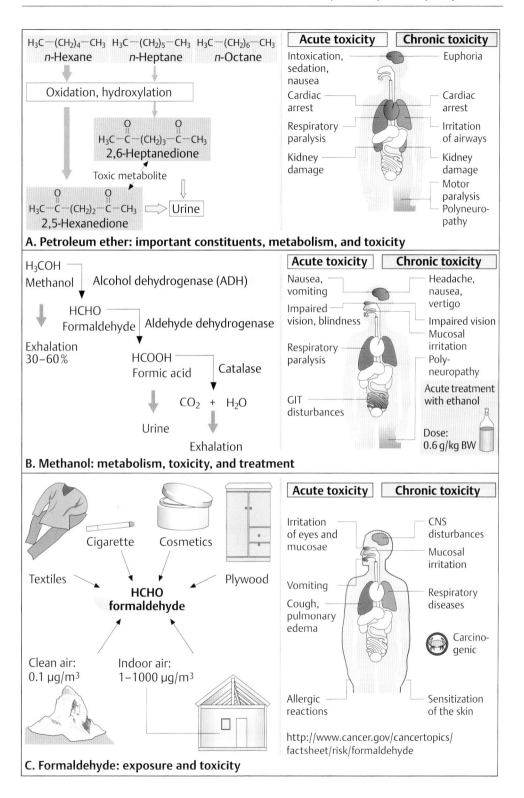

A. Petroleum ether: important constituents, metabolism, and toxicity

$H_3C-(CH_2)_4-CH_3$ *n*-Hexane $H_3C-(CH_2)_5-CH_3$ *n*-Heptane $H_3C-(CH_2)_6-CH_3$ *n*-Octane

Oxidation, hydroxylation

2,6-Heptanedione

Toxic metabolite

2,5-Hexanedione → Urine

Acute toxicity	Chronic toxicity
Intoxication, sedation, nausea	Euphoria
Cardiac arrest	Cardiac arrest
Respiratory paralysis	Irritation of airways
Kidney damage	Kidney damage
	Motor paralysis
	Polyneuro-pathy

B. Methanol: metabolism, toxicity, and treatment

H_3COH Methanol — Alcohol dehydrogenase (ADH)

HCHO Formaldehyde | Aldehyde dehydrogenase

Exhalation 30–60%

HCOOH Formic acid Catalase

CO_2 + H_2O

Urine

Exhalation

Acute toxicity	Chronic toxicity
Nausea, vomiting	Headache, nausea, vertigo
Impaired vision, blindness	Impaired vision
	Mucosal irritation
Respiratory paralysis	Poly-neuropathy
GIT disturbances	Acute treatment with ethanol
	Dose: 0.6 g/kg BW

C. Formaldehyde: exposure and toxicity

Cigarette Cosmetics

Textiles Plywood

HCHO formaldehyde

Clean air: 0.1 µg/m³

Indoor air: 1–1000 µg/m³

Acute toxicity	Chronic toxicity
Irritation of eyes and mucosae	CNS disturbances
	Mucosal irritation
Vomiting	Respiratory diseases
Cough, pulmonary edema	
	Carcino-genic
Allergic reactions	Sensitization of the skin

http://www.cancer.gov/cancertopics/ factsheet/risk/formaldehyde

◼ Cyclic Hydrocarbons

Monocyclic Aromatic Hydrocarbons

The aromatic hydrocarbons *benzene, toluene,* and *xylene* are important industrial solvents and raw materials in the chemical industry. They are detected everywhere in both outdoor and indoor environments.

Benzene

Occurrence (A). Benzene gets into the environment from industrial sources and as a natural constituent of crude oils and petroleum ethers (2–5% of the fuel). Up to 90% of emissions are due to motor vehicle traffic. Benzene concentrations in polluted areas near coking plants, refineries, and gasoline stations are typically 100–300 µg/m^3, while in rural and urban areas concentrations are usually between 1 and 10 µg/m^3. Indoor environments may also contain considerable amounts from tobacco smoke.

Absorption, distribution, and elimination (B). Benzene is well absorbed after inhalation and ingestion, and also through the skin. Initial uptake through the lungs is about 80%, depending on breathing intensity. When inhalation and exhalation have reached equilibrium, uptake drops to 50%. Uptake from the gastrointestinal tract is 100%. Benzene distribution in the body depends on the lipid content of the organs. Redistribution leads to long-term accumulation of benzene in the fatty tissue and bone marrow. Apart from steady elimination through the lungs, benzene is metabolized and excreted in the urine, mainly as sulfate and glucuronic acid conjugates (20–50% of the benzene).

Metabolism (C). Benzene is metabolized by cytochrome P450-dependent enzymes to a reactive epoxide, a considerable amount of which is converted to phenol by nonenzymatic means. Depending on the dose, other metabolic pathways may also be used (e.g., formation of glutathione conjugates, hydroquinone). The metabolite *S*-phenylmercapturic acid is used for monitoring workplace exposures.

Acute and chronic toxicity. The toxic effects of benzene have become known as a result of excessive occupational exposures; thanks to safety measures, these are no longer observed today. Prominent signs of acute inhalation exposure to solvent vapors of benzene include nonspecific reversible symptoms, such as fever and impaired vision, and also central nervous system symptoms (**D**). Benzene concentrations above 25 g/m^3 for more than 30 min are life-threatening and cause unconsciousness, arrhythmias, and impaired respiration.

Toxicological assessment of benzene includes the chronic effects on the hematopoietic system. Nonspecific symptoms, such as vertigo, headache, and hemorrhages are considered to be the result of bone marrow damage. Hematological parameters may be affected in different ways; thrombocytopenia is considered an early symptom. The carcinogenic effect of benzene (induction of leukemia) has been known for a long time; the first reports date back to the early 1900s. Epidemiological studies on heavily exposed workers revealed typical myeloid leukosis. Many effects have been confirmed in experimental animals: changes in cells and chromosomes like those found in exposed workers have been observed. In addition, changes in the immune responses have been detected.

Therapy. Treatment of acute poisoning is symptomatic; blood counts should be monitored after chronic exposure.

Guidance values. The carcinogenicity of benzene is well known.

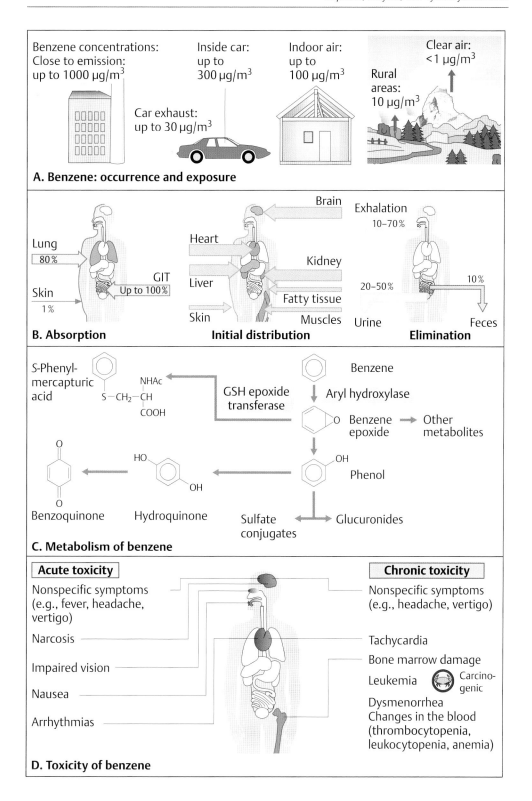

A. Benzene: occurrence and exposure

Benzene concentrations:
Close to emission: up to 1000 µg/m³

Car exhaust: up to 30 µg/m³

Inside car: up to 300 µg/m³

Indoor air: up to 100 µg/m³

Clear air: <1 µg/m³

Rural areas: 10 µg/m³

B. Absorption

Lung 80%

Skin 1%

GIT Up to 100%

Initial distribution

Brain

Heart

Kidney

Liver

Fatty tissue

Skin

Muscles

Elimination

Exhalation 10–70%

Urine 20–50%

Feces 10%

C. Metabolism of benzene

S-Phenyl-mercapturic acid

GSH epoxide transferase

Benzene

Aryl hydroxylase

Benzene epoxide → Other metabolites

Phenol

Benzoquinone   Hydroquinone

Sulfate conjugates ⇌ Glucuronides

D. Toxicity of benzene

Acute toxicity

Nonspecific symptoms (e.g., fever, headache, vertigo)

Narcosis

Impaired vision

Nausea

Arrhythmias

Chronic toxicity

Nonspecific symptoms (e.g., headache, vertigo)

Tachycardia

Bone marrow damage

Leukemia   Carcinogenic

Dysmenorrhea Changes in the blood (thrombocytopenia, leukocytopenia, anemia)

Toluene (A)

Occurrence. Toluene is used as a solvent (benzene substitute) and is an important raw material for chemical syntheses. Major emitters are oil refineries, motor vehicles, and various toluene-containing materials, such as paints; the latter may be responsible for indoor concentrations of 0.2 mg/m^3. Typical outdoor concentrations range between 0.01 and 0.1 mg/m^3 in centers of population and along roads.

Absorption, elimination, and metabolism. Toluene is absorbed up to about 50% after inhalation, and almost completely after ingestion. About 20% is eliminated via the lungs, and 80% is metabolized to benzoic acid and conjugates with glycine, sulfates, and glucuronic acid, and then excreted by the kidneys.

Acute and chronic toxicity. After inhalation of toluene, narcotic effects predominate; high concentrations irritate mucosae and eyes. Chronic exposure leads to nonspecific, depressive central nervous symptoms (vertigo, headaches, and prolonged reaction time). Liver and kidney disorders have been reported after frequent inhalation of large amounts of toluene (> 800 mg/m^3). Changes in blood count, like those characteristic for benzene, are not found. Toluene is not genotoxic. Epidemiological studies have not provided any evidence for carcinogenicity in humans. Teratogenic effects of high toluene concentrations have been described in some animal species.

Guidance values. The WHO guideline value for toluene in the general population is 8 mg/m^3 over a 24-h period.

Xylene (B)

Occurrence. Xylene (dimethylbenzene) is used as a solvent in paints and glues. It is a component of petroleum ether, together with benzene and toluene. The main sources of emission are refineries and motor vehicles. Xylene used for technical purposes is usually a mixture of the three isomers o-, m-, and p-xylene and also contains up to 15% ethylbenzene. Background concentrations of these ubiquitous compounds range from 0.1 µg/m^3 in rural areas to 50 µg/m^3 in centers of population. Concentrations measured indoors can reach up to 300 µg/m^3 (m- and p-xylene each).

Uptake, metabolism, and elimination. Xylene enters the body mainly by inhalation (60% absorption, depending on breathing) and ingestion (complete absorption). After oxidation of one methyl group and conjugation, the resulting entity is metabolized and excreted by the kidneys; only 5% is exhaled.

Acute and chronic toxicity. Xylene vapors acutely irritate the mucosae of the upper airways and the eyes. At high concentrations, xylene has a narcotic effect. Chronic exposure leads to nonspecific central nervous symptoms, such as headache, insomnia, and poor concentration. Damage to the liver, kidneys, myocardium, and hemopoietic system, accompanied by leukopenia and anemia, have been observed. Alcohol enhances the depressing effect of xylene on the central nervous system (as it does with other solvents). Epidemiological studies related to xylene exposure have not been reported. There is no evidence for a carcinogenetic effect of xylene (as a mixture of isomers). Fetotoxic effects have been observed in experiments with mice and rats.

Therapy. Treatment after inhalation of toluene and xylene is symptomatic; after ingestion, primary detoxification consists of administering activated charcoal and a purgative.

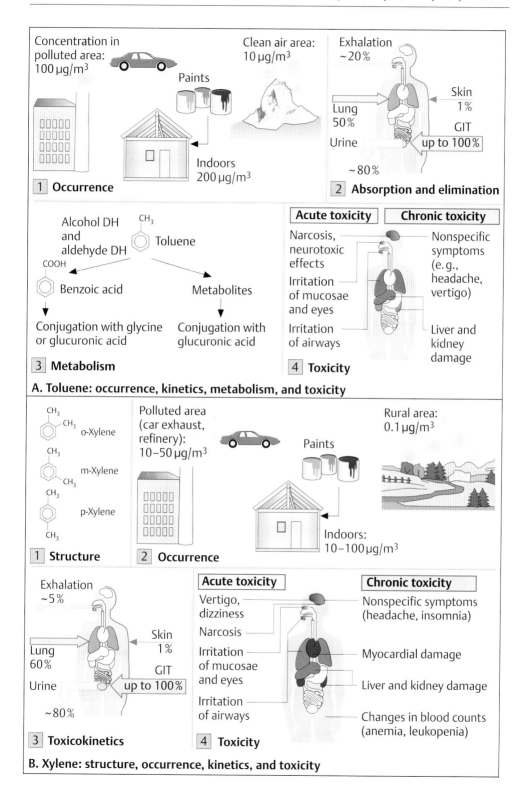

1 Occurrence

Concentration in polluted area: $100\,\mu g/m^3$

Clean air area: $10\,\mu g/m^3$

Paints

Indoors $200\,\mu g/m^3$

2 Absorption and elimination

Exhalation ~20%

Lung 50%

Urine ~80%

Skin 1%

GIT up to 100%

3 Metabolism

Alcohol DH and aldehyde DH

CH₃ Toluene

COOH Benzoic acid

Metabolites

Conjugation with glycine or glucuronic acid

Conjugation with glucuronic acid

4 Toxicity

Acute toxicity	Chronic toxicity
Narcosis, neurotoxic effects	Nonspecific symptoms (e.g., headache, vertigo)
Irritation of mucosae and eyes	
Irritation of airways	Liver and kidney damage

A. Toluene: occurrence, kinetics, metabolism, and toxicity

1 Structure

CH₃ CH₃ o-Xylene

CH₃ CH₃ m-Xylene

CH₃ CH₃ p-Xylene

2 Occurrence

Polluted area (car exhaust, refinery): $10–50\,\mu g/m^3$

Rural area: $0.1\,\mu g/m^3$

Paints

Indoors: $10–100\,\mu g/m^3$

3 Toxicokinetics

Exhalation ~5%

Lung 60%

Urine ~80%

Skin 1%

GIT up to 100%

4 Toxicity

Acute toxicity	Chronic toxicity
Vertigo, dizziness	Nonspecific symptoms (headache, insomnia)
Narcosis	
Irritation of mucosae and eyes	Myocardial damage
	Liver and kidney damage
Irritation of airways	Changes in blood counts (anemia, leukopenia)

B. Xylene: structure, occurrence, kinetics, and toxicity

Polycyclic Aromatic Hydrocarbons

Occurrence (A). Polycyclic aromatic hydrocarbons (PAHs) are largely formed by incomplete combustion of organic material and consist of a mixture of several hundred different compounds. These nonvolatile compounds are ubiquitous. They are found, for example, in car exhaust, soot, and tar fumes, and also in the smoke from food preservation and cigarettes. Since the mass ratios of different PAHs to one another (PAH profiles) are similar depending on the temperature, only a few PAHs (or just one: benzo[a]pyrene, BaP) are usually measured as indicators. PAHs have been detected in all environmental media. They affect humans primarily by polluting food (smoked fish and meat) and the air we breath, and also the soil (legacy hazardous sites). The concentration of PAHs in the air (excluding nitroarenes) varies considerably: up to 4 ng/m^3 in rural areas, and up to 40 ng/m^3 in centers of population without specific pollution sites. Indoors, PAHs are often more concentrated, for example, near roads and industrial emissions, and also due to tobacco smoke: 10–100 ng benzo[a]pyrene can be measured in the smoke of just *one* cigarette.

Uptake, metabolism, and elimination (B). Since PAHs are largely bound to dust particles, their uptake after inhalation depends on the fate of these particles. If the particles are not exhaled, the PAHs are deposited in the throat or respiratory tract and then absorbed in the intestinal tract (~10%) or from the terminal respiratory tract, where they are partly metabolized; they are metabolized more extensively in the liver. After intestinal absorption, the redistribution of PAHs from blood and muscle into fatty tissue takes place within a few days.

PAHs are metabolically activated to epoxides by cytochrome P450-dependent enzymes and induce their own metabolism. After conversion to diol epoxides, the metabolites bind covalently to DNA and thus induce tumors, or are metabolized to glutathione conjugates or to sulfates and glucuronides. In humans, the formation of DNA adducts has been detected mainly in the lungs, in lymphocytes, and in the placenta; however, it correlates only partially with the carcinogenicity of PAHs. Metabolites that are eliminated in the bile undergo enterohepatic recycling or are excreted by the kidneys.

Acute and chronic toxicity (C). PAHs acutely inhibit the growth of all organs; they also cause local skin pigmentation. However, the chronic effects of PAHs are of importance as they lead to carcinogenesis. As early as 1775, Sir Percivall Pott reported on the increased occurrence of cancer in London chimney-sweeps. The carcinogenicity of specific PAHs has been demonstrated in animal experiments. Inhalation of benzo[a]pyrene and dibenzo[a,h]anthracene, in particular, may cause tumors in the lungs. It is assumed that several other PAHs have a similar effect. Frequently, however, only local carcinogenic effects have been observed after cutaneous application, and the individual compounds differed considerably with respect to potencies. No carcinogenic effects have been detected for some representatives of this class of compounds. The decisive factor in determining whether or not a compound acts as a carcinogen is its metabolism in the liver. However, depending on the original compound, this process is influenced in many ways by both intoxication and detoxification.

Since exposure usually occurs by means of PAH-containing mixtures of pyrolytic products, the aim is to reduce the daily intake by minimizing the occurrence of these (**D**).

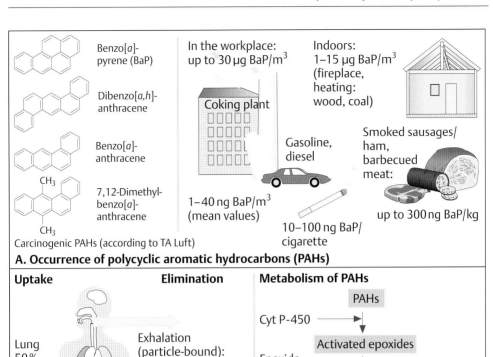

Benzo[*a*]-pyrene (BaP)

Dibenzo[*a,h*]-anthracene

Benzo[*a*]-anthracene

7,12-Dimethyl-benzo[*a*]-anthracene

Carcinogenic PAHs (according to TA Luft)

In the workplace:
up to 30 µg BaP/m^3

Coking plant

1–40 ng BaP/m^3
(mean values)

Gasoline, diesel

10–100 ng BaP/cigarette

Indoors:
1–15 µg BaP/m^3
(fireplace, heating: wood, coal)

Smoked sausages/ham, barbecued meat:

up to 300 ng BaP/kg

A. Occurrence of polycyclic aromatic hydrocarbons (PAHs)

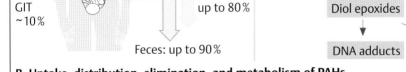

Uptake   **Elimination**   **Metabolism of PAHs**

Lung 50%

Skin

GIT ~10%

Exhalation (particle-bound): up to 50%

Metabolites in urine: up to 80%

Feces: up to 90%

PAHs

Cyt P-450 →

Activated epoxides

Epoxide hydrolase → → Conjugates, phenols

Dihydrodiols

Cyt P-450 → → Conjugates

Diol epoxides

→ Conjugates

DNA adducts

B. Uptake, distribution, elimination, and metabolism of PAHs

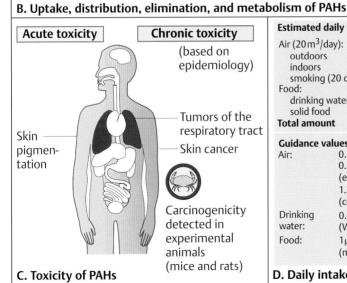

Acute toxicity	**Chronic toxicity**

(based on epidemiology)

Skin pigmentation

Tumors of the respiratory tract

Skin cancer

Carcinogenicity detected in experimental animals (mice and rats)

C. Toxicity of PAHs

Estimated daily intake of BaP

Air (20 m^3/day):
outdoors	1–100 ng
indoors	5–500 ng
smoking (20 cigarettes)	400 ng

Food:
drinking water (2 L)	1–4 ng
solid food	100 500 ng
Total amount about	**1500 ng**

Guidance values

Air:	0.1 mg BaP/m^3
	0.1 mg dibenzo[*a,h*]anthracene/m^3 (emission according to TA Luft)
	1.3 ng BaP/m^3 (concentration according to LAI)
Drinking water:	0.01 µg BaP/L (WHO guideline)
Food:	1 µg BaP/kg (meat products regulations)

D. Daily intake and guidance values

Halogenated Aliphatic Hydrocarbons

Basics. Among the halogen compounds containing fluorine, chlorine, or bromine, the chlorinated organic compounds are particularly important in toxicology. Chlorine is extremely reactive, and chlorine-containing compounds are therefore used in the chemical industry as reactive starting materials or intermediates. Unlike polyhalogenated *cyclic* compounds (see p. 112), which are the subject of international concern because of their global distribution and persistence in the environment, chlorinated *aliphatic* compounds are of immediate importance because of their acute and chronic toxic effects on parenchymatous organs. These effects are facilitated by the high vapor pressure of these compounds, which enhances their uptake and elimination. Other factors are various metabolic reactions, the products of which then determine the type and extent of the toxic effects. Even substances that are chemically closely related are metabolized differently, and hence also have different toxicities. The genotoxic effects of certain metabolites are accompanied by carcinogenic effects and therefore pose a special problem. Current risk assessments of chlorinated organic compounds take this into account (**A**). Polychlorinated alkanes, alkenes, and alkynes are largely used as *solvents* because of their good lipid-dissolving properties (**B**). Uptake is predominantly by inhalation; dermal or oral exposures are rare (accidents or attempted suicides). The high vapor pressure of these compounds usually produces rapid, concentration-dependent narcotic effects, the duration of which is determined by the speed of exhalation.

Trichloromethane (Chloroform)

Like other chlorinated hydrocarbons, trichloromethane ($CHCl_3$) has been in use since 1847 as an anesthetic. Because of its toxic effects, primarily on the liver and kidneys, other halogenated compounds with wider therapeutic ranges are currently used for anesthesia, e.g., halothane (see p. 108).

Absorption and metabolism. Upon absorption after inhalation, ingestion, or uptake through the skin, trichloromethane is metabolically activated in the liver. The secondary product trichloromethanol is converted to phosgene by dehydrochlorination; this reactive metabolite causes damage to cells and cellular components (**C**).

Acute toxicity (D). Symptoms of poisoning with inhaled trichloromethane include excitation, unconsciousness, and respiratory paralysis. Of particular importance is the cardiotoxic effect after exposure to high concentrations of a trichloromethane–air mixture (> 2.5 v/v), which causes sudden cardiac arrest due to the sensitization to catecholamines. Exposure for several hours causes a drop in blood pressure and shock. Examination of the liver reveals toxic hepatitis with centrilobular necroses, similar to poisoning with tetrachloromethane. In severe cases, acute liver atrophy with hepatic coma sets in. After dermal exposure, ulcers and inflammation of the skin may develop.

Chronic toxicity (D). The liver and kidneys are especially sensitive. The maximum workplace concentrations take this into consideration. Trichloromethane has genotoxic effects, and it is carcinogenic in experimental animals. Like other chlorinated methane derivatives, trichloromethane is considered to be a possible human carcinogen.

Therapy. Intensive monitoring of vital signs is essential. Treatment of poisoning by ingestion consists of rapid detoxification by induction of vomiting and gastric lavage; poisoning by inhalation calls for fresh air and hyperventilation therapy. In case of a fire, it is important that first aid workers wear protective masks (to prevent toxic pulmonary edema if phosgene is formed).

Compound	Threshold value (mL/m³)	Carcinogen	Suspected carcinogen
Chloroethane	–	–	3B
Chloroethene	–	+ (in humans)	1
1,1-Dichloroethane	100	–	–
1,1-Dichloroethylene	2	–	3B
1,2-Dichloroethane	–	+ (in humans)	2
1,2-Dichloroethylene	200	–	–
1,1,1-Trichloroethane	200	–	–
1,1,2-Trichloroethane	10	–	3B
1,1,2-Trichloroethylene	50	+ (in humans)	1
Tetrachloroethylene	–	–	3B

A. Toxicities and guidance values of halogenated hydrocarbons

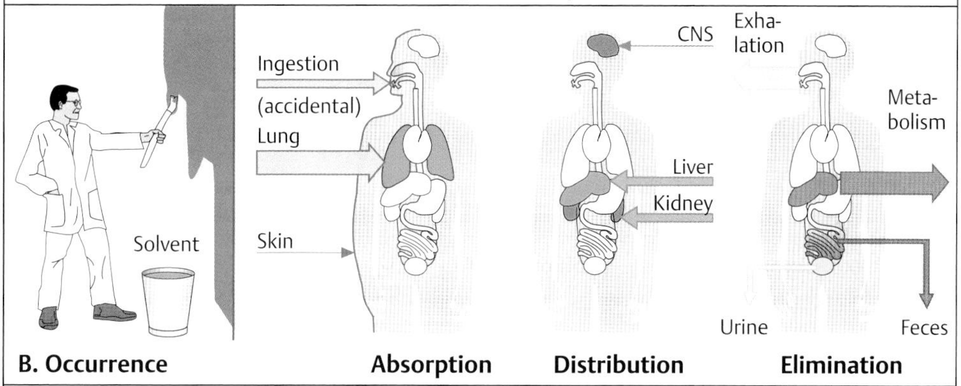

Solvent
Ingestion
(accidental)
Lung
Skin
CNS
Exha-
lation
Liver
Kidney
Meta-
bolism
Urine
Feces
Absorption
Distribution
Elimination

B. Occurrence

Liver
Hydroxy-
lation
Dehydro-
chlorination
$CHCl_3$
$HO-CCl_3$
$COCl_2$
Trichloro-
methane
Trichloro-
methanol
Phosgene
Cell damage
(e.g., in the pulmonary
epithelium)

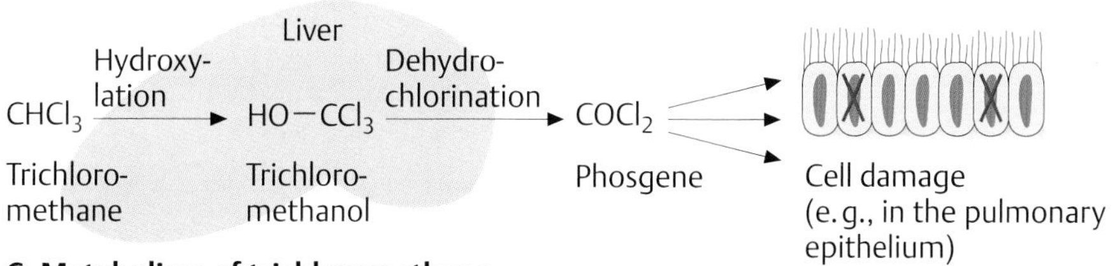

C. Metabolism of trichloromethane

Acute toxicity
Unconsciousness
Respiratory paralysis
Drop in blood pressure
Arrhythmias
Cardiac arrest
Toxic hepatitis
Necrosis, ulcers
Chronic toxicity
Liver damage
Kidney damage
Carcinogenic

D. Toxicity of trichloromethane

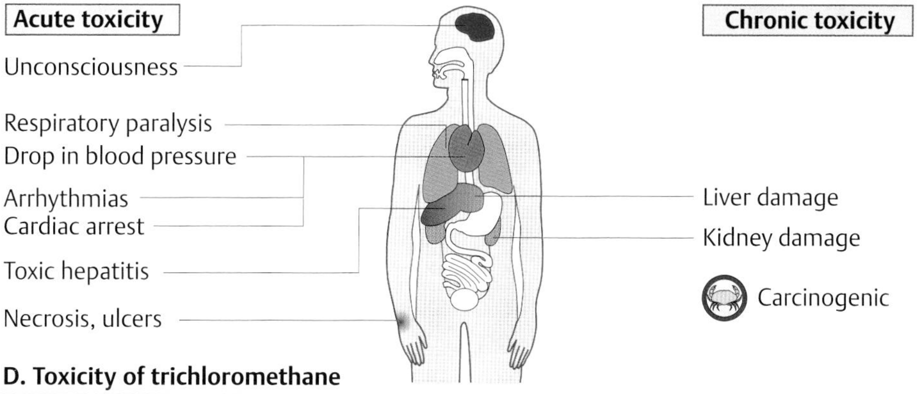

Tetrachloromethane (Carbon Tetrachloride)

Occurrence. Tetrachloromethane (CCl_4), like trichloromethane, has excellent lipid-dissolving properties; it was once employed as a fire extinguisher and a commonly used cleaning agent in households. Despite its high toxicity, it is still used in industry for cleaning machinery (**A**).

Severe poisonings by tetrachloromethane, including those with a lethal outcome, occurred frequently in the past. After signs of hepatotoxicity similar to those seen with other halogenated hydrocarbons were found, investigations into the effects of tetrachloromethane provided an exemplary explanation of the underlying mechanisms of organ damage.

Absorption, distribution, metabolism, and elimination (A). After ingestion or inhalation, tetrachloromethane is distributed to the central nervous system, liver, kidneys, and fatty tissue. It is also partly eliminated via the lungs. As a prerequisite of any organotoxic effects, the compound must be metabolized in the body (toxin generation). After dehalogenation of tetrachloromethane, a free trichloromethyl radical ($\bullet CCl_3$) is formed in the liver by the mixed-function oxidases. The free radical binds to macromolecules in the cells and reacts with the unsaturated fatty acids of membrane lipids (**B**). The liver's capacity for toxin generation declines markedly after repeated exposure, and acute toxic doses are finally tolerated as long as they are taken up slowly enough. By incorporating a hydrogen atom, the free radical forms trichloromethane, which can be detected as a metabolite (in addition to carbon monoxide, carbon dioxide, and traces of hexachloroethane).

Mechanism of action. Oxidative damage of membranes is thought to play an important role in the cytotoxic effects of chlorinated organic compounds. The result is that the cells first lose electrolytes (potassium ions), then release enzymes, and finally die. Furthermore, mutagenic secondary products may form by lipid peroxidation.

Acute and chronic toxicity. As with other chloroalkanes, central nervous effects predominate, such as headache, dizziness, nausea, and vomiting. The cardinal symptom is liver dysfunction associated with rapid increases in alanine aminotransferase (ALT) and aspartate aminotransferase (AST), icterus, and liver coma, followed by severe kidney damage (tubular necrosis) with anuria and uremia (**C**). Symptoms after chronic exposure to small amounts of tetrachloromethane include paresthesia and vertigo. Minor changes in liver function parameters are nonspecific and difficult to distinguish from other causes.

Therapy. Treatment is the same as for trichloromethane; ingestion of more than 1.5 mL/kg BW requires hyperventilation treatment (see p. 102).

Chloromethane (Methyl Chloride) and Dichloromethane (Methylene Chloride)

Occurrence and metabolism. Chloromethane has been used as a cooling agent (boiling point 22 °C), and dichloromethane is primarily used as a technical solvent. Monochloromethane disintegrates in the body into HCl and methanol. A glutathione-dependent pathway of dichloromethane metabolism leads to carbon dioxide. In low concentrations, however, it is mainly converted by oxidation to carbon monoxide (CO), which is formed depending on dose and time and binds to hemoglobin.

Toxicity (D). Both substances lead to nonspecific effects and disturbances of the central nervous system. Furthermore, chloromethane is fetotoxic, and dichloromethane is slightly irritating to the mucosae and has pronounced narcotic and hepatotoxic effects. Both substances are suspected carcinogens in humans.

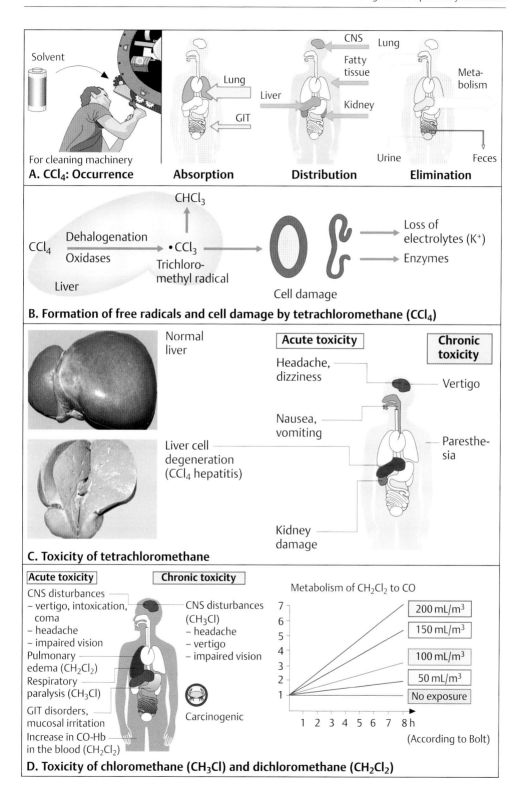

A. CCl₄: Occurrence **Absorption** **Distribution** **Elimination**

For cleaning machinery

Solvent

Lung
GIT

CNS Lung
Fatty tissue
Liver
Kidney

Lung
Meta-bolism

Urine Feces

B. Formation of free radicals and cell damage by tetrachloromethane (CCl₄)

CCl_4 → Dehalogenation Oxidases (Liver) → $\cdot CCl_3$ Trichloro-methyl radical → $CHCl_3$

Cell damage → Loss of electrolytes (K⁺), Enzymes

C. Toxicity of tetrachloromethane

Normal liver

Liver cell degeneration (CCl₄ hepatitis)

Acute toxicity

Headache, dizziness

Nausea, vomiting

Kidney damage

Chronic toxicity

Vertigo

Paresthe-sia

D. Toxicity of chloromethane (CH₃Cl) and dichloromethane (CH₂Cl₂)

Acute toxicity

CNS disturbances
– vertigo, intoxication, coma
– headache
– impaired vision
Pulmonary edema (CH₂Cl₂)
Respiratory paralysis (CH₃Cl)
GIT disorders, mucosal irritation
Increase in CO-Hb in the blood (CH₂Cl₂)

Chronic toxicity

CNS disturbances (CH₃Cl)
– headache
– vertigo
– impaired vision

Carcinogenic

Metabolism of CH_2Cl_2 to CO

200 mL/m³
150 mL/m³
100 mL/m³
50 mL/m³
No exposure

1 2 3 4 5 6 7 8 h

(According to Bolt)

Trichloroethylene (Trichloroethene)

This solvent, used extensively for industrial purposes, causes narcosis and euphoria similar to trichloromethane. It has been used in the past as a narcotic and abused for sniffing. It is clearly carcinogenic to humans.

Toxicokinetics and metabolism. Trichloroethylene and other chlorinated alkenes are converted to epoxides (oxiranes) by monoxygenases in a rate-determining biotransformation step. These highly reactive compounds bind to cellular macromolecules and may be responsible for chronic damage to the liver and other organs. Unlike trichloromethane, trichloroethylene at low concentrations has only minor hepatotoxic effects. It is metabolized to several acutely sedating and narcotic, nonhepatotoxic substances, such as chloral hydrate, trichloroethanol, and trichloroacetic acid. Trichloroethanol is the main metabolite of trichloroethylene in humans, and it is excreted in the urine (**A**). It is therefore used in occupational medicine for monitoring exposure. Other glutathione-dependent trichloroethylene metabolites are associated with tumor formation in animal experiments (lung, liver, and kidney tumors).

Tetrachloroethylene (Tetrachloroethene)

Occurrence and exposure. Tetrachloroethylene is the solvent most commonly used for dry cleaning; it is also used industrially for degreasing and in the synthesis of chlorofluorocarbons (CFCs). In the past, the large number of dry cleaning facilities alone caused considerable air pollution (e.g., up to 15 000 t/year in Germany). Nowadays tetrachloroethylene must be used in a closed system: the residues are distilled, and tetrachloroethylene is condensed and purified over activated charcoal. Because of industrial emissions, solvent loss (1%), and discharge from clothing, tetrachloroethylene is nevertheless ubiquitous in the general population (**B**). The main pathways of pollution are indoor and outdoor air as well as food, and sometimes also the soil and groundwater close to industrial plants. Accumulation of this lipophilic compound in fatty food can be prevented by storing food separately from the sources of contamination.

Toxicokinetics and metabolism. Tetrachloroethylene is largely exhaled unchanged. Its metabolism is similar to that of trichloroethylene and involves the formation of tetrachlorooxirane (epoxide) and the metabolite trichloroacetic acid (which is eliminated in the urine and has a half-life of 100 h), and also a glutathione-dependent pathway that is thought to be responsible for organ toxicity.

Acute and chronic toxicity. Acute symptoms are nonspecific and include headache, nausea, narcosis, and skin lesions (**C**). High doses cause pulmonary edema, gastrointestinal disorders, and damage to liver and kidneys. Similar symptoms are found after chronic exposure.

Fears arose in the general public after liver and kidney tumors had been detected in experimental animals exposed to tetrachloroethylene. Tumors in humans exposed to high concentrations cannot be unequivocally attributed to tetrachloroethylene because of mixed exposures in most cases. The suspicion remains that the compound is potentially carcinogenic in humans.

Regulations. The clean air legislation that has come into force in most industrialized countries specifies a maximum concentration in air ($0.1 \, \mathrm{mg/m^3}$) for closed spaces immediately adjacent to dry cleaning facilities: for example, the 8-h threshold of exposure in Germany is currently 340–350 $\mathrm{mg/m^3}$.

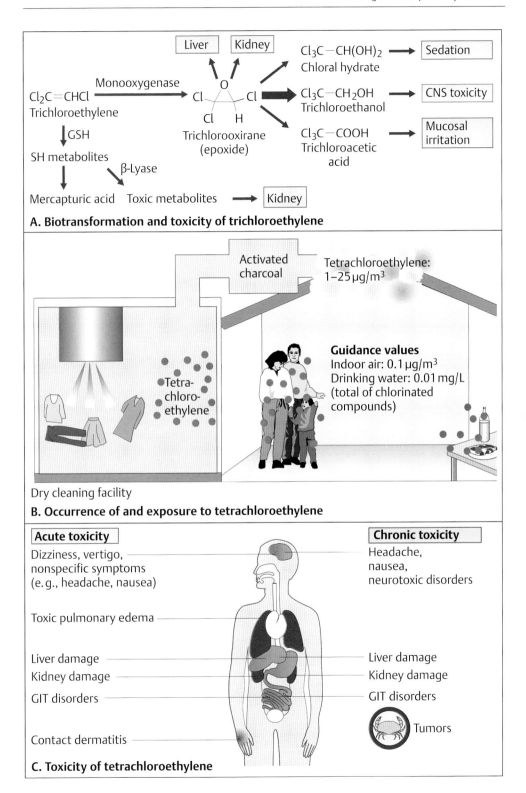

A. Biotransformation and toxicity of trichloroethylene

Dry cleaning facility

B. Occurrence of and exposure to tetrachloroethylene

C. Toxicity of tetrachloroethylene

▪ Other Halogenated Ethanes and Ethylenes

Vinyl Chloride

Toxicokinetics and metabolism. Biotransformation of the monomer vinyl chloride (VC, also known as chloroethene) to VC epoxide (chlorooxirane) deserves special attention (**A**). The activated product is considered the "ultimate" carcinogen responsible for the induction of tumors by VC. Conjugation with glutathione leads to detoxification of the toxic metabolite. Unfortunately, this physiological pathway of detoxification provides no adequate protection against alkylation of cellular macromolecules; therefore, even low concentrations of VC may cause tumors. Today, fully automated control and closed production plants prevent exposure to VC during production processes, and any exposure of employees can be monitored by personal dosimeters. During incineration, there is no re-formation of the monomeric VC from the polymeric end product, polyvinyl chloride (PVC); nevertheless, acid equivalents, aromatic hydrocarbons, and polychlorinated dibenzodioxins and dibenzofurans are released during thermal disposal of PVC-containing waste. These emissions can be kept under control by specific incineration conditions and filtering (**B**) (see also p. 55).

Acute and chronic toxicity. Mucosal irritation and narcotic effects due to vapors have occurred in individuals exposed to VC, and also gastrointestinal disorders and polyneuropathies, such as numbness in the extremities. The occurrence of arrhythmias has prevented the use of VC as an anesthetic; hepatosplenomegaly, skin lesions (scleroderma), and changes in the liver have been observed. VC is carcinogenic to humans (hemangiosarcoma of the liver) (**C**).

▪ Vinylidene Chloride (1,1-Dichloroethylene)

The compound is also used for the production of polymers. Unlike VC, it is highly hepatotoxic. Its metabolism is similar to that of VC. The compound is a suspected carcinogen; animal experiments have yielded inconsistent results (**D**).

▪ Halothane (2-Bromo-2-chloro-1,1,1-trifluoroethane)

Halothane was the first inhalation anesthetic that was easy to control and had relatively low systemic toxicity. However, it may have a hepatotoxic effect (even causing dystrophy), especially when the liver has already been damaged (**D**). The halogenated hydrocarbons isoflurane and enflurane are better tolerated.

▪ 1,1,1- and 1,1,2-Trichloroethane

The important solvent 1,1,1-trichloroethane is practically nontoxic; it is used in correction fluid (Tipp-Ex, White-Out). By contrast, its positional isomer 1,1,2-trichloroethane is hepatotoxic and nephrotoxic (like trichloromethane) and also irritates the mucosae and airways (**D**).

▪ 1,1,2,2-Tetrachloroethane

In the past, this solvent has been commonly used in the textile industry. It has the highest acute toxicity of all the chlorinated ethanes, and, like 1,1,2-trichloroethane and trichloromethane, it is hepatotoxic. Inhalation causes acute central nervous effects, such as headache, and also nausea, tachycardia, and mucosal irritation. Following chronic exposure, liver and kidney dysfunction, icterus, and ascites may occur, as well as polyneuropathies (**D**). Ingestion of 3 mL may lead to liver dystrophy (similarly to poisoning by tetrachloromethane).

▪ 1,2-Dichloroethane and 1,2-Dibromoethane

Both compounds are ubiquitous in lead-containing fuels, where they are used as lead scavengers. They have an alkylating effect and are carcinogenic in experimental animals.

Therapy

After ingestion of high doses, primary detoxification has priority; further treatment is symptomatic.

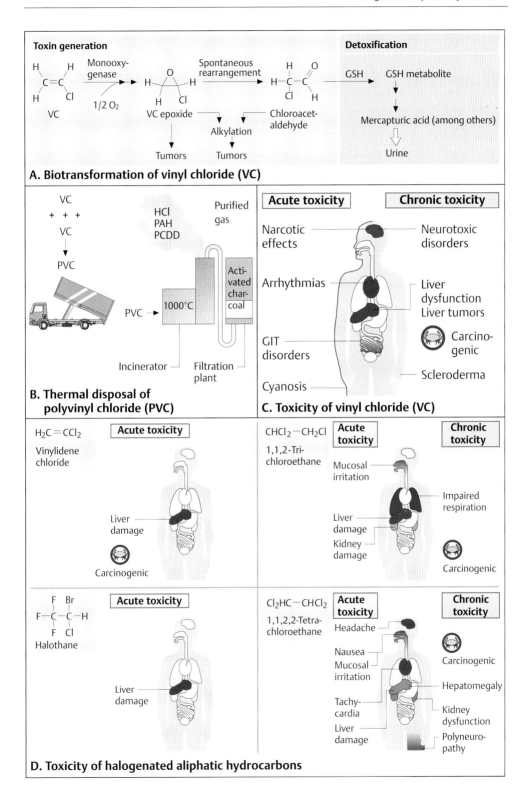

Toxin generation

VC → (Monooxygenase, $1/2\,O_2$) → VC epoxide → (Spontaneous rearrangement) → Chloroacetaldehyde

VC epoxide / Chloroacetaldehyde → Alkylation → Tumors

VC epoxide → Tumors

Detoxification

Chloroacetaldehyde → GSH → GSH metabolite → Mercapturic acid (among others) → Urine

A. Biotransformation of vinyl chloride (VC)

VC + VC + VC → PVC

PVC → Incinerator (1000°C) → HCl, PAH, PCDD → Filtration plant (Activated charcoal) → Purified gas

B. Thermal disposal of polyvinyl chloride (PVC)

C. Toxicity of vinyl chloride (VC)

Acute toxicity	Chronic toxicity
Narcotic effects	Neurotoxic disorders
Arrhythmias	Liver dysfunction / Liver tumors
GIT disorders	Carcinogenic
Cyanosis	Scleroderma

$H_2C = CCl_2$
Vinylidene chloride

Acute toxicity

Liver damage

Carcinogenic

$F-C-C-H$ (F, F / Br, Cl)
Halothane

Acute toxicity

Liver damage

$CHCl_2 - CH_2Cl$
1,1,2-Trichloroethane

Acute toxicity

Mucosal irritation
Liver damage
Kidney damage

Chronic toxicity

Impaired respiration
Carcinogenic

$Cl_2HC - CHCl_2$
1,1,2,2-Tetrachloroethane

Acute toxicity

Headache
Nausea
Mucosal irritation
Tachycardia
Liver damage

Chronic toxicity

Carcinogenic
Hepatomegaly
Kidney dysfunction
Polyneuropathy

D. Toxicity of halogenated aliphatic hydrocarbons

Chlorofluorocarbons

Basics. The toxicity of chlorofluorocarbons (CFCs) in plants, animals, and humans is generally low. However, CFCs are thought to be responsible for the reduced amount of ozone in the atmosphere (the ozone hole; see ozone depletion, p. 152).

Since CFCs in the troposphere are not washed out by precipitation, they persist there for a very long time (> 75 years). A worldwide restriction of their production was agreed in the Montreal Protocol in 1987. Partly halogenated compounds (hydrochlorofluorocarbons, HCFCs) and nonchlorinated compounds (hydrofluorocarbons, HFCs) have been developed as alternatives. HCFCs have a very low ozone-depleting potential, and HFCs have none at all (**A**).

A special nomenclature has been introduced for low-molecular weight CFCs with a maximum of four carbon atoms. According to this nomenclature, the letter R (for refrigerant) is followed by a three-digit number: the first digit indicates the number of C atoms minus one, the second digit indicates the number of H atoms plus one, and the third digit indicates the number of F atoms. Other nomenclatures are also in use.

Low-molecular-weight CFCs (e.g., $CFCl_3$, CF_2Cl_2) are used mostly as blowing agents, aerosol propellants in spray cans (e.g., inhalation aerosols), and refrigerants in cooling systems. (They are best known by their trade names, e. g., Freon and Frigen.) With respect to toxicology, the use of these agents is generally recognized as safe. However, organ damage and even death have been observed in individuals with excessive exposure to certain broncholytic sprays designed for inhalation, and also in persons exposed to large amounts as a result of sniffing.

Polytetrafluoroethylene (Teflon) is employed as a nonstick coating in cooking pots and frying pans for normal household use. When Teflon is heated for technical purposes (e.g., during welding), fluorine compounds are formed; they may cause irritation of the airways. Similar symptoms may arise from the excessive use of Teflon spray cans.

Absorption, metabolism, and elimination. CFCs are rapidly and almost completely absorbed via the lungs. However, they are also quickly exhaled in a CFC-free atmosphere. CFCs are distributed via the blood plasma to the organs and quickly pass into the central nervous system due to their lipophilic properties (**B**).

Small amounts of CFCs can be degraded in the liver by mixed-function oxidases (P450 monooxidases) to acetic acid derivatives. The resulting degradation products are excreted in the urine. Unchanged CFCs are almost completely exhaled (**B**).

Toxicity. *Acute toxicity* is considered low for all these substances. Uptake of large amounts of CFCs causes reversible central nervous symptoms, such as mild anesthesia, lethargy, or impaired coordination. After IV administration of epinephrine following the uptake of high CFC doses, cardiac sensitization (arrhythmias) has been observed in humans (**C**).

Chronic toxicity in animals and humans is considered very low for all CFCs (**C**). In experimental animals, application of very high doses caused a reduction in body weight and plasma lipids, in addition to central nervous symptoms, but only after 2 years of exposure.

Teratogenic, mutagenic, and carcinogenic effects of CFCs, including HCFCs and HFCs, have not been reported. Exceptions include chlorofluoromethane and 2,2-dichloro-1,1,1-trifluoroethane.

Therapy. No treatment is required after *ingestion* of small amounts of CFCs. When ingested in larger amounts, activated charcoal and sodium sulfate (Glauber's salt) should be administered. Fresh air is essential in case of *inhalation*; administration of epinephrine and catecholamines is not recommended as they may cause arrhythmia.

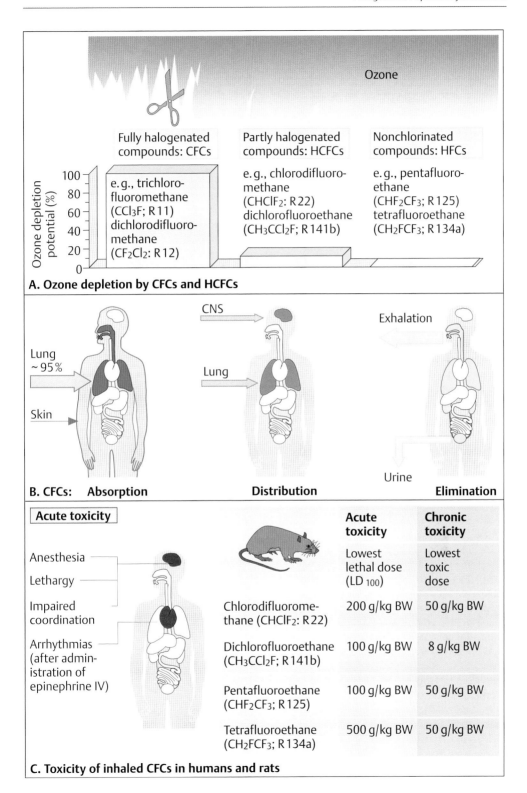

A. Ozone depletion by CFCs and HCFCs

Fully halogenated compounds: CFCs

e.g., trichloro-fluoromethane (CCl₃F; R 11) dichlorodifluoro-methane (CF₂Cl₂: R 12)

Partly halogenated compounds: HCFCs

e.g., chlorodifluoro-methane (CHClF₂: R 22) dichlorofluoroethane (CH₃CCl₂F; R 141b)

Nonchlorinated compounds: HFCs

e.g., pentafluoro-ethane (CHF₂CF₃; R 125) tetrafluoroethane (CH₂FCF₃; R 134a)

B. CFCs: Absorption Distribution Elimination

C. Toxicity of inhaled CFCs in humans and rats

Acute toxicity

Anesthesia
Lethargy
Impaired coordination
Arrhythmias (after administration of epinephrine IV)

	Acute toxicity	Chronic toxicity
	Lowest lethal dose (LD 100)	Lowest toxic dose
Chlorodifluorome-thane (CHClF₂: R 22)	200 g/kg BW	50 g/kg BW
Dichlorofluoroethane (CH₃CCl₂F; R 141b)	100 g/kg BW	8 g/kg BW
Pentafluoroethane (CHF₂CF₃; R 125)	100 g/kg BW	50 g/kg BW
Tetrafluoroethane (CH₂FCF₃; R 134a)	500 g/kg BW	50 g/kg BW

■ Halogenated Cyclic and Polycyclic Hydrocarbons

Basics. Halogenated cyclic and polycyclic hydrocarbons persist for very long times both in the air and in the soil. Because of their global distribution and accumulation in the human body, they play an important role as environmental chemicals with hazardous waste characteristics.

■ Halogenated Cyclic Hydrocarbons

Chlorinated Benzenes and Phenols

Application. Aromatic chlorinated compounds have been used worldwide in pest control because of their insecticidal, fungicidal, and bactericidal properties (see p. 193).

Acute and chronic toxicity. *Chlorobenzene* (**A**) in high doses causes central nervous disorders and degenerative changes of the liver and kidneys. The toxicity of *dichlorobenzene* varies depending on the position of the chlorine atom: *o-dichlorobenzene* causes primarily mild anesthesia, whereas *p-dichlorobenzene* is primarily a mucosal irritant. Changes in the blood count and damage to the lungs, liver, and kidneys are observed at high concentrations. Incineration of chlorine-containing compounds generates *m-dichlorobenzene*, which is therefore found everywhere in the air, soil, and water. Typical outdoor concentrations of *m*-dichlorobenzene in rural areas are around $0.1\,\mu g/m^3$ and in centers of population up to $1\,\mu g/m^3$. In this dose range, there is no information available on human exposures to this compound of low acute toxicity. In animal experiments, high dosages were hepatotoxic and promoted tumor development in rats. There was no evidence for mutagenic and teratogenic effects. *Trichlorobenzenes* irritate the eyes, mucosae, and airways, and *tetrachlorobenzenes* cause chromosomal aberrations after chronic exposure.

   Hexachlorobenzene (HCB) is also ubiquitous because of its extensive use as a fungicide; background concentrations of $0.1–0.5\,ng/m^3$ are detected everywhere. HCB present in dusts and air mixtures irritates the eyes, skin, mucosae, and the respiratory tract. Narcotic effects

occur as well. Heated chlorine-containing vapors (explosive!) may lead to pulmonary edema. Liver damage has been observed after chronic exposure. The use of HCB-treated cereals in Turkey caused mass poisoning accompanied by skin eruptions, enlargements of liver and thyroid gland, and even death. Tumors were observed after exposure to toxic doses. HCB induces cytochrome P450-dependent enzyme systems and is excreted in the feces.

Halogenated phenols. These are used as disinfectants and are highly corrosive. They also occur as intermediates during the synthesis of other chlorinated hydrocarbons. Inflammatory, light-sensitive dermatosis (including chloracne) as well as disorders of the liver, kidneys, and hematopoietic system have been observed in humans after dermal exposure to *2,4,6-trichlorophenol*. In experimental animals exposed to high doses (500–1000 mg/kg BW), trichlorophenol had a carcinogenic effect. *Pentachlorophenol (PCP)* is an insecticide and fungicide that has been used for a long time as a wood preservative. PCP is rapidly absorbed through the skin and converted in the liver to glucuronides that are eliminated in the urine (**B**). In the target organs—liver and kidneys—the highest concentrations have been found after exposure by ingestion or inhalation. The predominating acute symptoms (*wood preservative syndrome*) are nonspecific and include vertigo, nausea, and vomiting (**C**). Many symptoms are thought to be caused by contamination of the technical product with dibenzodioxins and dibenzofurans. There is limited evidence that PCP is genotoxic, but high doses have been shown to be carcinogenic in mice.

Therapy. Treatment is symptomatic; primary detoxification is needed in cases of acute poisoning by ingestion. First aid providers should wear protective clothing, as these compounds are easily absorbed through the skin.

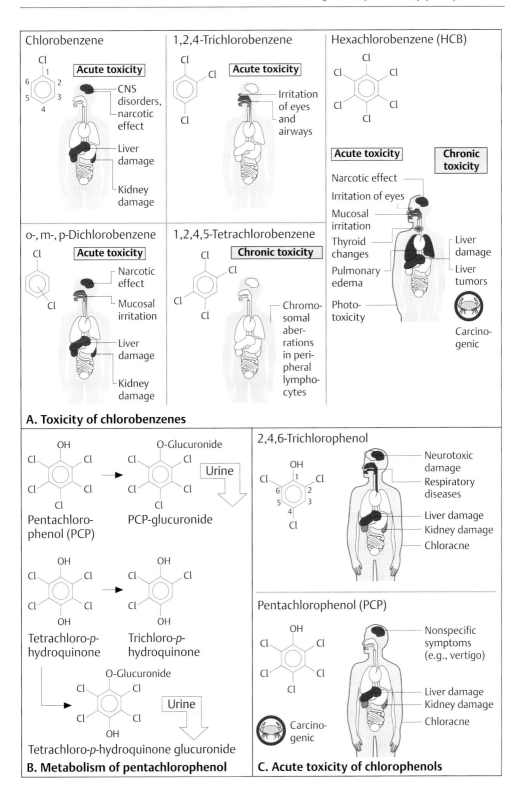

A. Toxicity of chlorobenzenes

Chlorobenzene

Acute toxicity
- CNS disorders, narcotic effect
- Liver damage
- Kidney damage

1,2,4-Trichlorobenzene

Acute toxicity
- Irritation of eyes and airways

Hexachlorobenzene (HCB)

Acute toxicity / Chronic toxicity
- Narcotic effect
- Irritation of eyes
- Mucosal irritation
- Thyroid changes
- Pulmonary edema
- Photo-toxicity
- Liver damage
- Liver tumors
- Carcino-genic

o-, m-, p-Dichlorobenzene

Acute toxicity
- Narcotic effect
- Mucosal irritation
- Liver damage
- Kidney damage

1,2,4,5-Tetrachlorobenzene

Chronic toxicity
- Chromo-somal aber-rations in peri-pheral lympho-cytes

B. Metabolism of pentachlorophenol

Pentachloro-phenol (PCP) → PCP-glucuronide → Urine

Tetrachloro-*p*-hydroquinone → Trichloro-*p*-hydroquinone

Tetrachloro-*p*-hydroquinone glucuronide → Urine

C. Acute toxicity of chlorophenols

2,4,6-Trichlorophenol
- Neurotoxic damage
- Respiratory diseases
- Liver damage
- Kidney damage
- Chloracne

Pentachlorophenol (PCP)
- Nonspecific symptoms (e.g., vertigo)
- Liver damage
- Kidney damage
- Chloracne
- Carcino-genic

■ Halogenated Polycyclic Hydrocarbons I

Polychlorinated Biphenyls

Chemistry. The polychlorinated biphenyls (PCBs) are a group of nonpolar chlorinated compounds that differ in their chlorine content and the positions of the chlorine atoms attached to the benzene rings (**A**). In total, 209 individual compounds (congeners) are possible. Since 1929, country-specific PCB mixtures of different compositions have been produced industrially (e.g., in Europe under the trade names Aroclor, Clophen, Phenoclor; usually with a chlorine content of 40–60%). Certain congeners (Nos. 28, 52, 101, 138, 153, and 180) are used as indicators for the total PCB content (**A**).

Occurrence and exposure. The industrially valuable chemical and physical properties of PCBs have lead to their wide application, for example, as hydraulic oils, lubricants, flame retardants, and insulators in transformers. The use of PCBs has been restricted or banned in many industrialized countries since the 1970s because of their persistence in the air, soil, and water. Nevertheless, they continue to exist in paints, sealants, adhesives, and plastic as a source of outdoor and indoor exposure. Between 0.003 ng PCB/m^3 (in clean air areas) and 20 ng PCB/m^3 are found in outdoor air; in PCB-polluted indoor environments, values over 10 000 ng PCB/m^3 may be found.

Toxicokinetics. The main pathway of exposure for humans is by ingestion of PCBs with fat-rich food (**B**) and also, in individual cases (indoor pollution), by inhalation. After redistribution in the body, PCBs are metabolized in the liver depending on their level of chlorination, thus reducing their toxicity. Highly chlorinated PCBs, in particular, accumulate in organs and body fat (~2 mg PCB/kg fat). Breast milk may contain up to 1 mg PCB/kg milk fat; since 1981, the contamination of breast milk has been declined by about 50%. The elimination of various congeners is very slow, with half-lives ranging between 1 and 10 years.

Acute and chronic toxicity. Technical mixtures of PCBs have relatively little acute toxicity, but impurities introduced during synthesis may increase the toxicity considerably. The effects of PCBs in humans have been documented as the result of poisonings at the workplace and two accidental mass poisonings with highly contaminated rice oil in Japan (Yusho disease, 1968) and Taiwan (Yu Cheng disease, 1979). The main signs were skin lesions and various nonspecific symptoms as well as impaired immune reactions and liver dysfunction. Miscarriages were observed in Yusho patients; babies born alive were underweight and showed distinct lesions of the skin and mucosae (**C**). The intensity of (mostly sex-independent) symptoms and PCB concentrations measured in the blood were positively correlated. For the most part, however, the effects observed were explained by contamination with polychlorinated dibenzofurans and other chlorinated compounds. A sensitive parameter of chronic PCB exposure is the induction of cytochrome P450-dependent enzyme systems; it is used in animal experiments for studying the toxicity of PCB mixtures and that of individual congeners. The threshold concentration for other toxic effects (e.g., fetotoxicity) are considerably higher. PCB mixtures have dose-related effects in rats and mice, where they act as tumor promoters and liver carcinogens. Carcinogenic effects in humans have not been definitively established.

Exposure and guidance values. Humans are chronically exposed to PCBs as ubiquitous hazardous waste components. The average daily uptake of 0.1 µg PCB/kg BW with food amounts to about 10% of the acceptable daily intake (ADI) value set by the World Health Organization (WHO). The guideline values apply to indoor exposure (**D**).

Therapy. Treatment is symptomatic. Detoxification is required in cases of acute poisoning after ingestion.

Basic structure of PCBs

PCB No.	Indicator congeners	Portion present in Clophen (%) A30	A60
28	2,4,4'-Trichlorobiphenyl	8	
52	2,2',5,5'-Tetrachlorobiphenyl	2	<1
101	2,2',4,5,5'-Pentachlorobiphenyl	<1	5
138	2,2',3,4,4',5'-Hexachlorobiphenyl		12
153	2,2',4,4',5,5'-Hexachlorobiphenyl		10
180	2,2',3,4,4',5,5'-Heptachlorobiphenyl		7

A. Chemistry of polychlorinated biphenyls (PCB)

PCB	28	52	101	138	153	180	Total PCB
Sea fish (North Sea)	<0.01	<0.01	<0.01	<0.01	0.01	<0.01	0.1 mg/kg fresh weight
River eel	0.24	<0.1	>0.1	0.2	0.2	<0.1	2.2 mg/kg fresh weight
Rye (cereal)	(–)	<0.01	<0.01	<0.01	<0.01	(–)	<0.01 mg/kg dry weight
Beef, dairy products	<0.01	0.01	<0.01	<0.02	<0.02	<0.01	0.14 mg/kg fat
Breast milk	<0.01	0.01	<0.01	0.24	0.33	0.18	1.4 mg/kg fat

B. Occurrence and distribution of PCB congeners in food in industrialized countries

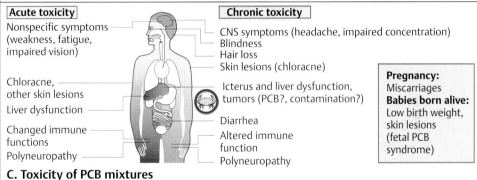

Acute toxicity

Nonspecific symptoms (weakness, fatigue, impaired vision)

Chloracne, other skin lesions
Liver dysfunction
Changed immune functions
Polyneuropathy

Chronic toxicity

CNS symptoms (headache, impaired concentration)
Blindness
Hair loss
Skin lesions (chloracne)
Icterus and liver dysfunction, tumors (PCB?, contamination?)
Diarrhea
Altered immune function
Polyneuropathy

Pregnancy: Miscarriages
Babies born alive: Low birth weight, skin lesions (fetal PCB syndrome)

C. Toxicity of PCB mixtures

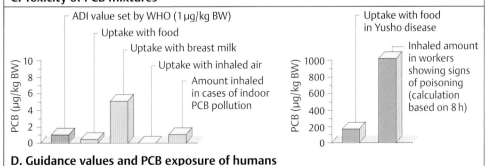

ADI value set by WHO (1 µg/kg BW)
Uptake with food
Uptake with breast milk
Uptake with inhaled air
Amount inhaled in cases of indoor PCB pollution

Uptake with food in Yusho disease
Inhaled amount in workers showing signs of poisoning (calculation based on 8 h)

D. Guidance values and PCB exposure of humans

◼ Halogenated Polycyclic Hydrocarbons II

Polychlorinated Dibenzodioxins and Dibenzofurans 1

Chemistry. The family of polychlorinated dibenzodioxins and dibenzofurans (PCDD/PCDFs) is a large one, including 210 isomers (**A**). *Dioxin* is the general term used for the many different members of the PCDD/PCDF family. The toxic potential of these isomers varies by a factor of 1000 to 10 000. All compounds with substitutions in positions 2, 3, 7, and 8 are toxicologically important; the most toxic substance in this group is 2,3,7,8-tetrachlorodibenzo-*p*-dioxin (2,3,7,8-TCDD), and the entire family is often incorrectly referred to as 2,3,7,8-TCDD. To assess the toxicity of the congeners relevant to human health, *toxicity equivalency factors (TEF)* have been established by using different end points (**A**). This makes it possible to determine the relative toxicity of a known congener mixture in comparison to 2,3,7,8-TCDD (which has a TEF of 1); the relative toxicity is then expressed in toxicity equivalents (TE). Brominated congeners of this family are assessed in the same way.

Occurrence and exposure. Advances in chemical analysis have made it possible to discover the sources of the worldwide contamination with PCDD/PCDFs (**A**). These substances are unintentionally generated during production of certain chemical compounds, for example, during the synthesis of certain chlorine-containing organic chemicals, such as pentachlorophenol or chlorophenoxyacetic acid herbicides.

In 1976, an industrial accident in a factory in Seveso (Italy) during the manufacture of biocides made headlines. Large quantities of 2,3,7,8-TCDD (which later became known as "Seveso dioxin") were generated in a thermal runaway reaction. The total amount of dioxin released was about 1 kg. Today's ubiquitous contamination of the environment with dioxins (**B**) is caused by impurities in biocides and PCBs and by combustion processes in which, depending on the temperature, PCDD/PCDFs may form from organic and inorganic sources in the presence of chlorine. PCDD/PCDFs are detected in the vehicle exhaust gases, in the soot from domestic chimneys, and in cigarette smoke. The most important sources of continuous contamination of the environment leading to bioaccumulation in the food chain have been the industrial processes of waste incineration and scrap metal recovery (**B**). In industrialized countries, total PCDD/PCDF emissions (e.g., ~2 kg estimated in Germany in 1990), particularly the contribution from waste incineration (40% in the past), have been significantly reduced by elaborate flue gas purification systems. In Germany, for example, since 1993, the limiting emission value for flue gas from waste incinerators has been 0.1 ng TE/m^3.

Intoxications. About 1000 cases of PCDD/PCDF poisoning due to industrial accidents have been reported worldwide, some of them involving very high workplace exposures. In cases of acute exposure, mucosal irritation and nonspecific symptoms were observed, in addition to polyneuropathy and disorders of lipid metabolism, disturbed heme synthesis, and liver dysfunction (**C**). The exclusive cardinal symptom for very high exposure is chloracne, which may persist for years. Following the Seveso disaster (the highest reported exposure to 2,3,7,8-TCDD worldwide), chloracne in unprotected body areas was reported predominantly in children. There was no clear correlation between the occurrence of chloracne and the body load of the individual: the TCDD concentrations measured in the blood of chloracne patients at the time of the accident ranged from 1700 to more than 56 000 ng/kg body fat. Since the true level of exposure due to accidents like the one in Seveso is usually unknown, clear dose–response relationships for the effects of TCDD poisoning are very difficult to establish. Specifically, the dioxin poisonings in Seveso did not lead to any fatalities, the chloracne resolved in all cases and there was no significant increase in the rate of cancer among those exposed.

Selected PCDDs	TEF
2,3,7,8-TCDD	1
1,2,3,7,8-PeCDD	1
1,2,3,4,7,8-HxCDD	0.1
1,2,3,6,7,8-HxCDD	0.1
1,2,3,7,8,9-HxCDD	0.1
1,2,3,4,7,8,9-HpCDD	0.01
OCDD	0.0001

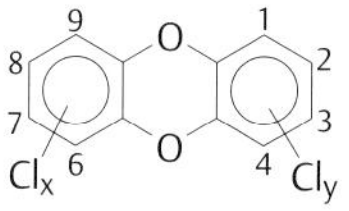

Polychlorodibenzo-*p*-dioxins (PCDDs)

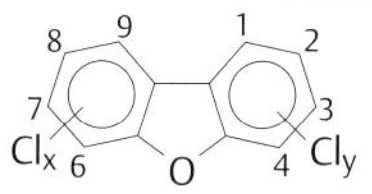

Polychlorodibenzo-furans (PCDFs)

Number of chlorine atoms	PCDD isomers	PCDF isomers
1	2	4
2	10	16
3	14	28
4	23	38
5	14	28
6	10	16
7	2	4
8	1	1

Selected PCDFs	TEF
2,3,7,8-TCDF	0.1
2,3,4,7,8-PeCDF	0.5
1,2,3,7,8-PeCDF	0.05
x,2,3,7,8,x-HxCDF	0,1
1,2,3,4,6,7,8-HpCDF	0.01
1,2,3,4,7,8,9-HpCDF	0.01
OCDF	0.0001

A. Structural formulas and toxicity of PCDD/PCDFs

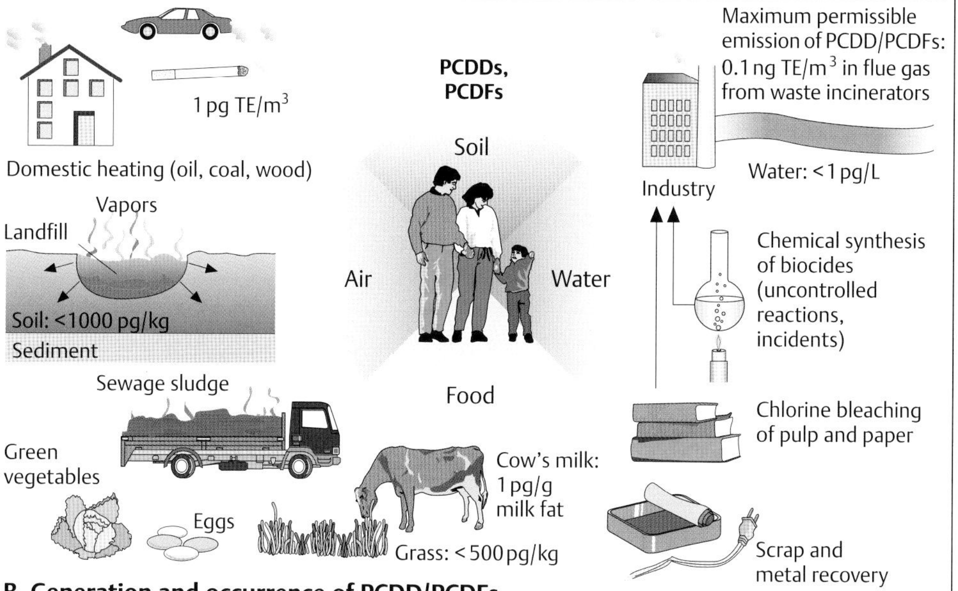

Domestic heating (oil, coal, wood)

1 pg TE/m^3

PCDDs, PCDFs

Soil

Air

Water

Vapors

Landfill

Soil: <1000 pg/kg

Sediment

Green vegetables

Sewage sludge

Eggs

Food

Grass: <500 pg/kg

Cow's milk: 1 pg/g milk fat

Maximum permissible emission of PCDD/PCDFs: 0.1 ng TE/m^3 in flue gas from waste incinerators

Industry

Water: <1 pg/L

Chemical synthesis of biocides (uncontrolled reactions, incidents)

Chlorine bleaching of pulp and paper

Scrap and metal recovery

B. Generation and occurrence of PCDD/PCDFs

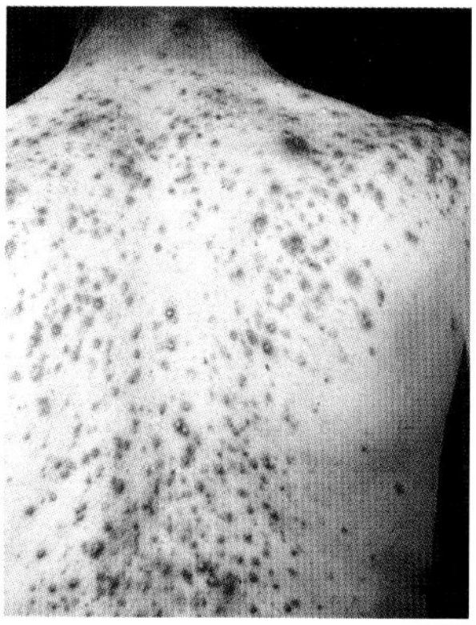

Acute toxicity

Polyneuropathy
Chloracne
Irritation of airways
Thyroid dysfunction

Changes in blood count
Liver dysfunction
Hypoglycemia
Disorders of lipid metabolism
Diarrhea
Impaired immune system
Reproductive disorders
Nonspecific symptoms (weakness, fatigue, weight loss)

Chloracne on a patient's back

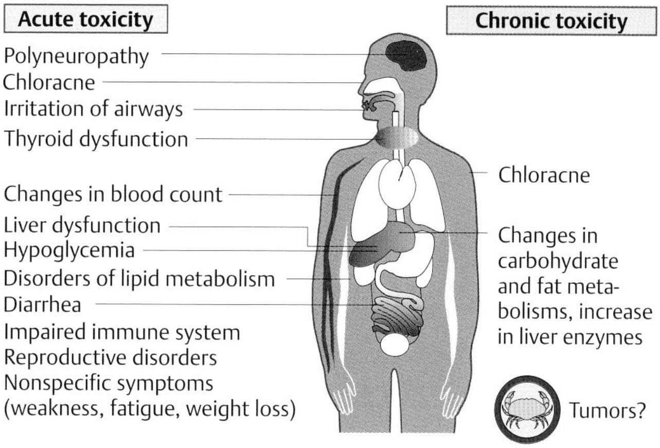

Chronic toxicity

Chloracne

Changes in carbohydrate and fat metabolisms, increase in liver enzymes

Tumors?

C. Toxicity of PCDD/PCDFs

Halogenated Polycyclic Hydrocarbons III

Polyhalogenated Dibenzodioxins and Dibenzofurans 2

Uptake, metabolism, distribution, and elimination. PCDD/PCDFs are semivolatile; they are predominantly transported and distributed when bound to dust. This determines the exposure pathways in humans (**A**): less than 1 % of the total daily uptake of PCDD/PCDFs is inhaled, and dermal absorption is also low. In Germany, the total amount taken up by an individual (~ 1.3 pg TE/kg BW per day) is determined by the intake of fatty food (fish, meat, dairy products, and eggs). Vegetables contribute only a little to the total daily uptake because PCDD/PCDFs are poorly transported by roots.

Absorption, metabolism, and elimination of PCDD/PCDFs decrease with increasing chlorine content. Dioxins and furans behave differently. 2,3,7,8-TCDD is distributed very slowly, and it is largely eliminated via the bile and the intestinal tract. Its half-life in humans is therefore 5–7 years; in other species, particularly rodents, the half-life of 2,3,7,8-TCDD is just a few weeks. For all PCDD/PCDFs, the highest concentrations are found in the liver and fatty tissue. Because of their high solubility in fat and their long half-lives, PCDD/PCDFs also tend to accumulate in breast milk (**A**).

Exposure in the general population lies within the range of the tolerable daily intake (TDI) of 1 pg TE/kg BW. In Germany, for example, the average amount of PCDD/PCDFs accumulated in a person's body is around 40 ng TE/kg body fat, of which about 6 ng is 2,3,7,8-TCDD (for comparison, the international value is 4–20 ng TCDD/kg body fat). The high PCDD/PCDF concentrations in breast milk have been a cause for concern: on average, 30 ng TE/kg milk fat used to be found. This load has declined recently, as is the case with other persistent chlorinated hydrocarbons. Generally, significant differences between regions with different exposures have not been found, and uptake from contaminated soil, dust, or air tends to be of minor importance. However, with increasing maternal age, PCDD/PCDFs accumulate in the fatty tissue and breast milk; the infant may therefore take up TCDD equivalents from the breast milk in amounts (> 100 pg TE/kg BW) that may exceed many internationally established limits for prevention and intervention. However, a considerable proportion of the toxic constituents of PCDD/PCDFs is only incompletely absorbed or is eliminated extremely rapidly, thus making it unlikely that there is any acute or chronic danger to the health of the infant from breastfeeding.

Risk assessment. The ADI values for PCDD/PCDFs are based on animal experiments, and they include safety factors. The World Health Organization (WHO) established 10 pg TE/kg BW as the value for intervention. The TDI values of different countries differ by a factor of more than 1000 (**B**); the values range from 0.006 to 10 pg/kg per day. Differences result from using different TEFs and from the interpretation of data obtained exclusively from animal experiments. Today, a better estimate of the effects on human health is possible by comparing the PCDD/PCDF levels in the body fat of individuals with high exposure at the workplace and those in the general population with low exposure (**C**).

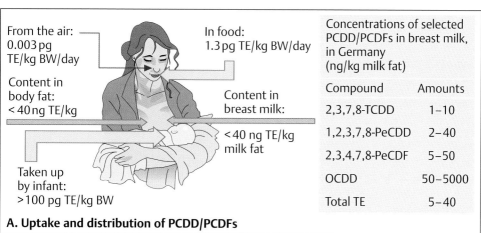

From the air:
0.003 pg
TE/kg BW/day

In food:
1.3 pg TE/kg BW/day

Content in
body fat:
< 40 ng TE/kg

Content in
breast milk:
< 40 ng TE/kg
milk fat

Taken up
by infant:
>100 pg TE/kg BW

Concentrations of selected PCDD/PCDFs in breast milk, in Germany (ng/kg milk fat)	
Compound	Amounts
2,3,7,8-TCDD	1–10
1,2,3,7,8-PeCDD	2–40
2,3,4,7,8-PeCDF	5–50
OCDD	50–5000
Total TE	5–40

A. Uptake and distribution of PCDD/PCDFs

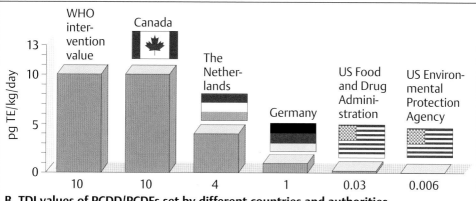

WHO intervention value

Canada

The Netherlands

Germany

US Food and Drug Administration

US Environmental Protection Agency

pg TE/kg/day

| 10 | 10 | 4 | 1 | 0.03 | 0.006 |

B. TDI values of PCDD/PCDFs set by different countries and authorities

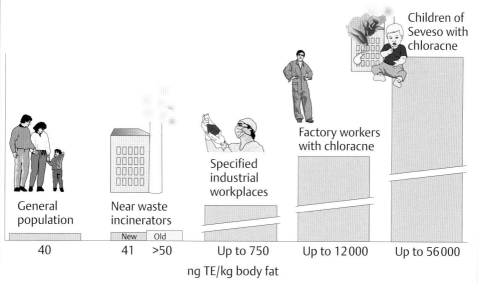

Children of Seveso with chloracne

Factory workers with chloracne

Specified industrial workplaces

General population

Near waste incinerators

New   Old

| 40 | 41 | >50 | Up to 750 | Up to 12000 | Up to 56000 |

ng TE/kg body fat

C. Concentrations of PCDD/PCDFs in human fatty tissue

■ Halogenated Polycyclic Hydrocarbons IV

Polyhalogenated Dibenzodioxins and Dibenzofurans 3

Mechanisms of action. There are various hypotheses on the molecular mechanisms for the various toxic effects of PCDD/PCDFs, the most studied of which relate to 2,3,7,8-TCDD. The defining step in causing an effect is recognized to be the binding of the molecule to the *Ah receptor* (**A**). This selectively binding protein was first discovered in the cytosol of mouse hepatocytes, and it may be involved in the effects on the skin (hyperkeratosis and metaplasia of the sebaceous glands). It causes the expression of P450-dependent enzymes, such as aryl hydroxylase, and is considered to be the inducing receptor for TCDD. It is called the aryl hydrocarbon (Ah) receptor since it also binds nonhalogenated hydrocarbons, such as benzo[*a*]pyrene. It has also been detected in other animal species, and in organs other than the liver. However, it is important to note that many of the reported toxic effects (e.g., the large species- and sex-specific differences in lethality) cannot be explained by receptor binding alone (**B**).

Immunotoxicity, reproductive toxicity, mutagenicity, and carcinogenicity. Immunosuppressive effects of 2,3,7,8-TCDD on lymphoid organs (thymus) have been found during the growth period of various animal species. Teratogenic effects have also been reported in mice, with reproductive toxicity being observed only in the maternal toxic dose range. PCDDs and PCDFs are not considered genotoxic.

2,3,7,8-TCDD is carcinogenic in experimental animals (**C**). Daily oral administration of 2,3,7,8-TCDD to rats over a period of 2 years caused tumors mainly in the liver and respiratory tract at the highest dosage level of 100 ng/kg BW; 10 ng/kg resulted in changes of individual organs, and 1 ng/kg had no effect (NOAEL) (**C**). Similar studies were performed with other animal species, with similar effects.

Epidemiology. In several epidemiological studies, individuals were examined who had come into contact with TCDD alone or with congener mixtures, either in the workplace or during industrial accidents. From recent epidemiological studies, there is evidence of an increased incidence of soft-tissue sarcomas in people with high exposures. The most extensive study included over 5000 chemical workers in the United States who had been exposed to TCDD for various periods of time during the manufacture of 2,4,5-trichlorophenol, 2,4,5-trichlorophenoxyacetic acid, hexachlorophene, and related compounds. The serum of workers with less then 1 year of exposure contained 233 pg TCDD/g fat, and the serum of workers with more than 1 year of exposure contained 418 pg TCDD/g fat. On average, only 7 pg TCDD/g fat were detected in the general population or nonexposed workers (**D**). Compared with the total cancer mortality, this corresponds to a 1.5-fold increase in risk for exposed workers. However, for soft-tissue sarcomas the incidence in highly exposed workers was 9.2 times higher.

Studies in the highly polluted area of Seveso have not revealed a relationship between the exposure of the inhabitants and the frequency of death due to cancer, as compared with a control group. For certain types of cancer, however, interpretation of the data is difficult because of the relatively short latency period, the small number of cases, and the unreliable estimates of exposure. In many countries, the risk for the general population is considered very small given the current daily exposure.

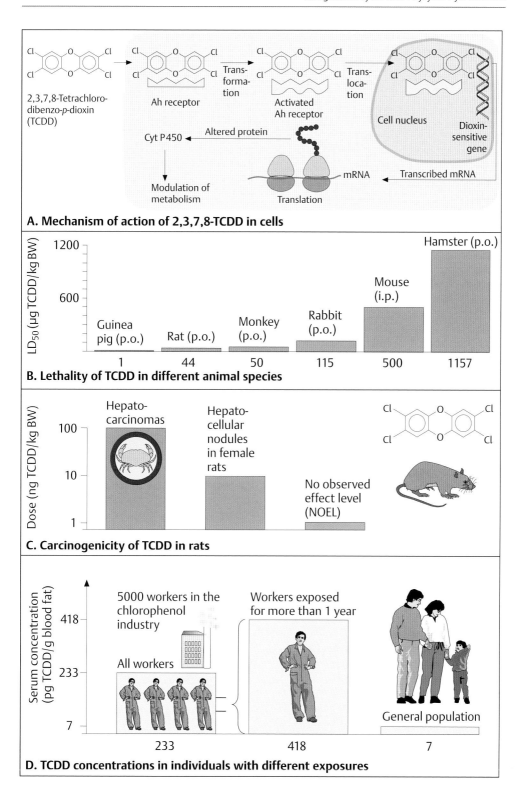

A. Mechanism of action of 2,3,7,8-TCDD in cells

B. Lethality of TCDD in different animal species

C. Carcinogenicity of TCDD in rats

D. TCDD concentrations in individuals with different exposures

◼ Dust and Particle-Bound Emissions

Sources and Effects

Basics (A). Dust in the workplace has long been recognized as a cause of acute and chronic bronchopulmonary diseases (e.g., miller's asthma in bakers, silicosis and grinder's disease in miners, and siderosis in welders). In addition to the acutely irritating, allergenic, and fibrotoxic effects of dusts, the carcinogenic properties of dust from wood and fibers (e.g., asbestos) are of great importance. The dusts present in indoor and outdoor environments carry metals, organic pollutants, and allergens; hence, it is not only in the workplace that they are toxicologically relevant. Ubiquitous compounds, such as PAHs, PCBs, and PCDD/PCDFs, condense on dust particles and are absorbed via the bronchi and lungs. When deposited together with the dust, these substances may enter the food chain in the same way as heavy metals.

Epidemiology. In the 1960s and 1970s, the winter smog periods in London and New York led to increased morbidity and mortality due to high concentrations of dust particles and gaseous air pollutants (see p. 134). Today, we know that smog with a high portion of airborne dust poses a health risk, especially to elderly and sick people.

Toxicokinetics (B). When airborne dust is inhaled, it deposits at various sites in the respiratory tract. The chemical properties and the particle size of the dust vary with the humidity of the breath and thus play a decisive role: large dust particles ($\geq 3\,\mu m$ inhaled through the nose) are deposited in the postnasal space, while smaller particles reach the bronchi and the pulmonary alveoli. Fine dust ($\sim 0.5\,\mu m$) is rarely deposited; it is largely exhaled. When the bronchial mucosa is intact, the deposited dust particles are relatively quickly exported from the airways and mostly eliminated via the gastrointestinal tract. Existing damage to the ciliated epithelium by pollutants (e.g., irritant gases, tobacco smoke) may lead to a loss of mucociliary clearance. Some of the particles (e.g., soot) accumulate in the lungs, and any dissolved constituents (e.g., cadmium) are transported by the blood to other organs or are partly eliminated by metabolic processes.

Toxic effects (C). The effects of dust are varied; they depend on its chemical composition and the concentration of particles in the inhaled air. Pulmonary function may be directly affected, and resistance to infections may decline because of impaired ciliary clearance. The toxicity of absorbed substances (metals, organic compounds) must be considered separately. Synergistic effects of exposure to various substances in combination with dust are also possible; for example, inhalation of PAHs from exhaust gas together with soot particles resulted in an increase in tumor formation in experimental animals (combination effect).

In Germany, for example, the limiting value for fine dust in the air in the workplace is generally $6\,mg/m^3$ air; the typical dust content of outdoor air is 100 times lower. Guidance values for the general population (as set by the World Health Organization) take into account the damaging local effects of airborne dust ($70\,\mu g/m^3$) in combination with sulfur dioxide ($125\,\mu g/m^3$ in 24 h). Below these concentrations, any negative effect on human health is unlikely; however, this is difficult to establish, in view of the variable inter-individual exposure to indoor pollutants (tobacco smoke, workplace).

Prevention. Measures to remove dust from industrial waste gases have significantly reduced emissions. Today, the use of adequate filtering has lead to a reduction in airborne dust below $10\,mg/m^3$ (in 1960, it was $\sim 500\,mg/m^3$ in industrialized countries), and pollution by airborne dust and particle-bound substances in centers of population has declined accordingly.

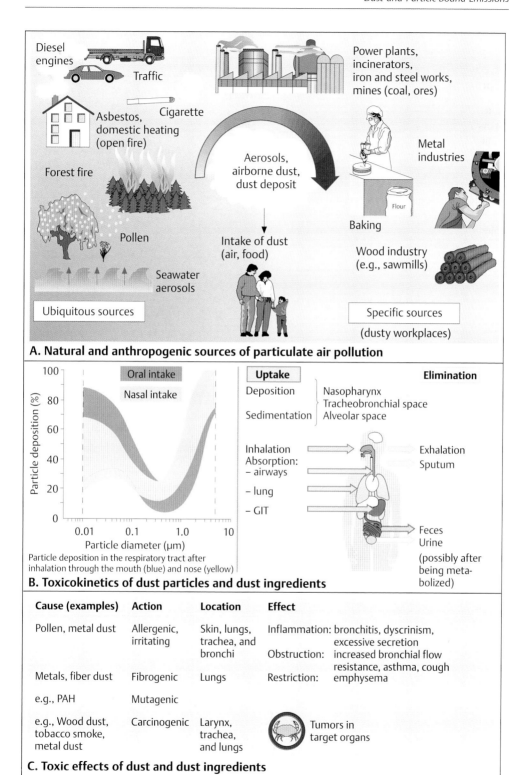

A. Natural and anthropogenic sources of particulate air pollution

B. Toxicokinetics of dust particles and dust ingredients

Particle deposition in the respiratory tract after inhalation through the mouth (blue) and nose (yellow)

Cause (examples)	Action	Location	Effect	
Pollen, metal dust	Allergenic, irritating	Skin, lungs, trachea, and bronchi	Inflammation:	bronchitis, dyscrinism, excessive secretion
			Obstruction:	increased bronchial flow resistance, asthma, cough
Metals, fiber dust	Fibrogenic	Lungs	Restriction:	emphysema
e.g., PAH	Mutagenic			
e.g., Wood dust, tobacco smoke, metal dust	Carcinogenic	Larynx, trachea, and lungs	Tumors in target organs	

C. Toxic effects of dust and dust ingredients

▧ Nitroso Compounds

Importance and Classification

Basics. *N*-Nitroso compounds play an important role as environmental carcinogens. They may be taken up by ingestion, inhalation, or through the skin. Various *N*-nitroso compounds are also produced in the body.

Some pharmaceuticals, such as nitrosocimetidine (the nitrosated form of the gastrointestinal therapeutic agent cimetidine), are mutagenic and carcinogenic. Aminophenazone is metabolized to the highly carcinogenic compound *N*-nitrosodimethylamine and is therefore no longer used.

To avoid the burden of endogenously formed *N*-nitroso compounds, pharmaceutical drugs containing nitrosatable groups are now tested at the level of preclinical toxicology studies for their potential to be nitrosated.

N-Nitroso compounds are divided into *N*-nitrosamides and *N*-nitrosamines according to their chemical structure (**A**).

N-Nitrosamides

Exposure and effect. Nitrosamides (*N*-nitroso *N*-methylureas) are formed exogenously as well as endogenously by the nitrosation of amides. In some regions of China (e.g., the Fuzhou area in Fujian province), very high concentrations of *N*-nitrosamides (up to 80 µg/kg) have been detected in food prepared from fish. The nitrosamides had obviously formed in an acidic milieu (~ pH 2), as the original product had a distinctly lower nitrosamide content (2–6 µg/kg). In experiments with rats, ulcers and adenocarcinomas were observed in the stomach after 16 weeks of oral administration of this nitrosamide-containing fish product. The nitrosamide concentrations measured in the gastric juice of gastritis patients from this region correlated well with the severity of the gastritis. *N*-Nitrosamides are thought to be responsible for the high rate of gastric cancer and subsequent death in these regions.

Data obtained from animal experiments have indicated the carcinogenic effect of nitrosamides. For example, studies have demonstrated the induction of urinary bladder carcinoma in rats by *N*-butyl-(4-hydroxybutyl)nitrosamides.

Following acute poisoning, the characteristic effects are ulcers with massive bleeding in the gastrointestinal tract and, as a delayed reaction, damage to bone marrow stem cells with pronounced leukopenia.

Mechanism of action. In an aqueous milieu, nitrosamides spontaneously decompose into electrophilic intermediates: alkyldiazohydroxide and a diazonium ion (**B**). These may react with nucleophilic groups of DNA, RNA, and proteins, the alkylation of which has mutagenic and carcinogenic effects.

N-Nitrosamines I

Formation. After bacterial decomposition of meat and fish products, the addition of nitrite pickling salt (see p. 214), followed by heating over an open fire, leads to nitrosation of large amounts of biogenic amines (see p. 213). Fish protein decomposes very rapidly, and the nitrosamine content of cured fish products is therefore critical (**C**). Nitrosation occurs faster with less alkaline amines than with more alkaline amines, because the highly alkaline amines are almost completely protonated in a slightly acidic environment. Secondary amines (**D**) are nitrosated faster than tertiary amines. When primary amines are nitrosated, unstable molecules with alkylating effects are formed.

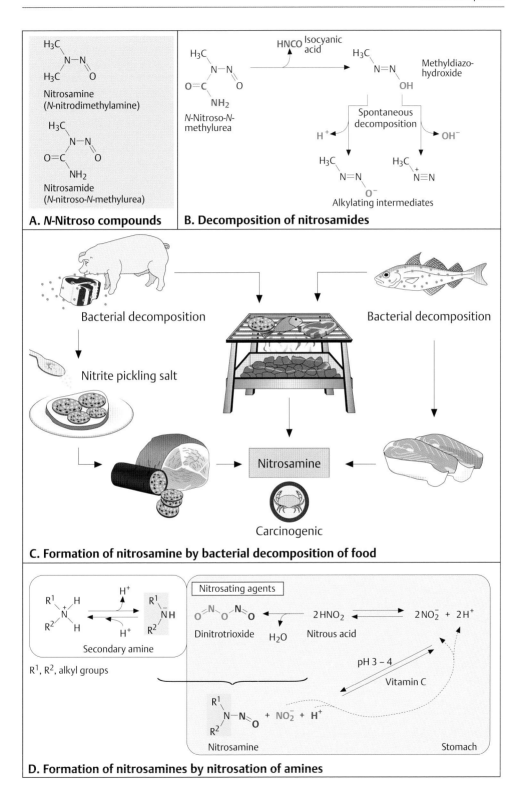

A. _N_-Nitroso compounds

B. Decomposition of nitrosamides

C. Formation of nitrosamine by bacterial decomposition of food

D. Formation of nitrosamines by nitrosation of amines

125

N-Nitrosamines II

Exposure and uptake. *Exogenous exposure* to nitrosamines from food has markedly declined in Europe during recent years. On average, the adult oral intake of nitrosamines is now less than 0.5 µg/day. Years ago, the nitrosamine content was particularly high in beer (up to 6.8 µg/L) and cured meat products (up to 12 µg/kg). Manufacturing procedures have now changed, with the abandonment of hot-air drying of barley for malt production, and the addition of ascorbic acid during meat processing; beer now contains less than 1.2 µg/L of nitrosamines, and they are rarely detectable in meat products.

Ingested nitrosamines are largely absorbed in the upper part of the small intestine.

Uptake due to nicotine consumption. Smokers have a considerable burden of nitrosamines. Large amounts of tobacco-specific nitrosamines are formed during the fermentation of the tobacco leaves, by nitrosation of nicotine and other alkaloids (**A**). Smoking 40 cigarettes results in an intake of approximately 40–160 µg of nitrosamines. The consumption of *snuff* or *chewing tobacco* may lead to a daily intake of up to 400 µg nitrosamines. Tobacco-specific nitrosamines are inhaled by smokers with the mainstream (~1–4 µg *N*-nitrosodimethylamine per filterless cigarette), and they are released in 20- to 100-fold higher concentrations with the gas phase of the sidestream. This causes a considerable nitrosamine burden (up to 0.6 µg/h) for passive smokers (**B**).

Uptake through the skin. Various nitrosamines are rapidly taken up through the skin. For the assessment of occupational exposure, the non-volatile compounds, such as *N*-nitrosodiethanolamine, are therefore as important as the volatile ones. Following the cutaneous exposure of workers to materials contaminated with nitrosamines, up to 40 µg of nitroso compounds were detected in the urine within 24 h.

Endogenous formation. In the acidic environment of the stomach, nitrosamines form from amines and nitrosating compounds (nitrites, oxides of nitrogen, dinitrogen trioxide, nitrosyl halogenides). The nitrosation reaction is inhibited by vitamin C (see p. 215). Nitrite is added to meat products in the form of nitrite pickling salt (99.5 % sodium chloride, 0.5 % sodium nitrite)—a maximum of 150 mg pickling salt/kg meat product. This is done for preservation (inhibition of bacterial growth) and for flavoring and coloring (the heat-stabile nitrosomyoglobin gives the meat a pinkish red color). The nitrite also effectively inhibits the growth of clostridial bacteria (*Clostridium botulinum*), the metabolite of which (botulinum toxin) is a dangerous poison.

Cured meat products and other foods therefore contain considerable amounts of nitrites (**C**). Nitrates are also present in large amounts in numerous other foods (e.g., nitrate-fertilized leafy vegetables, processed cheese). They are easily transformed to nitrites by reduction in the oral cavity, gastrointestinal tract, and bacterially infected urinary tract.

Since bacteria (e.g., *E. coli, Proteus vulgaris*) and macrophages catalyze the reduction of nitrate and the formation of nitrosamines from nitrites and amines, patients with chronic urinary tract infection are at greater risk for nitrosamine-induced tumors of the urinary tract.

Because individual parameters play an important role, it is difficult to assess the burden that endogenous nitrosamines pose to humans.

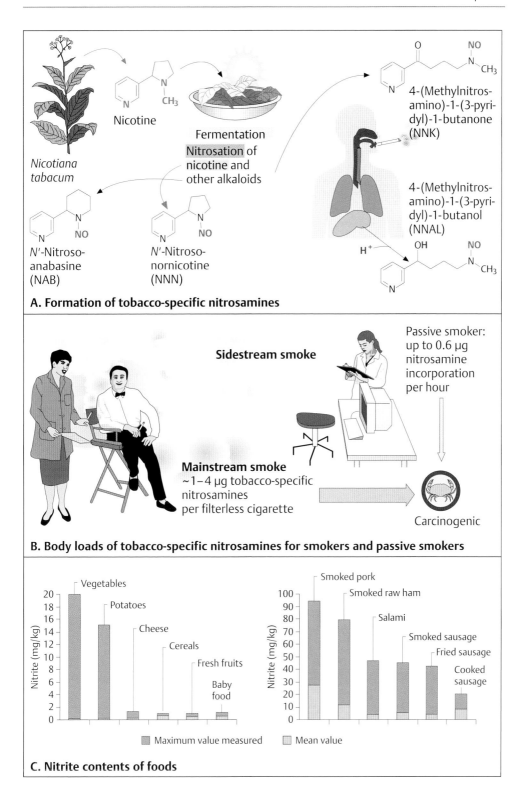

A. Formation of tobacco-specific nitrosamines

B. Body loads of tobacco-specific nitrosamines for smokers and passive smokers

C. Nitrite contents of foods

N-Nitrosamines III

Metabolism and elimination. Many nitrosamines are more than 99% metabolized during the first passage through the intestinal wall and the liver (first pass effect). The capacity to metabolize them is exhausted at very high doses (> 40 µg/kg body weight).

The biotransformation of N-nitrosodibutylamine (NDBA) to N-nitrosobutyl-(3-carboxypropyl)amine results in the formation of a carcinogen; this metabolite induces bladder cancer (**A**).

The main detoxification pathway is oxidative denitrosation mediated by the cytochrome P450 system. Most short-chain N-alkylnitrosamines are metabolized to carbon dioxide and then exhaled. Water-soluble hydroxyalkylnitrosamines are largely excreted by the kidneys.

Detoxification of 4-(methylnitrosamino)-1-(3-pyridyl)-1-butanol occurs by pyridine-N-oxidation or by reduction of the carbonyl group and glucuronidation; the resulting metabolite is excreted by the kidneys.

Alcohol (ethanol) seems to reduce the rate of nitrosamine metabolism, thus causing not only a longer turnover time but also a shift in organotropism. Nitrosamines and their metabolites also appear in the breast milk.

Effects. Larger doses (> 30 µg/kg BW) of nitrosamines are cytotoxic and cause necrosis.

Nitrosamine compounds are thought to have teratogenic, mutagenic, and carcinogenic effects.

Various metabolites of nitrosamines methylate DNA, RNA, and proteins even in small doses and may therefore induce tumors. Out of approximately 300 nitrosamine compounds examined, about 90% are carcinogenic in experimental animals.

Tumors induced by nitrosamines occur predominantly in the esophagus, stomach, liver, kidneys, and respiratory tract.

A single exposure to dimethylnitrosamine (2 mg/kg BW) by inhalation caused mucoepidermal tumors of the nasal mucosa in about one-third of the animals treated. Long-term administration of dimethylnitrosamine (0.13 µg/kg food) induced liver carcinomas in rats. Oral administration of nitrosoethylamine in smaller doses caused cancer in rodents.

Daily administration of diethylnitrosamine (5 mg/kg BW) in the drinking-water over a period of 150 days induced multiple well-differentiated hepatocellular carcinomas in the liver of rats (**B**).

Various tobacco-specific nitrosamines (see p. 126) are potent carcinogens in animal experiments. In epidemiological studies, tumors of the oral cavity, lungs, and esophagus of smokers were attributed to exposure to 4-methylnitrosamino-1-(3-pyridyl)-1-butanol (NNAL), a metabolite of 4-(methylnitrosamino)-1-(3-pyridyl)-1-butanone (NNK) (see p. 126, **A**).

Nitrosamines are converted to carcinogenic compounds by biotransformation. The toxin-generating step is α-C-hydroxylation mediated by cytochrome P450. The resulting unstable α-hydroxynitrosamine decomposes into methyldiazohydroxide and further into a diazonium or carbenium cation intermediate, while splitting off formaldehyde (**C**). These cation intermediates can methylate proteins, DNA, and RNA and are the ultimate carcinogens.

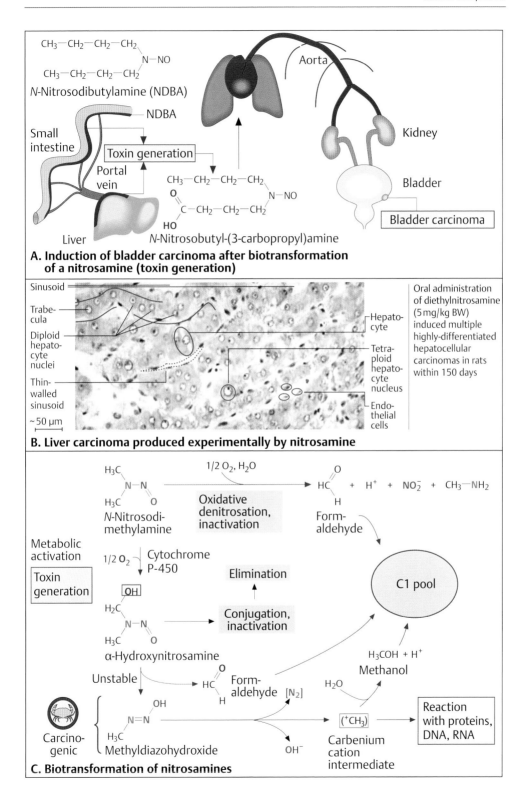

A. Induction of bladder carcinoma after biotransformation of a nitrosamine (toxin generation)

N-Nitrosodibutylamine (NDBA)

NDBA

Small intestine

Portal vein

Toxin generation

N-Nitrosobutyl-(3-carbopropyl)amine

Liver

Aorta

Kidney

Bladder

Bladder carcinoma

B. Liver carcinoma produced experimentally by nitrosamine

Sinusoid

Trabe-cula

Diploid hepato-cyte nuclei

Thin-walled sinusoid

~50 μm

Hepato-cyte

Tetra-ploid hepato-cyte nucleus

Endo-thelial cells

Oral administration of diethylnitrosamine (5 mg/kg BW) induced multiple highly-differentiated hepatocellular carcinomas in rats within 150 days

C. Biotransformation of nitrosamines

N-Nitrosodi-methylamine

$1/2\ O_2$, H_2O

Oxidative denitrosation, inactivation

Formaldehyde

HC + H^+ + NO_2^- + CH_3-NH_2

Metabolic activation

Toxin generation

$1/2\ O_2$ Cytochrome P-450

α-Hydroxynitrosamine

Elimination

Conjugation, inactivation

C1 pool

$H_3COH + H^+$ Methanol

Unstable

Formaldehyde

$[N_2]$

H_2O

Carcino-genic

Methyldiazohydroxide

OH^-

$(^+CH_3)$

Carbenium cation intermediate

Reaction with proteins, DNA, RNA

■ Aromatic Amino and Nitro Compounds

Basics. Aromatic amino and nitro compounds are used in the synthesis of dyes, drugs, and pesticides, in plastics processing, and in the coloration of hair and fur. They are also employed in the manufacture of explosives. Almost 90 % of aromatic amines and around 70 % of aromatic nitro compounds are considered carcinogenic. Tobacco smoke contains several of these compounds.

Many aromatic amino and nitro compounds are potent blood poisons leading to the formation of methemoglobin. Poisonings involving the formation of methemoglobin are often associated with alcohol intolerance, similar to the well-known effect of the drug Antabuse (disulfiram, see p. 206).

■ Arylamines

These are aromatic compounds with alkaline characteristics due to substitution of a hydrogen atom with an amine (NH_2) group. There are monocyclic arylamines, such as *aniline*, and bicyclic arylamines, such as *4-aminodiphenyl* (**A**). Aniline is used in the manufacture of dyes, pharmaceuticals, and biocides. As early as 1895 it was known that aniline is partly responsible for the development of bladder cancer in workers in the color and dye industry.

Uptake, distribution, metabolism, and elimination. Arylamines are extremely well absorbed by the gastrointestinal and respiratory tracts, and also partly through the skin; they are then distributed throughout the body. Elimination of monocyclic arylamines takes place primarily through metabolism in the kidneys, while bicyclic arylamines are excreted in the feces. Their elimination half-lives range between 2 h and 4 days, depending on the compound.

Toxic effect. Arylamines are metabolically activated in the body. *N*-Hydroxylation of monocyclic arylamines leads to toxin generation via the cytochrome P450 system; the toxic metabolites phenylhydroxylamine and nitrosobenzene play a role in the formation of methemoglobin (cyanosis) (**B**). Arylamines are detoxified in the liver by cytosolic *N*-acetyltransferase or by *N*-glucuronidation. Individuals with rapid acetylation are less sensitive to the poisonous effects than those with slow acetylation.

After direct protonation (formation of electrophilic intermediates), phenylhydroxylamine reacts in the bladder with nucleophilic centers in DNA to form DNA adducts (**C**). This adduct formation serves as a measure of the extent of activation of arylamines to genotoxic metabolites. The target organ for these substances is the urinary bladder, where tumors will develop.

Acute and chronic toxicity. Acute toxicity of monocyclic arylamines is primarily characterized by the formation of methemoglobin (**B**, **D**). Chloroaniline has the strongest cyanotic effect. The uptake of minute amounts of alcohol enhances the effect. Aniline and toluidine may cause acute bladder irritation.

Chronic toxicity is characterized by anemia and autonomic disturbances (**D**). The hair dye *p*-phenylenediamine may cause contact dermatitis and asthma attacks, and also edema and kidney failure when ingested. Benzidines (**A**) are toxic to the liver and kidneys (**D**).

Most arylamines are considered mutagenic and carcinogenic. 4-Aminodiphenyl, benzidine, 2-naphthylamine, and 4-chloro-*o*-toluidine cause bladder cancer in humans.

Therapy. Administration of activated charcoal and Glauber's salt (sodium sulfate). Methemoglobinemia of more than 40 % requires administration of redox dyes, such as toluidine blue or methylene blue (**E**).

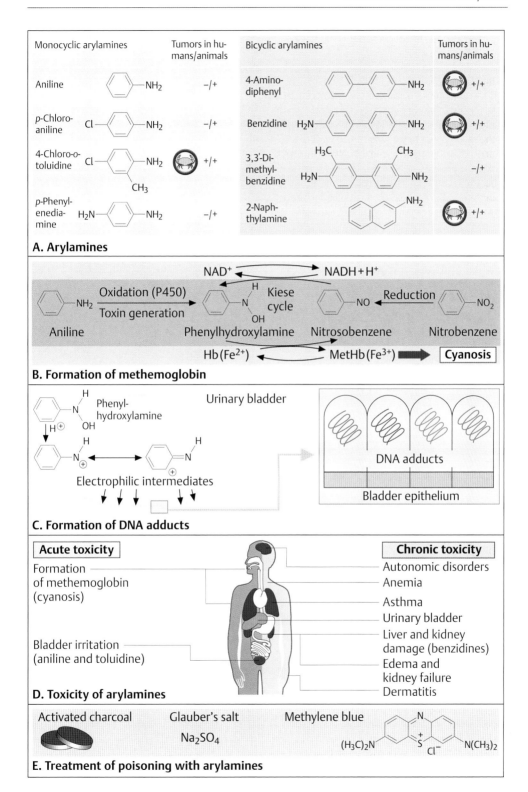

A. Arylamines

B. Formation of methemoglobin

C. Formation of DNA adducts

D. Toxicity of arylamines

E. Treatment of poisoning with arylamines

Nitroaromatic Compounds

Nitroaromatic compounds (**A**) are used in the manufacture of dyes, pesticides, and pharmaceuticals. Some solid monocyclic nitroaromates (e.g., 2,4,6-trinitrotoluene, TNT) explode upon impact or ignition; other explosive compounds are generated when they are mixed with oxidizing or reducing agents, such as nitrobenzenes and nitrotoluenes. 1-Nitronaphthalene is used industrially, and 2,4,7-trinitrofluorene-9-one is employed in photocopying machines. 4-Nitrobiphenyl has been detected in diesel exhausts.

Uptake, distribution, and elimination. Nitroaromatic compounds are well absorbed via the gastrointestinal and respiratory tracts, and also through the skin. They are partly stored in fatty tissue.

Monocyclic nitroaromates are primarily eliminated by the kidneys.

Acute and chronic toxicity. Nitroaromatic compounds are reduced by bacteria in the intestine, or in the liver by nitroreductases, to more poisonous amino and *N*-hydroxylamino compounds that lead to the formation of methemoglobin. Their toxicity is therefore similar to that of aromatic amines (see p. 130). 1,2-Dinitrobenzene has a strong cyanotic effect.

Nitroaromatic compounds cause dermatitis upon contact with the skin, conjunctivitis and corneal lesions upon contact with the eyes, and also painful gastric spasms and diarrhea when ingested. Chronic toxicity in humans is predominantly characterized by liver damage and a characteristic change in skin and nail color (yellow) and hair color (brownish red). Excessive exposure to TNT results in aplastic anemia and cataracts (TNT cataract; **B**).

Thus far, the carcinogenicity of nitroaromatic compounds has been demonstrated only in experimental animals; e.g., tumors are induced in rats exposed to *dinitrotoluene* (lung tumors), *2-nitrotoluene* (skin tumors), *1-chloro-4-nitrobenzene* (spleen and liver tumors), *1-nitronaphthalene* and *4-nitrobiphenyl* (urinary bladder tumors), and *2,4,7-trinitrofluorene-9-one* (lung and skin tumors).

For the nitroaromates mentioned above, the LD_{50} in rats ranges from 120 mg/kg (1-nitronaphthalene) to 22 000 mg/kg (2,4,7-trinitrofluorene-9-one). Almost all nitroaromates are mutagenic.

Heterocyclic Aromatic Amines

Heterocyclic aromatic amines (HAAs) (**A**) are generated during the grilling, frying, or heating of protein-rich food, such as 2-amino-1-methyl-6-phenylimidazo[4,5-*b*]pyridine (PhIP) in barbecued beef (up to 16 ng/g), roast beef (0.6 ng/g), barbecued chicken (39 ng/g), barbecued lamb (43 ng/g), and barbecued fish (up to 70 ng/g).

The HAAs, such as PhIP and 2-amino-3-methyl-9 H-pyrido[2,3-*b*]indole (MeAαC), have also been detected in the tar fraction of cigarettes (MeAαC and PhIP, ~2 ng/cigarette), in wine (PhIP, ~30 ng/L), and in beer (PhIP, ~15 ng/L).

All HAAs so far tested had mutagenic effects and were carcinogenic in experimental animals.

In the liver, HAAs are *N*-hydroxylated, glucuronated, and then excreted in the bile. Bacterial β-glucosidases in the colon cleave off the glucuronide. The resulting hydroxylamine is converted by ornithine acetyltransferase (OAcT) in the mucosa to the reactive compound *N*-acetoxyarylamine, which reacts with nucleophilic centers in DNA (**C**). Most HAAs are colon carcinogens, and among them PhIP and MeIQx were found in food at very high levels.

Epidemiological studies have indicated that colon cancer occurs more often in Western countries than in developing countries, possibly as a result of increased meat and fish consumption resulting in an increased risk of colon cancer.

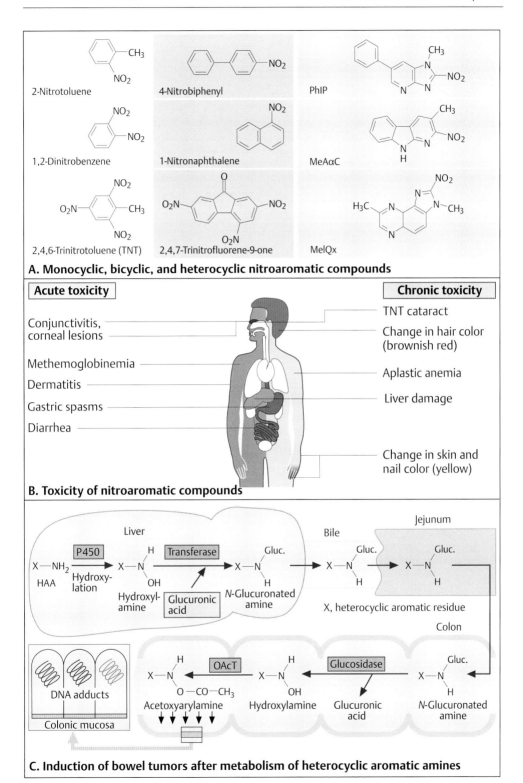

A. Monocyclic, bicyclic, and heterocyclic nitroaromatic compounds

2-Nitrotoluene

4-Nitrobiphenyl

PhIP

1,2-Dinitrobenzene

1-Nitronaphthalene

MeAαC

2,4,6-Trinitrotoluene (TNT)

2,4,7-Trinitrofluorene-9-one

MelQx

Acute toxicity

Conjunctivitis, corneal lesions

Methemoglobinemia

Dermatitis

Gastric spasms

Diarrhea

Chronic toxicity

TNT cataract

Change in hair color (brownish red)

Aplastic anemia

Liver damage

Change in skin and nail color (yellow)

B. Toxicity of nitroaromatic compounds

Liver

P450

Transferase

Bile

Jejunum

$X—NH_2$

HAA

Hydroxy-lation

$X—N$ H OH

Hydroxyl-amine

Glucuronic acid

Gluc.

$X—N$ H N-Glucuronated amine

Gluc.

$X—N$ H

Gluc.

$X—N$ H

X, heterocyclic aromatic residue

Colon

DNA adducts

Colonic mucosa

OAcT

$X—N$ H O—CO—CH_3

Acetoxyarylamine

$X—N$ H OH

Hydroxylamine

Glucosidase

Glucuronic acid

Gluc.

$X—N$ H N-Glucuronated amine

C. Induction of bowel tumors after metabolism of heterocyclic aromatic amines

133

▪ Gaseous Compounds

Air Pollution and Smog

Five substances or groups of substances are thought to be responsible for around 98% of all air pollution (**A**). The main causes of the pollution are traffic (60%), industries, domestic heating, and power plants. A special kind of air pollution is called "smog" (**B**).

Acid smog (winter smog, London smog) (C). The term *acid smog* is based on what happened in London during the smog catastrophe of 1952. At that time, cold and damp weather prevailed and prevented the exchange of air (atmospheric inversion layer, low wind speed). This created extremely high concentrations of sulfur dioxide (SO_2; up to 1.3 mL/m^3 air) and—after oxidation in the atmosphere or reaction with water—also sulfurous acid (H_2SO_3) and sulfuric acid (H_2SO_4), combined with a high concentration of suspended particles (soot). These special weather conditions caused the deaths of about 4000 people in 2 weeks (**D**).

Sulfur dioxide. This gas (SO_2) is formed during the combustion of sulfur-containing materials (coal, gasoline, heating oil, diesel fuel), during the roasting of ore, and also in small amounts during the manufacture of cement. When inhaled, SO_2 is partly absorbed in the upper airways; when inhaled through the mouth and with a high respiratory volume per minute (e. g., during sports), most of it gets into the lungs. The absorbed SO_2 persists for days in the body because it binds to proteins.

Effect. An increase in airway resistance is characteristic of the exposure to SO_2, presumably as the result of reversible inhibition of parasympathetic control over the tonus of respiratory smooth muscles. In addition, SO_2 causes or aggravates various disorders of the respiratory tract (**E**).

Studies using experimental animals have demonstrated that chronic SO_2 exposure causes chronic bronchitis with mucosal hypertrophy. Short exposure to high concentrations of SO_2 reduced the frequency of ciliary action in the mucosa of the upper airways; the effect was reversible. Chronic exposure to SO_2, however, caused the mucosal membrane to thicken and thus indirectly inhibited particle transport toward the throat.

Even minor exposure to SO_2 (> 0.25 mL/m^3) is dangerous to predisposed individuals, particularly those suffering from asthma, because of a pre-existing increased airway resistance.

SO_2 and its secondary products (sulfurous acid and ammonium sulfate), together with nitric acid (HNO_3, secondary product of oxides of nitrogen), are the major causes of forest decline in Europe ("Waldsterben"). This *acid rain* affects the leaves and roots of trees, and can also destroy buildings and stone monuments (**F**). Despite a marked reduction in the atmospheric concentrations of acid compounds in recent years, the extent of forest damage has hardly changed.

Photochemical smog (summer smog, Los Angeles smog). The term *Los Angeles smog* reflects the fact that this type of smog was discovered and described for the first time in Los Angeles.

The main components of photochemical smog are ozone (see p. 144), nitrogen oxides (NO_x), aldehydes, peroxyacetyl nitrates (which are of minor importance), and hydrocarbons (HC, see p. 104). Photo-oxidants are formed in the atmosphere under the influence of sunlight. The rate of formation depends on the concentration of pollutants that have accumulated and is particularly high when air exchange is poor. This frequently occurs in the sunny and traffic-congested city of Los Angeles, which is located in a basin. Under certain weather conditions there is often little exchange of air (**F**).

Effect. Photochemical oxidants have an irritating effect on the mucosa of the eyes and respiratory tract, and they affect sports performance. A connection between the motor vehicle densities in nearby cities and damage to the plants in the surrounding areas has been demonstrated. Nevertheless, an influence of photochemical smog on the mortality rate of the population has not yet been proven convincingly.

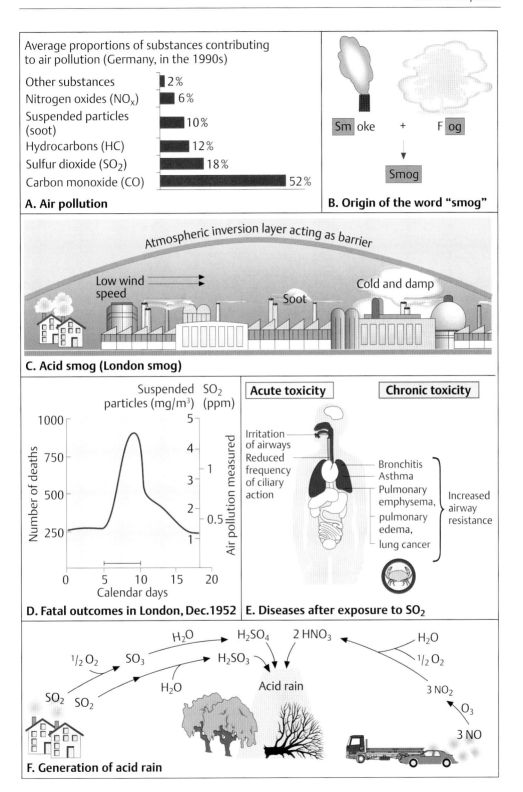

Average proportions of substances contributing to air pollution (Germany, in the 1990s)

Other substances	2%
Nitrogen oxides (NO$_x$)	6%
Suspended particles (soot)	10%
Hydrocarbons (HC)	12%
Sulfur dioxide (SO$_2$)	18%
Carbon monoxide (CO)	52%

A. Air pollution

Sm oke + F og → Smog

B. Origin of the word "smog"

Atmospheric inversion layer acting as barrier

Low wind speed

Soot

Cold and damp

C. Acid smog (London smog)

Suspended particles (mg/m³) SO$_2$ (ppm)

Number of deaths

Calendar days

D. Fatal outcomes in London, Dec. 1952

Acute toxicity   **Chronic toxicity**

Irritation of airways
Reduced frequency of ciliary action

Bronchitis
Asthma
Pulmonary emphysema, pulmonary edema, lung cancer

Increased airway resistance

Air pollution measured

E. Diseases after exposure to SO$_2$

$\frac{1}{2}O_2$ SO$_3$ $\xrightarrow{H_2O}$ H_2SO_4 $2 HNO_3$ $\xleftarrow{H_2O}$ $\frac{1}{2}O_2$

SO$_2$ SO$_2$ $\xrightarrow{H_2O}$ H$_2$SO$_3$

Acid rain

3 NO$_2$
O$_3$
3 NO

F. Generation of acid rain

Nitrogen Oxides

Nitrogen oxides (NO, NO_2, N_2O, N_2O_5, NO_3, collectively known as NO_x) are contained at high concentrations in the exhaust gas of motor vehicles (up to $1000 \, mL/m^3$) and in tobacco smoke (up to $300 \, mL/m^3$). They are used in the manufacturing of dyes, nitrocellulose, and fertilizers.

Pure NO (nitric oxide; a colorless gas; olfactory threshold ~$0.1 \, mL/m^3$; density $1.25 \, g/L$) has no irritating effect, but its absorption leads to methemoglobin formation, platelet aggregation, and vasodilatation (**A**). NO is rapidly oxidized in the environment to nitrogen dioxide (NO_2 or N_2O_4) (**B**).

Effect. NO_2 is a reddish brown gas (density, $1.45 \, g/L$). It is an irritant gas causing toxic pulmonary edema, pulmonary emphysema, and pulmonary fibrosis, presumably as the result of lipid peroxidation (**C**). Deficiency of vitamin E enhances this effect. Damage to elastin and collagen in the connective tissue of the lungs has been demonstrated. Exposure of rats to NO_2 at $0.5 \, mL/m^3$ for 4 h, or at $1 \, mL/m^3$ for 1 h, caused disintegration of mast cells in the lungs. The damage may be repaired within 24 h, or it may be the beginning of an acute inflammatory reaction. In humans and animals, exposure to more than $2 \, mL/m^3$ of NO_2 leads to clinically measurable restrictions in pulmonary function (reduced compliance, increased airway resistance, and increased rate of respiration); initially, the respiratory volume per minute remains unchanged. Chronic or acute NO_2 exposure is thought to pave the way for bacterial or viral colonization of the lungs.

Therapy. Inhalation of cortisone to prevent the development of pulmonary edema (**D**), and symptomatic treatment.

Aldehydes

Aldehydes (see p. 94) are quantitatively important products in the photo-oxidation of hydrocarbons and their reaction with oxygen species (see p. 146). In the atmosphere above cities, about 50% of aldehydes have been identified as formaldehyde and 5% as acrolein. In Germany, the formaldehyde emission from motor vehicles before the introduction of catalysts was about $35\,000$ t/year. Industry in Germany uses around $500\,000$ t/year.

Effect. Formaldehyde (a colorless, pungent gas) easily dissolves in water and irritates the mucosa of the upper airways. In experimental animals, formaldehyde ($3.5 \, mL/m^3$) induced malignant tumors in the nasal mucosa; this finding has not yet been confirmed in humans, although there is a risk of developing an allergy. Formaldehyde is rapidly degraded in the environment.

The unsaturated aldehyde acrolein ($> 0.6 \, mL/m^3$) has an even stronger irritating effect on the mucosae than formaldehyde. The induction of liver enzymes was observed in rats exposed to acrolein. Both aldehydes reduce the compliance of the lungs and increase the airway resistance. Since formaldehyde and acrolein have synergistic effects, the total aldehyde content is usually determined without further specification.

Acid smog and photochemical smog induce or aggravate various disorders of the lungs and upper airways (see SO_2, p. 134). However, numerous studies have documented that (passive) smoking plays a more dominant role in these disorders than atmospheric air pollution.

Respiratory Poisons

Suffocating gases. This heterogeneous group (N_2, NO_x, CO_2, CO, SO_2, HCN, and H_2S) includes gases that are largely ineffective toxicologically but, at high concentrations, suppress the oxygen content of respiratory air—sometimes to below the minimum required for survival (10–15% O_2).

Noble gases and nitrogen. The noble gases (also known as rare or inert gases, though they are neither) have no toxicological effects, but nitrogen (N_2) has a narcotic effect at high concentrations. This can lead to fatal accidents during diving, when divers go too deep ($> 60 \, m$) while using compressed air (rapture of the deep) (**E**).

Nitrous Oxide (Dinitrogen Monoxide, Laughing Gas)

Nitrous oxide (N_2O) is a narcotic that temporarily displaces the essential O_2 content in the lungs. It is eliminated extremely rapidly.

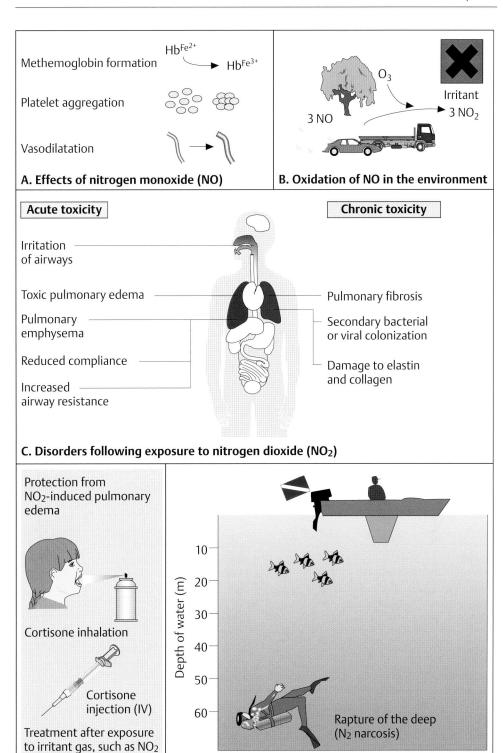

Methemoglobin formation $Hb^{Fe2+} \rightarrow Hb^{Fe3+}$

Platelet aggregation

Vasodilatation

A. Effects of nitrogen monoxide (NO)

O_3

Irritant

$3\,NO$ → $3\,NO_2$

B. Oxidation of NO in the environment

Acute toxicity

Chronic toxicity

Irritation
of airways

Toxic pulmonary edema

Pulmonary
emphysema

Reduced compliance

Increased
airway resistance

Pulmonary fibrosis

Secondary bacterial
or viral colonization

Damage to elastin
and collagen

C. Disorders following exposure to nitrogen dioxide (NO₂)

Protection from
NO₂-induced pulmonary
edema

Cortisone inhalation

Cortisone
injection (IV)

Treatment after exposure
to irritant gas, such as NO₂

D. Treatment

Depth of water (m)

10

20

30

40

50

60

Rapture of the deep
(N₂ narcosis)

E. Effect of high partial pressure of nitrogen (N₂)

Carbon Dioxide

Carbon dioxide (CO_2) is heavier than air and therefore accumulates close to the ground (e.g., in fermentation rooms). High CO_2 content in mines and tunnels has frequently caused accidents. Depending on the dose, CO_2 leads to respiratory acidosis (> 3 % v/v), stimulates the respiratory center via chemoreceptors (3–5 % v/v) (**A**), and has a narcotic effect (> 5 % v/v). Continuous exposure to elevated CO_2 concentrations leads to increased deposition of carbonate in the matrix of the bones.

Carbon Monoxide

Carbon monoxide (CO) is a colorless, odorless, and tasteless gas, i. e., there are no warning signs (density, 0.97 kg/L). Large quantities of CO are produced by microorganisms in the oceans and through oxidation of methane (marsh gas) in the troposphere. Traces of CO are generated in the body by a secondary pathway of pyrrole metabolism. Similarly, CO is formed by degradation of chlorophyll from leaves. It is also generated by incomplete oxidation of hydrocarbons. Numerous accidents have been caused by poorly functioning furnaces or by running a combustion engine in a closed garage (producing up to 10 % CO when idling). Intentionally diverting the car exhaust into the interior of the car is frequently chosen as a method of suicide. Introduction of regulated three-way catalytic converters has dramatically reduced the discharge of carbon monoxide per kilometer driven (~ 2 g CO/km instead of 60 g/km) (**B**).

Effect. After inhalation, CO diffuses quickly from the alveoli into the capillaries. Its elimination by exhalation is also rapid. CO occupies the sixth coordination position of the central iron atom (Fe^{2+}) in the four heme groups of the hemoglobin molecule and competes with O_2 for the same binding site. Since CO has a 200- to 300-fold higher affinity to Fe^{2+} than O_2 does (**C**), the portion of carboxyhemoglobin (CO-Hb) formed at a CO concentration of only 0.1 % (v/v) in inhaled air is 50 %, i. e., hemoglobin's oxygen transport capacity is halved. However, when some of the heme molecules of hemoglobin are occupied by CO, the remaining heme molecules release less O_2 into the tissue (negative cooperativity), thus further reducing an effective oxygen supply to the organs. CO_2, which occupies a different binding site from CO, is more readily dissolved in deoxygenated blood (Haldane effect). The overall result is that organs are insufficiently supplied with oxygen, while CO_2 accumulates in the blood. Furthermore, CO seems to bind to cytochromes, thus directly inhibiting the activity of these membrane-bound hemoproteins.

The effect of CO is determined by the amount taken up and the oxygen requirement of individual organs (**D**). Organ damage is caused by the combination of oxygen deficiency, accumulation of CO_2 (formation of HCO_3^- in the blood), and metabolic lactate acidosis, as well as by direct damage to myoglobin and cytochromes. The symptoms correlate with the carboxyhemoglobin content of the blood (**E**).

In pregnant women, CO rapidly penetrates the placenta. In smoking mothers, it leads to persistent neurological damage to the fetus, although any damage to the mother may still be reversible. Severe CO poisoning causes microscopically detectable alterations in the fetal brain and may also lead to persistent or late damage in adults (**F**).

Detection. Spectroscopic determination of the amount of carboxyhemoglobin is performed with lysed blood, after first reducing oxyhemoglobin (O_2-Hb) to hemoglobin by means of sodium dithionite because its absorption is similar to that of CO-Hb. Poisoned patients look rather grayish pale due to the reduced circulation, but autopsy findings reveal a cherry-red color of the muscles.

Therapy. The poisoned person is removed from the contaminated area. Oxygen is administered to facilitate the dissociation of CO from hemoglobin, and bicarbonate is given to counteract acidosis (**G**). If the carboxyhemoglobin level is more than 25 %, hyperbaric O_2 (at three times atmospheric pressure) is applied; the amount of oxygen dissolved in the plasma is then almost 5 % (v/v), which is sufficient to supply the organs with oxygen.

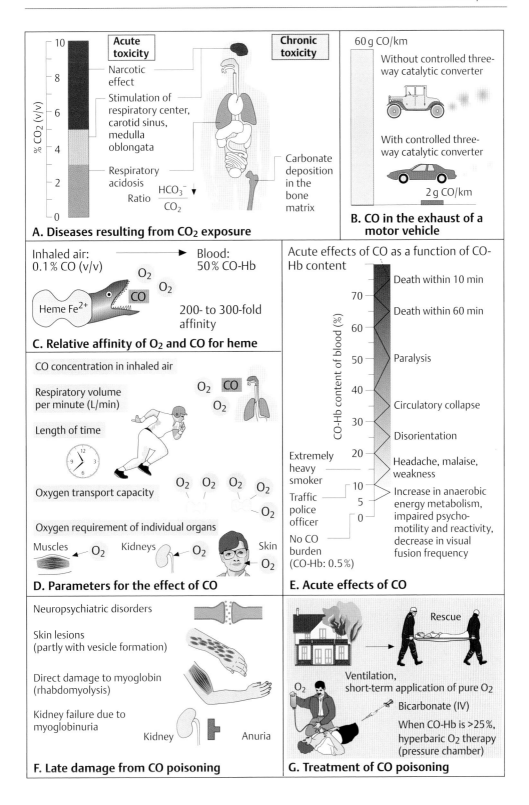

A. Diseases resulting from CO₂ exposure

10
8
6
4
2
0

% CO₂ (v/v)

Acute toxicity

Narcotic effect

Stimulation of respiratory center, carotid sinus, medulla oblongata

Respiratory acidosis

Ratio $\dfrac{HCO_3^-}{CO_2}$ ↓

Chronic toxicity

Carbonate deposition in the bone matrix

B. CO in the exhaust of a motor vehicle

60 g CO/km

Without controlled three-way catalytic converter

With controlled three-way catalytic converter

2 g CO/km

C. Relative affinity of O₂ and CO for heme

Inhaled air: 0.1 % CO (v/v) → Blood: 50 % CO-Hb

Heme Fe²⁺

200- to 300-fold affinity

D. Parameters for the effect of CO

CO concentration in inhaled air

Respiratory volume per minute (L/min)

Length of time

Oxygen transport capacity

Oxygen requirement of individual organs

Muscles   Kidneys   Skin

E. Acute effects of CO

Acute effects of CO as a function of CO-Hb content

CO-Hb content of blood (%)

70 — Death within 10 min

Death within 60 min

60

50 — Paralysis

40

30 — Circulatory collapse

Disorientation

20 — Headache, malaise, weakness

Extremely heavy smoker

10

Traffic police officer   5

0 — Increase in anaerobic energy metabolism, impaired psycho-motility and reactivity, decrease in visual fusion frequency

No CO burden (CO-Hb: 0.5 %)

F. Late damage from CO poisoning

Neuropsychiatric disorders

Skin lesions (partly with vesicle formation)

Direct damage to myoglobin (rhabdomyolysis)

Kidney failure due to myoglobinuria

Kidney   Anuria

G. Treatment of CO poisoning

Rescue

Ventilation, short-term application of pure O₂

Bicarbonate (IV)

When CO-Hb is >25 %, hyperbaric O₂ therapy (pressure chamber)

Hydrogen Cyanide and Cyanide Salts

Hydrogen cyanide (HCN, hydrocyanic acid) is a colorless liquid or gas (density, 0.68 kg/L; melting point, $-14\,^\circ$C; boiling point, $26\,^\circ$C). At pH 7.4, only 1.6% of HCN is dissociated, i.e., it is a very weak acid (pk_a 9.2). It easily diffuses through the cell membrane and is one of the most rapidly acting poisons.

Most humans smell the characteristic odor of bitter almonds very easily, but some are unable to detect it at all because of genetic predisposition.

The toxic effect is due to the cyanide anion (CN^-). Cyanides are used for metal hardening and as solvents during precious metal refining. They have also played a role as poisons for suicide and homicide (including genocide by the use of cyanide in gas chambers). Hydrogen cyanide and cyanide salts are formed (in addition to CO) by incomplete combustion of all nitrogen-containing substances (e.g., plastics such as polyurethane and polyacrylnitrile, as well as wool and silk). CN^- is also generated in the body from cyanogenic glycosides or nitriles (**A**), although there is little danger of poisoning by consuming bitter almonds. For this to occur, adults would have to eat about 50 bitter almonds (equivalent to ~ 0.2 g of cyanide) and children about 10. By contrast, there have been numerous cases of neuropathy as a result of poisoning after improper (nontraditional) preparation of manioc roots (cassava, a cyanogenic food plant from South America and southern Africa).

Unless due caution is exercised, the use of sodium nitroprusside (nitroferricyanide) in the treatment of hypertensive crisis may lead to alarming conditions when large amounts of CN^- are cleaved off in the body (particularly if the dose has been increased as a result of tachyphylaxis).

Effect. HCN is taken up via the lungs, while cyanide salts are ingested and converted to HCN in the acidic milieu of the stomach before being absorbed. In the cells, CN^- binds with high affinity, although reversibly, to the iron atom (Fe^{3+}) of mitochondrial cytochrome aa_3 (cytochrome c oxidase) and other metalloenzymes (**B**). Because of the inhibition of the electron transport chain, oxygen cannot be activated (ATP deprivation, internal suffocation, lactic acidosis). The first symptoms after oral uptake of cyanides are observed within a few minutes (15–60 min after ingestion of bitter almonds or flax seeds). After the inhalation of cyanide, the first symptoms occur within a few seconds. At concentrations of 200–300 mL/m^3 air the effect of HCN is rapid and lethal, and a concentration of 100 mL/m^3 is life-threatening.

Acute effects include throat irritation (in the case of HCN), dyspnea, reddening of the skin and mucosae (no O_2 consumption, arterialization of venous blood), malaise, spasmodic vomiting, disturbed conduction of the heart, respiratory paralysis, and death. Oxygen deficiency (resulting from respiratory paralysis) and acidosis may induce persistent or late damage (e.g., to the nervous system) (**C**).

Because of the high endogenous detoxification capacity (0.1–1 mg CN/kg per hour), chronic poisoning only occurs when CN^- uptake rises continuously or when there are genetic disorders of cyanide detoxification (hereditary retinal degeneration, trophic neuropathy).

Endogenous detoxification. This takes place by intracellular coupling with sulfane sulfur (**D**). This detoxification step is mediated by the intramitochondrial enzyme rhodanase and generates rhodanide (SCN^-), which is then excreted by the kidneys. Because of the high turnover rate, large amounts of CN^- can be detoxified (see above), although it is limited by the small amount of sulfur available within cells.

Therapy. Sulfur substitution: sodium thiosulfate ($Na_2S_2O_3$; 10–20 mL of a 10% solution) IV is used as an antidote. Since this causal treatment is too slow for severe poisonings, hemoglobin is first converted to methemoglobin (target amount: ⅓ HbFe^{3+}), which is achieved by IV injection of 4-dimethylaminophenol (4-DMAP; 3 mg/kg BW). The CN^- anion then binds rapidly and with high affinity to the Fe^{3+} of methemoglobin and so is diverted from the cytochromes (**E**).

Less effective and less easy to control is inhalation of amyl nitrite. Treatment with hydroxocobalamin is suitable for use in smoke inhalation victims (for severe gas poisoning due to fire, see p. 138).

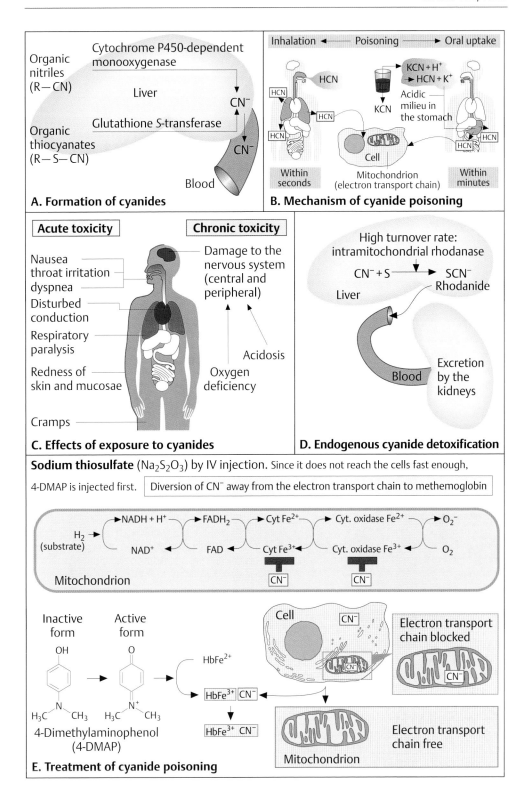

A. Formation of cyanides

Organic nitriles (R—CN)

Cytochrome P450-dependent monooxygenase

Liver

Glutathione S-transferase

Organic thiocyanates (R—S—CN)

CN^-

CN^-

Blood

B. Mechanism of cyanide poisoning

Inhalation ◄——— Poisoning ———► Oral uptake

HCN

$KCN+H^+$
$HCN+K^+$

KCN

Acidic milieu in the stomach

HCN

Cell

Within seconds

Mitochondrion (electron transport chain)

Within minutes

C. Effects of exposure to cyanides

Acute toxicity

Chronic toxicity

Nausea throat irritation dyspnea

Disturbed conduction

Respiratory paralysis

Redness of skin and mucosae

Cramps

Damage to the nervous system (central and peripheral)

Acidosis

Oxygen deficiency

D. Endogenous cyanide detoxification

High turnover rate: intramitochondrial rhodanase

$CN^- + S$ ——► SCN^- Rhodanide

Liver

Blood

Excretion by the kidneys

Sodium thiosulfate ($Na_2S_2O_3$) by IV injection. Since it does not reach the cells fast enough,

4-DMAP is injected first. | Diversion of CN^- away from the electron transport chain to methemoglobin

H_2 (substrate)

NADH + H$^+$ ► FADH$_2$ ► Cyt Fe^{2+} ► Cyt. oxidase Fe^{2+} ► O_2^-

NAD$^+$ ◄ FAD ◄ Cyt Fe^{3+} ◄ Cyt. oxidase Fe^{3+} ◄ O_2

Mitochondrion

CN^- CN^-

Inactive form

Active form

OH

O

HbFe^{2+}

HbFe^{3+} CN^-

Cell CN^-

Electron transport chain blocked

CN^-

HbFe^{3+} CN^-

Electron transport chain free

4-Dimethylaminophenol (4-DMAP)

Mitochondrion

E. Treatment of cyanide poisoning

Organic cobalt compounds, such as dicobalt edetate (Co$_2$-EDTA, Kelocyanor), or inorganic cobalt compounds are now no longer used because of their severe side effects.

Hydrogen Sulfide

Hydrogen sulfide (H$_2$S) is a colorless, flammable gas formed during the reaction of mineral acids with sulfides of heavy metals, as well as during the decomposition of protein (sewer gas contains up to 10% H$_2$S). Considerable amounts of H$_2$S are also formed during the papermaking process. In addition, H$_2$S accumulates in cellars, canals, and containers. The warning sign—an offensive smell of rotten eggs (sensitivity threshold ~ 0.025 mL/m^3)—diminishes as the result of rapid habituation. First aid helpers attempting to rescue victims from poisoned areas are therefore prone to accidents.

Effect (A). Concentrations of more than 10–50 mL/m^3 cause irritation, possibly pulmonary edema, and intracellular hypoxia; the mechanisms are unknown. Concentrations of more than 500 mL/m^3 cause unconsciousness and quick development of central respiratory paralysis. H$_2$S is rapidly oxidized in the body and eliminated as sulfate.

After chronic exposure (e.g., of workers in synthetic fiber manufacturing facilities), corneal damage, increased airway resistance, pulmonary edema, pneumonia, and myocardial degeneration have been observed.

Therapy. Nonspecific measures (keeping the airways free, correction of acidosis).

Fumigants

Some gaseous compounds are used as fumigants for controlling insects, rodents, and other pests in areas that cannot be reached otherwise. Fumigants are very dangerous poisons, and in many industrialized countries their sale is restricted and their use requires a permit (**B**). Details of how to carry out fumigation procedures are described in national legislation and regulations. For example, ships in transit may be fumigated only with phosphine, containers in transit may be treated only with phosphine or methyl bromide, and ethylene oxide may be used only in fumigation chambers.

In industrialized countries, widely used fumigants include the following (**C**):

Methyl bromide (bromomethane). In the 1960s, the use of this insecticide (a colorless, nonflammable gas; boiling point 4.5 °C; density 3 kg/L) caused more lethal accidents in California than the use of organophosphates (see p. 200). The extremely poisonous methyl bromide is commonly mixed with chloropicrin, a potent irritant that serves as a warning agent. The target organ of the systemic effects of methyl bromide is the central nervous system. A likely mechanism of action for poisoning of the central nervous system is the reaction with endogenous sulfhydryl groups. Dithiol compounds (e.g., dimercaptopropanol, dimercaptosuccinic acid [DMSA]) are being considered as possible agents for treatment.

Hydrogen cyanide and formaldehyde. For details, see p. 140 and pp. 94, 136, respectively.

Ethylene oxide (Oxirane). This is a colorless gas (boiling point 11 °C; density 1.5 kg/L) with a high olfactory threshold (at ~ 700 mL/m^3). It is a strong irritant, and it forms explosive mixtures with air. Ethylene oxide is mutagenic and carcinogenic.

Phosphorus hydrides: hydrogen phosphide (PH$_3$), phosphines, and phosphine-producing pesticides. Phosphine is the common name for hydrogen phosphide (a colorless, heavy gas; formerly called phosphorus [tri]hydride). In the presence of traces of water, the gas is slowly released from aluminum phosphide tablets. It is a metabolic poison and neurotoxin that is more toxic than methyl bromide but considered safer to handle.

The following fumigants are also used: vinyl cyanide (acrylonitrile, CH$_2$CHCN), carbon disulfide (CS$_2$), tetrachloromethane (carbon tetrachloride, CCl$_4$, see p. 104), trichloronitromethane (CCl$_3$NO$_2$), and ethylene dibromide (1,2-dibromoethane, CH$_2$BrCH$_2$Br$_2$), and dibromochloropropane (ClCH$_2$CHBrCH$_2$Br).

Detection. The gaseous compounds mentioned above can be determined quantitatively by means of gas chromatography or infrared spectroscopy, and semiquantitatively using colorimetric indicator tubes (Draeger tubes).

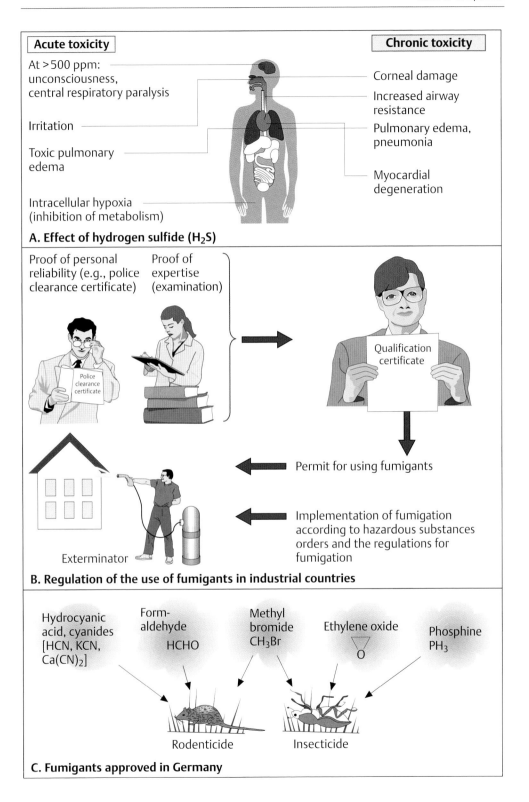

Acute toxicity

At >500 ppm: unconsciousness, central respiratory paralysis

Irritation

Toxic pulmonary edema

Intracellular hypoxia (inhibition of metabolism)

Chronic toxicity

Corneal damage

Increased airway resistance

Pulmonary edema, pneumonia

Myocardial degeneration

A. Effect of hydrogen sulfide (H$_2$S)

Proof of personal reliability (e.g., police clearance certificate)

Proof of expertise (examination)

Police clearance certificate

Qualification certificate

Permit for using fumigants

Implementation of fumigation according to hazardous substances orders and the regulations for fumigation

Exterminator

B. Regulation of the use of fumigants in industrial countries

Hydrocyanic acid, cyanides [HCN, KCN, Ca(CN)$_2$]

Formaldehyde HCHO

Methyl bromide CH$_3$Br

Ethylene oxide O

Phosphine PH$_3$

Rodenticide

Insecticide

C. Fumigants approved in Germany

Vehicle Exhaust Gases

Basics

Gases. The following gases are detected after combustion of fuel in gasoline or diesel engines: nitrogen (N_2, ~71%), carbon dioxide (CO_2, ~18%), water vapor (H_2O, ~8%), argon (Ar, ~1%), and oxygen (O_2, ~1%). Together they amount to more than 99% (w/w) of the total vehicle exhaust. The residual portion (**A**) is made up by *restricted components*, such as carbon monoxide (CO), nitrogen oxides (NO_x), hydrocarbons (HCs), and particles, and by *non-restricted components*, such as sulfur dioxide (SO_2), hydrogen, aldehydes, ketones, and other compounds. Several substances are regulated by law, and the reduction of these necessarily also reduces other substances. In a wider sense, sulfur compounds in exhaust gases are thus restricted by means of the sulfur content of fuels, which is relevant for diesel fuel.

European Union Guideline 94/12. This guideline strictly regulates vehicle exhaust emissions. A car equipped with a gasoline engine may currently emit no more than 2.2 g of CO and 0.5 g of total HCs+NO_x per kilometer driven, and a car with a diesel engine may emit only 1.0 g of CO, 0.7 g of total HCs+NO_x, and 0.08 g of particles per kilometer driven. Because of the short reaction times of air/fuel mixtures (from 10 ms when idling to 1 ms at high rotational speed), vehicle exhaust also contains unburned hydrocarbons and lead compounds (from gasoline engines) as well as sulfur compounds and particles (from diesel engines). The amounts of individual gases and particles in the exhaust depend on many parameters, for example, the type of fuel and its additives, the proportion of combustion air, the engine parameters (such as adjustment of the ignition), or the function and type of the engine. A reduction of all toxic components in vehicle exhaust can be achieved by treating the exhaust gas in a catalytic converter.

Function of a Catalytic Converter for Vehicle Exhaust Gases (B)

Reduction in emissions of CO, HCs, and NO_x. These emissions are reduced by using a catalytic converter. This consists of a honeycombed carrier layer (made of ceramics or metal), to which an intermediate layer (wash coat) is applied to enlarge the surface; this layer contains activity-increasing additives (promoters). On top of this comes the catalytically active layer, consisting of platinum and rhodium (in a 5:1 ratio, possibly also containing some palladium), where the chemical reactions are catalyzed (e.g., the conversions of CO, HCs, and NO_x) (**C**). Since lead damages the catalytic surface layer, lead-free fuel must be used. CO and hydrocarbons are converted in the presence of O_2, while NO_x requires reducing conditions. The O_2 content in the exhaust gas is continuously measured by means of a lambda probe so that the optimal air mixture can be adjusted accordingly.

Traffic. Motor vehicles are the main source of toxic emissions, i.e., CO, NO_x, and organic compounds. (Power plants are the main source of SO_2 emission.) Traffic and energy conversion are the major participants in producing CO_2, which —together with other greenhouse gases (e.g., methane, nitrous oxide, ozone, CFCs, H_2O vapor)—is responsible for the greenhouse effect. The amount released into the air is about 20 kg CO_2 for every 100 km driven.

Greenhouse Effect

Each year, all combustion processes combined emit 7.5 billion tons of CO_2 into the Earth's atmosphere. The effect of increased CO_2 concentrations (**D**) is that the thermal radiation normally reflected by the Earth is increasingly retained. This is thought to lead to global warming by 3–4 °C by 2050, thus causing global changes in the climate. Parts of the polar ice will melt, and sea levels will rise by around 0.5 m. This threatens the existence of some countries, such as the Maldives. In Europe, there will be no snow below 1500 m, thus triggering changes in run-off volumes and groundwater levels. It is feared that this will have global ecological consequences.

Reduction in CO_2 emissions (e.g., lower energy consumption, reduced traffic) can help to counteract the threat of climate change.

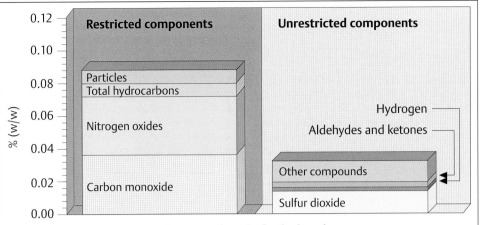

A. Composition of the residual portion (<1%) of vehicle exhaust

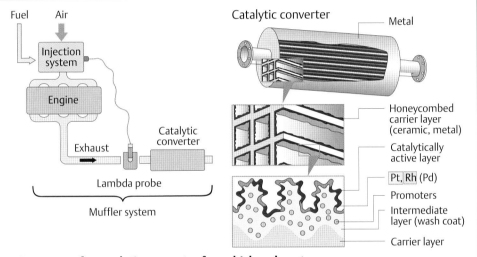

B. Structure of a catalytic converter for vehicle exhaust gases

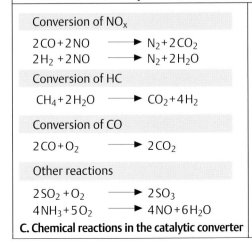

Conversion of NO$_x$

$$2CO + 2NO \longrightarrow N_2 + 2CO_2$$
$$2H_2 + 2NO \longrightarrow N_2 + 2H_2O$$

Conversion of HC

$$CH_4 + 2H_2O \longrightarrow CO_2 + 4H_2$$

Conversion of CO

$$2CO + O_2 \longrightarrow 2CO_2$$

Other reactions

$$2SO_2 + O_2 \longrightarrow 2SO_3$$
$$4NH_3 + 5O_2 \longrightarrow 4NO + 6H_2O$$

C. Chemical reactions in the catalytic converter

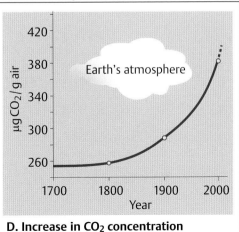

D. Increase in CO$_2$ concentration

Oxygen Species and Free Radicals

Formation and Effect

Reactive oxygen species and free radicals are characterized by their extreme reactivity and very short half-life. They are generated during (patho)physiological processes by all forms of life. *Free radicals* are chemically unstable atoms, molecules or ions that possess unpaired electrons, with a single unpaired electron occupying a molecular orbital. Radicals are therefore paramagnetic, i.e., they orient themselves in a magnetic field. Radicals are formed by the uptake or donation of an electron, or by cleavage of a covalent bond (**A**). *Reactive oxygen species* include (in order of decreasing reactivity): the hydroxyl radical ($\cdot$OH), singlet oxygen ($^1O_2$), the superoxide radical anion (O_2^-), and hydrogen peroxide (H_2O_2). Molecular oxygen (dioxygen, O_2) is largely nonreactive. In its triplet ground state ($^3O_2$), it is a biradical, i.e., the outermost molecular orbitals ($2\,p\pi^*$) each contain one unpaired electron with parallel spins. For ozone (O_3, another reactive oxygen species), see pp. 150–153.

Singlet oxygen. The exited state of O_2 is formed during several (patho)physiological processes (e.g., phagocytosis, prostaglandin biosynthesis). The outer electrons of $^1O_2$ have antiparallel spins. Two forms occur: $^1\Sigma_g^+O_2$ (the paired electrons occupy one molecular orbital each) and $^1\Delta_gO_2$ (the two electrons occupy the same $2\,p\pi^*$ orbital) (**B**).

Superoxide radical. The O_2^- radical is formed by reduction of molecular oxygen as a secondary product of mitochondrial respiration. As mitochondrial O_2^- production is proportional to oxygen tension, it plays an important role in oxygen toxicity. The O_2^- radical is primarily produced by phagocytes (e.g., during inflammation). This generation of reactive oxygen stimulates the phagocytosis of opsonized bacteria and the activity of complement factor C5a, leukotriene B4, and tumor promoters (e.g., phorbol myristyl acetate). The O_2^- radical is also liberated during enzymatic reactions (e.g., by xanthine oxidases in postischemic tissue).

Hydrogen peroxide. H_2O_2 is generated as a secondary product in enzymatic reactions mediated by various superoxide dismutases (e.g., monoamine oxidase): $2\,O_2^- + 2\,H^+ \rightarrow O_2 + H_2O_2$. It can also be generated by direct transfer of two electrons to molecular oxygen (**B**). H_2O_2 is a stable compound that acts in living cells as an oxidizing and reducing agent.

Hydroxyl radical. The $\cdot$OH radical is a powerful oxidant with a high rate constant of formation. It is generated in inflamed tissues in a reaction mediated by a transition metal. This reaction, in which Fe^{2+} is oxidized to Fe^{3+}, is known as the Fenton reaction (**B**). The $\cdot$OH radical is also produced during the reaction of H_2O_2 with nitrogen oxides. The Haber–Weiss reaction, in which an $\cdot$OH radical is formed while an O_2^- radical is consumed, occurs in vivo only at high H_2O_2 concentrations (**B**).

Alkoxy radicals (RO$\cdot$), peroxy radicals (ROO$\cdot$), and organic free radicals. These are formed during the metabolism of several foreign substances (xenobiotics). For example, the compounds 1,2-dibromoethane (a gasoline additive), tetrachloromethane (CCl_4), or paracetamol are metabolized into free radicals and may therefore cause damage to the body (**A, B**).

The formation of radicals in phagocytes is part of the body's defense system against infections. Phagocytes use the toxic potential of reactive oxygen species to kill phagocytosed bacteria (**B**).

Effects (B). Radicals and reactive oxygen species may have the following damaging effects: oxidation of unsaturated fatty acids, depolymerization of collagen, denaturation of enzymes, hemolysis, inactivation of neurotransmitters, destruction of mucopolysaccharides of the synovial fluid, destruction of protein structures (leading to increased allergenicity), and promotion of tumor development.

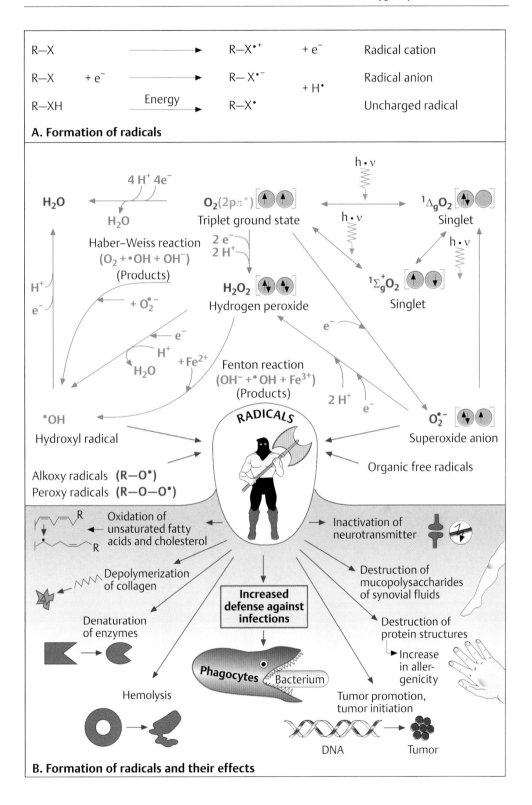

R—X $\longrightarrow$ R—X$^{\bullet +}$ + e$^-$ Radical cation

R—X + e$^-$ $\longrightarrow$ R—X$^{\bullet -}$ Radical anion
+ H$^{\bullet}$

R—XH $\xrightarrow{\text{Energy}}$ R—X$^{\bullet}$ Uncharged radical

A. Formation of radicals

H$_2$O $\longleftarrow$ 4 H$^+$ 4e$^-$ $\quad$ O$_2$(2pπ^*) Triplet ground state $\quad$ $^1\Delta_g$O$_2$ Singlet

H$_2$O

Haber–Weiss reaction
(O$_2$ + $^{\bullet}$OH + OH$^-$)
(Products)

H$^+$
e$^-$

+ O$_2^{\bullet -}$

H$_2$O$_2$ Hydrogen peroxide

$^1\Sigma_g^+$O$_2$ Singlet

e$^-$
H$^+$
H$_2$O

+ Fe^{2+}

Fenton reaction
(OH$^-$ + $^{\bullet}$OH + Fe^{3+})
(Products)

2 H$^+$
e$^-$

$^{\bullet}$OH
Hydroxyl radical

RADICALS

O$_2^{\bullet -}$
Superoxide anion

Alkoxy radicals **(R—O$^{\bullet}$)**
Peroxy radicals **(R—O—O$^{\bullet}$)**

Organic free radicals

Oxidation of
unsaturated fatty
acids and cholesterol

Inactivation of
neurotransmitter

Depolymerization
of collagen

Destruction of
mucopolysaccharides
of synovial fluids

Denaturation
of enzymes

**Increased
defense against
infections**

Destruction of
protein structures

Increase
in aller-
genicity

Hemolysis

Phagocytes Bacterium

Tumor promotion,
tumor initiation

DNA $\quad$ Tumor

B. Formation of radicals and their effects

147

Protective Mechanisms

Life in an oxygen-rich environment requires an effective defense system which prevents cellular damage associated with the generation of reactive oxygen species and free radicals (see p. 146). Living cells possess several enzymatic and nonenzymatic protective mechanisms that alleviate or prevent the damaging effects of reactive oxygen species and free radicals.

Enzymatic Protective Mechanisms (A)

Superoxide dismutases (SODs). These enzymes convert superoxide radical anions (O_2^-) into hydrogen peroxide (H_2O_2), thus protecting cells from dangerous superoxide levels (**A**). SODs are metalloenzymes; their catalytic center contains a transition metal ion (Cu, Zn, Fe, or Mn, depending on the species). In phylogenetic terms, SODs are very old proteins; they seem to have developed about a billion years ago to protect cells against the damaging effects of oxygen. The rate constant determined for the reaction of O_2^- with superoxide dismutase is 2×10^{-9} L mol^{-1} s^{-1}; hence, the reaction is so fast that it is limited only by the diffusion of substrate to the SOD. This means that O_2^- radicals produced in cells captured immediately at the site of formation. (The equilibrium concentration of O_2^- in the liver under normal conditions is only 10^{-11} to 10^{-12} mol/L.)

Catalase. Like superoxide dismutases, catalase catalyzes dismutation; it converts H_2O_2 into O_2 and H_2O (**A**). Catalase is an ubiquitous hemoprotein in mammalian tissues. In hepatocytes, it is largely present in peroxisomes.

Glutathione peroxidase. This tetrameric protein reduces H_2O_2 while consuming the tripeptide glutathione (GSH) (**A**). The catalytic center of the cytosolic form of the enzyme contains the essential trace mineral selenium. Under normal conditions, the activities of catalase and glutathione peroxidase keep the cellular H_2O_2 concentration at 10^{-7} to 10^{-9} mol/L. Unlike catalase, glutathione peroxidase also reacts with the hydroperoxides of unsaturated fatty acids, steroids, and nucleotides.

Glutathione S-transferases. These enzymes conjugate organic free radicals and reactive organic molecules with GSH. They are key enzymes for the formation of mercapturic acids and cysteinyl leukotrienes. As selenium-independent glutathione peroxidases, they can also react with the organic hydroperoxide (ROOH) already formed, but not with H_2O_2. A high intracellular GSH level is required to maintain cell functions. The GSH consumed during the enzymatic reactions mentioned above must therefore be recovered. NADPH-dependent glutathione reductase can convert glutathione disulfide (GSSG) to GSH: GSSG + NADPH + H$^+$ → 2 GSH + NADP$^+$. NADPH is recovered via the glucose 6-phosphate reaction.

Nonenzymatic Protective Mechanisms (B)

Ascorbic acid (vitamin C). This captures free radicals, in particular O_2^- and ˙OH, but also H_2O_2 and singlet O_2.

Vitamin A. Its precursor β-carotene (provitamin A) is found in the retina. It effectively quenches singlet O_2 and is a direct scavenger of free radicals.

α-Tocopherol. The lipophilic antioxidant α-tocopherol (vitamin E) reacts with peroxy and alkoxy radicals (e.g., in peroxidized membrane phospholipids) and thus prevents lipid peroxidation.

Taurine and uric acid. These water-soluble antioxidants can inactivate ˙OH, ROO˙, and singlet O_2.

Glutathione. The tripeptide glutathione (γ-Glu-Cys-Gly) plays an important role, not only in the enzymatic inactivation of radicals; it can also react nonenzymatically with radicals such as O_2^-, ˙OH, RO˙ und ROO˙, while forming oxidized glutathione (GSSG): R˙ + GSH → RH + GS˙; GS˙ + GS˙ → GSSG.

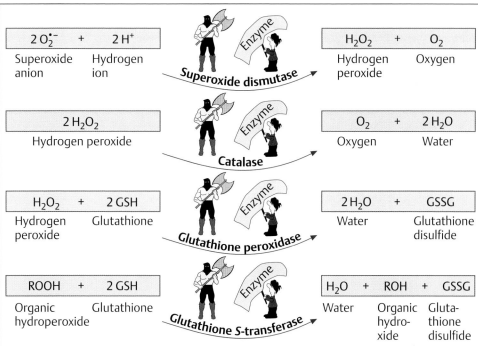

A. Enzymatic protective mechanisms against reactive oxygen species and free radicals

Substance	Structure	Function
Ascorbic acid (vitamin C)		Capture of $O_2^{\cdot-}$, $\cdot OH$, H_2O_2, and singlet O_2
Vitamin A		Capture of singlet O_2
α-Tocopherol (vitamin E)		Capture of $RO^{\cdot}$, $ROO^{\cdot}$
Uric acid		Capture of $\cdot OH$, $ROO^{\cdot}$, and singlet O_2
Taurine	H_2N H $H-C-C-SO_3H$ H H	Capture of $\cdot OH$, $ROO^{\cdot}$, and singlet O_2
Glutathione	γ-Glu-Cys-Gly	Capture of $O_2^{\cdot-}$, $\cdot OH$, $RO^{\cdot}$, $ROO^{\cdot}$

B. Nonenzymatic protective mechanisms against reactive oxygen species and free radicals

Ozone (O₃)

Ozone is a bluish, highly toxic gas (the dose–response curve is very steep). It is a very strong oxidant with high reactivity. Ozone is generated in the stratosphere through the reaction of molecular oxygen (O_2) with UV light. The O_3 concentration in the stratosphere is about 20 mg/m³ air, in the upper troposphere about 2–4 mg/m³, and in the lower troposphere, depending on the day, between 0.004 and 0.2 mg/m³ (**A**). The half-life of O_3 in the troposphere is short (7 min). Since ozone decomposes rapidly in buildings and is not produced there, its concentration is lower indoors than outdoors.

Uptake (A). During physical activity (e.g., work, sports), up to 90% of ozone is taken up by the lungs.

Distribution (A). Because of its high reactivity, ozone is rapidly metabolized while still in the lungs (in the pulmonary circulation, at the latest) by means of the antioxidant system (see p. 148).

Mechanism of action (B). Ozone is very damaging to cells. It induces oxidative changes in the lipids of cell membranes, in proteins (e.g., enzymes, structural and receptor proteins), and in hyaluronic acid, thus leading to loss of function (cell damage). The generation of hydroperoxides (ROOH) and their radicals (ROO', RO') as well as superoxide radicals (O_2^-) and hydroxyl ('OH) radicals increasingly leads to cell damage (see p. 146).

Acute toxicity (C). Inhalation of 2–10 mg O_3/m³ air for 1–2 h causes damage (often within 60 min) mainly to the conjunctiva of the eyes and the mucosae of the lower respiratory tract. The effects observed include severe lachrymation, changes in visual acuity, cyanosis, and pulmonary dysfunction (e.g., dyspnea, toxic pulmonary edema, decline in vital capacity). In humans, inhalation of only 0.2 mg/m³ ozone (for 1–2 h) may lead to uncomfortable irritation of the eyes, nose, and throat. It also reduces physical fitness: women who inhaled 0.26 mg/m³ (for several hours) showed an 11% decline in fitness. Children generally respond more to ozone than adults.

Chronic toxicity (C). In humans, chronic ozone inhalation (0.5–1 mg/m³) leads to emphysema and fibrotic changes of the pulmonary tissue, bronchiolitis, and the appearance of hyperplastic alveolar cells (type I). The inhibited formation of bactericidal O_2^- radicals in activated macrophages and the reduced ciliary action of the ciliary epithelium of the lungs is associated with an increased risk of infections. Because of increased pendelluft volume, pregnant women are often more sensitive to ozone. On the other hand, studies on asthmatics did not find evidence for an increased sensitivity to ozone.

Therapy (D). In cases of acute ozone poisoning (> 2 mg/m³), toxic pulmonary edema should be prevented by administering glucocorticoid spray. Apart from this, the treatment is symptomatic. Antioxidants (see p. 148) may be used to reduce ozone toxicity.

Critical assessment. No increased cancer risk has been observed even in professions particularly exposed to ozone, such as inert gas welders and operators of sun parlors or photocopying machines. Since the critical ozone level for triggering early symptoms in humans is 0.2 mg/m³, the international values (0.2 mg/m³) no longer contain a safety range. Such ozone concentrations are already ubiquitous in some regions; hence, there is no longer any leeway for further anthropogenic emission of ozone or its precursor substances.

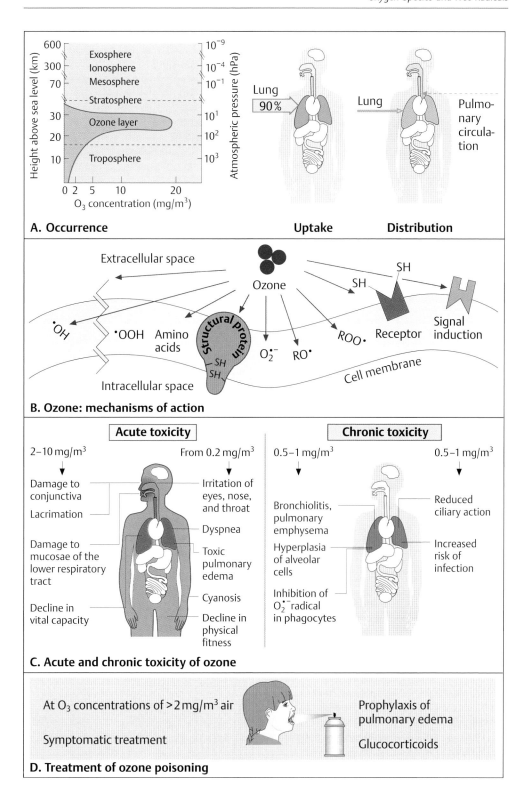

A. Occurrence — Uptake — Distribution

Lung 90%

Lung — Pulmonary circulation

Exosphere
Ionosphere
Mesosphere
Stratosphere
Ozone layer
Troposphere

Height above sea level (km)
Atmospheric pressure (hPa)
O_3 concentration (mg/m^3)

B. Ozone: mechanisms of action

Extracellular space
Ozone
SH
SH
$\cdot$OH
$\cdot$OOH   Amino acids
Structural protein
SH
SH
$O_2^{\cdot-}$ RO$^{\cdot}$
ROO$^{\cdot}$ Receptor
Signal induction
Intracellular space
Cell membrane

C. Acute and chronic toxicity of ozone

Acute toxicity

2–10 mg/m^3

Damage to conjunctiva

Lacrimation

Damage to mucosae of the lower respiratory tract

Decline in vital capacity

From 0.2 mg/m^3

Irritation of eyes, nose, and throat

Dyspnea

Toxic pulmonary edema

Cyanosis

Decline in physical fitness

Chronic toxicity

0.5–1 mg/m^3

Bronchiolitis, pulmonary emphysema

Hyperplasia of alveolar cells

Inhibition of $O_2^{\cdot-}$ radical in phagocytes

0.5–1 mg/m^3

Reduced ciliary action

Increased risk of infection

D. Treatment of ozone poisoning

At O_3 concentrations of >2 mg/m^3 air

Symptomatic treatment

Prophylaxis of pulmonary edema

Glucocorticoids

151

Ozone Depletion ("Ozone Hole")

In 1920, the British scientist Gordon Dobson demonstrated the existence of the ozone layer in the stratosphere where around 90% of the total ozone is found. In 1985, J. C. Farman et al. reported periodic ozone losses over the Antarctic since 1977 (the "ozone hole"). During the same period, a proportional increase in chlorine monoxide (ClO) was observed.

Harmless UVA radiation is essential for living organisms and reaches the Earth largely unhindered. By contrast, both *UVB radiation* and *UVC radiation* are biologically *harmful* because they induce DNA damage (see p. 298).

Formation and destruction of ozone (A). The ozone layer shields the Earth from harmful solar radiation by screening out the UVB and UVC rays. When oxygen rises into the atmosphere, the high-energy, short-wave UVC radiation cleaves molecular oxygen (O_2) into atomic oxygen (O), which rapidly reacts with O_2 to form ozone (O_3). The less energetic UVB radiation does not affect O_2, but it stimulates O_3 to decompose into O and O_2. The formation and destruction of ozone are in equilibrium (ozone cycle). Addition of chlorofluorohydrocarbons (CFCs) to the atmosphere disturbs this equilibrium.

Ozone depletion. The inactive and very stable (though largely nontoxic) CFCs, which are used as coolants and propellants, reach the lower layers of the atmosphere and remain there for up to 50 years. Near the equator, however, warm upward currents bring these CFCs into the stratosphere (**B2**). Here, under the influence of UV light, $CFCl_3$ reacts to form Cl and $CFCl_2$. Cl then reacts with O_3 to form reactive ClO and stable O_2. When ClO encounters another O atom, this leads to spontaneous formation of O_2 and a Cl atom, which again attacks an O_3 molecule (**B1**). These reactions continue until Cl is captured by H or N (e.g., formation of chlorine nitrate [$ClNO_3$]). Calculations have shown that a single Cl atom can destroy up to 1000 O_3 molecules.

The **ozone hole** is an Antarctic phenomenon and is more pronounced in the southern spring. Large-scale whirlwinds build up over the Antarctic continent. During the long winter (4 months of darkness) temperatures drop sharply here, and the *circumpolar vortex* becomes very strong. Cl and O_3 are drawn into the vortex, where they react more readily (**C**). The vortex additionally prevents the influx of ozone, which primarily forms around the equator. Over the Arctic, the circumpolar vortex does not reach high speeds, as it is slowed down by the landmasses surrounding the Arctic Ocean; hence no such reactions occur in the northern hemisphere. This explains why O_3, as of today, has declined by more than 50% over the Antarctic but only by about 5% over the Arctic. The cold winter winds cause ice crystals to form in the dry stratosphere of the Antarctic. The ice crystals make certain reactions possible: molecules which have previously bound Cl atoms react with the surface of the ice crystals and release Cl_2 gas. As soon as the sun returns in the spring, the Cl_2 molecules are cleaved into Cl atoms (**C**) so that the ozone layer can be attacked again (**B1**).

Other catalysts of ozone destruction include sulfur compounds (which reach the stratosphere as the result of volcanic eruptions, like Mount Pinatubo in 1991) and bromide.

Calculations have shown that a 1% decrease in ozone leads to a 4% increase in skin cancer. In countries close to the ozone hole (e.g., New Zealand), the potential risk is therefore increased. So far, studies have not yielded any evidence for harmful effects on the Antarctic phytoplankton, even though UVB radiation has increased by a factor of two. Ozone depletion can be minimized by using the nontoxic, chlorine-free CFCs that are now available.

Nitrogen monoxide (NO) stimulates the formation of ozone (**B1**), which leads to high ozone levels in regions with smog. When smog is transferred into clean air regions, even more ozone is formed there under the more intense UV radiation.

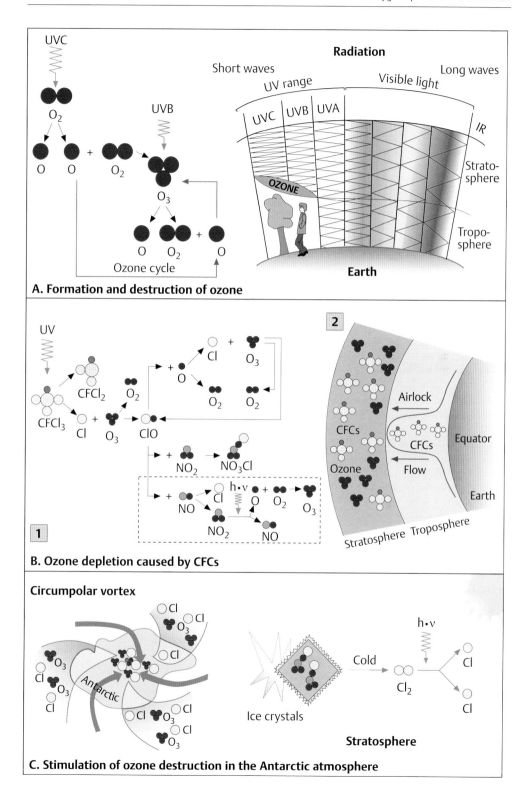

A. Formation and destruction of ozone

B. Ozone depletion caused by CFCs

C. Stimulation of ozone destruction in the Antarctic atmosphere

▪ Tobacco Smoke (Active and Passive Smoking)

History

Smoking is said to have been known in China more than 2000 years ago. In a document dated November 10, 1492, the explorer Christopher Columbus first mentioned that the natives of the West Indies (the Arawaks) smoked tobacco leaves wrapped in maize leaves ("tobagos").

In 1556, the French ambassador Jean Nicot brought the tobacco plant to France from Portugal. It is a member of the nightshade family (*Solanaceae*) and was named after him: *Nicotiana tabacum*. Tobacco plants arrived in Germany around 1600.

Mainstream and Sidestream Smoke (A)

Smoke that is actively inhaled into the lungs (e. g., when smoking a cigarette) is called mainstream smoke, or *active smoke*. Second-hand smoke (e.g., the smoke from a burning cigarette, or the exhaled mainstream smoke) is called sidestream smoke, or *passive smoke*. Active smokers inhale both mainstream and sidestream smoke. The two types of smoke differ in several physico-chemical properties, because sidestream smoke is the product of incomplete combustion. Slow smoldering at the edge of an ashtray provides far less oxygen to the burning cigarette than active smoking, and temperature differences of several hundred °C exist between the formation of active and passive smoke.

There are up to 4000 substances in mainstream smoke, and these are also present in various amounts in sidestream smoke. Both types of tobacco smoke contain volatile compounds (gaseous phase) and particles (particulate phase). During active smoking, potential carcinogens are thought to be contained mainly in the particulate phase. Active smokers who consume 20 cigarettes/day inhale up to 20 000 times more particle-bound, tobacco-specific nitrosamines (which are carcinogens) than passive smokers who inhale sidestream smoke for 8 h.

Nicotine (B)

Tobacco contains 0.2–5 % nicotine, an alkaloid that was isolated for the first time in 1828 by the German chemists L. Reimann and W. Posselt. Nicotine is a powerful poison. The lethal dose for humans starts at 50 mg, making it more toxic than arsenic or potassium cyanide.

Nicotine is rapidly absorbed via the bronchi and the lungs. It can be detected in the brain about 10 s after the first inhalation. Nicotine is quickly oxidized in the liver to form cotinine (see formula: the oxygen bond is shown in blue) and excreted in the urine (the elimination half-life is 2 h).

Effects of nicotine. By activating the parasympathetic nervous system, nicotine increases the production of gastric juice (which is why smoking is prohibited for patients with a peptic ulcer) and stimulates peristalsis (diarrhea). This explains why an early-morning cigarette promotes defecation and why beginners have diarrhea after their very first cigarette.

Activation of the sympathetic nervous system and the adrenal medulla (epinephrine secretion) may raise the heart rate. The increase in epinephrine secretion causes vasoconstriction (rise in blood pressure); it also increases the breakdown of fat and glycogen (elevated blood glucose levels suppress the sensation of hunger).

The release of vasopressin by the neurohypophysis (posterior lobe of hypophysis) has an antidiuretic effect and also causes a rise in blood pressure. Nicotine increases the respiratory rate and blood coagulability and leads to increased sensitivity by the stimulation of certain receptors. Sensitization of chemoreceptors stimulates the vomiting center.

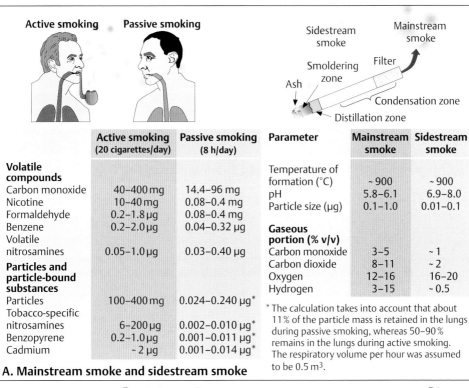

	Active smoking (20 cigarettes/day)	Passive smoking (8 h/day)	Parameter	Mainstream smoke	Sidestream smoke
Volatile compounds			Temperature of formation (°C)	~ 900	~ 900
Carbon monoxide	40–400 mg	14.4–96 mg	pH	5.8–6.1	6.9–8.0
Nicotine	10–40 mg	0.08–0.4 mg	Particle size (µg)	0.1–1.0	0.01–0.1
Formaldehyde	0.2–1.8 µg	0.08–0.4 mg			
Benzene	0.2–2.0 µg	0.04–0.32 µg	**Gaseous portion (% v/v)**		
Volatile nitrosamines	0.05–1.0 µg	0.03–0.40 µg	Carbon monoxide	3–5	~ 1
Particles and particle-bound substances			Carbon dioxide	8–11	~ 2
			Oxygen	12–16	16–20
Particles	100–400 mg	0.024–0.240 µg*	Hydrogen	3–15	~ 0.5
Tobacco-specific nitrosamines	6–200 µg	0.002–0.010 µg*			
Benzopyrene	0.2–1.0 µg	0.001–0.011 µg*			
Cadmium	~ 2 µg	0.001–0.014 µg*			

* The calculation takes into account that about 11 % of the particle mass is retained in the lungs during passive smoking, whereas 50–90 % remains in the lungs during active smoking. The respiratory volume per hour was assumed to be 0.5 m³.

A. Mainstream smoke and sidestream smoke

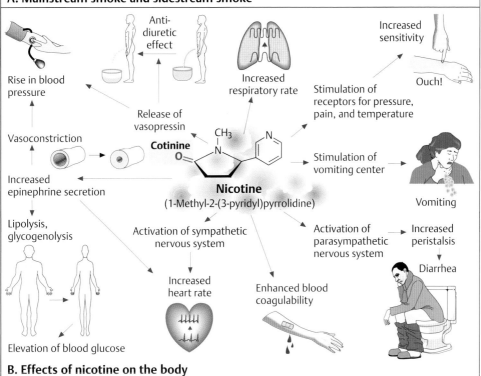

B. Effects of nicotine on the body

Damage Caused by Tobacco Smoke

Epidemiological studies have clearly documented a connection between cigarette smoking and an increased development of tumors of the lungs, trachea, larynx, oral cavity, esophagus, pancreas, kidneys, and urinary bladder.

The development of vascular diseases in smokers is mainly due to nicotine. Nicotine increases the levels of glucose and fatty acids in the blood, enhances platelet aggregation, promotes hypercoagulation, and lowers fibrinolysis.

Chronic exposure to nicotine leads to coronary heart disease, such as occlusion of coronary arteries and myocardial infarction. It also causes peripheral arterial occlusive disease (PAOD, also known as "smoker's leg") and cerebrovascular disease (cerebral infarction or stroke) (**A**).

The risk of developing coronary heart disease is 7 times higher for smokers consuming more than 40 cigarettes/day than it is for nonsmokers (**B1**).

However, nicotine is not the only substance responsible for the consequences of smoking: other substances contained in tobacco smoke are carcinogenic. These carcinogens include nitrosamines, formaldehyde, benzopyrene, acrolein, phenol, quinoline, benzene, vinyl chloride, metals, and many other compounds. Many substances in tobacco smoke are procarcinogens, that is, they are activated by the body to carcinogens and then form adducts with the DNA of cells (e.g., O^6-methylguanine). Formation of DNA adducts is thought to be the first step in the development of tobacco-induced tumors. The main portion of carcinogenic activity has to reside in the particulate phase, since the gaseous phase of tobacco smoke does not induce tumors in animal experiments (see p. 154, **A**).

The inhalation of particle-bound substances (tar) over many years leads to inactivation of the ciliary epithelium and inhibition of the mucociliary transport in the lungs. This results in chronic obstructive pulmonary disease (COPD; chronic bronchitis or "smoker's lung"). The deposition of these substances over decades leads to the development of tarry lungs (**A**) and bronchial carcinoma.

The risk of developing bronchial carcinoma is about 5 times higher for smokers consuming more than 40 cigarettes/day than it is for nonsmokers (**B2**).

Some studies indicate a slightly increased risk (by a factor of < 2), of developing bronchial carcinoma for nonsmoking spouses, when the other spouse smokes more than 40 cigarettes/day (**B3**). Other studies have not found an increased risk for passive smokers.

Smoking and Alcohol

The risk of developing *oral cancer* increases by a factor of 15 for individuals who smoke more than 40 cigarettes and consume more than 40 g alcohol per day, as compared with individuals who neither smoke nor drink (500 mL of beer contain ~ 16 g alcohol; 250 mL wine contain ~ 20 g). The risk of developing esophageal carcinoma increases by a factor of 150 for individuals who smoke more than 30 cigarettes and drink more than 120 g of alcohol per day (**B4**).

After 5–10 years, ex-smokers almost regain the risk level of nonsmokers of developing the above diseases (**B1–3**).

Smoking and Pregnancy

Smoking women who desire to have children must wait about three times longer to become pregnant than nonsmoking women. Children of smoking women have lower birth weights (~ 200 g less) than children of nonsmoking women. During the first 2 years of life, children exposed to passive smoke suffer about twice as often from respiratory diseases as children of nonsmokers. The fertility of women is reduced by half if their mothers smoked during the pregnancy.

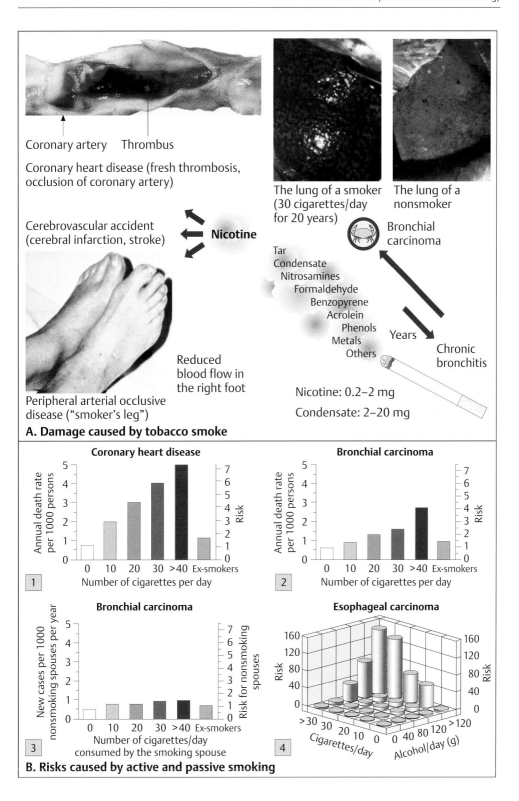

Coronary artery   Thrombus

Coronary heart disease (fresh thrombosis, occlusion of coronary artery)

Cerebrovascular accident (cerebral infarction, stroke)

Nicotine

Peripheral arterial occlusive disease ("smoker's leg")

Reduced blood flow in the right foot

The lung of a smoker (30 cigarettes/day for 20 years)

The lung of a nonsmoker

Bronchial carcinoma

Tar
Condensate
Nitrosamines
Formaldehyde
Benzopyrene
Acrolein
Phenols
Metals
Others

Years

Chronic bronchitis

Nicotine: 0.2–2 mg

Condensate: 2–20 mg

A. Damage caused by tobacco smoke

Coronary heart disease

Annual death rate per 1000 persons

Risk

0   10   20   30   >40 Ex-smokers
Number of cigarettes per day

1

Bronchial carcinoma

Annual death rate per 1000 persons

Risk

0   10   20   30   >40 Ex-smokers
Number of cigarettes per day

2

Bronchial carcinoma

New cases per 1000 nonsmoking spouses per year

Risk for nonsmoking spouses

0   10   20   30   >40 Ex-smokers
Number of cigarettes/day consumed by the smoking spouse

3

Esophageal carcinoma

Risk

Risk

>30 30   20   10   0
Cigarettes/day

0   40   80   120 >120
Alcohol/day (g)

4

B. Risks caused by active and passive smoking

◼ Mineral Fibers

Application

Mineral fibers, such as asbestos, have been used for more than 2000 years to increase the crushing strength of earthenware. The characteristic properties of asbestos are its resistance to heat and chemicals and its tensile strength. Mineral fibers have been used mainly for manufacturing low-friction coatings and for thermal and acoustic insulation (**A**). In the 1970s, the annual production worldwide reached approximately 5 million tons, about 200 000 t of which was used in Germany. By 2002, the use of mineral fibers in Germany had declined to less than 10 000 t/year. We distinguish between natural and artificial mineral fibers (**B**).

Natural Mineral Fibers

Gypsum fibers. These are among the most common natural fibers. They do not play an important role in toxicology because they are soluble in water.

Asbestos fibers. These consist of magnesium and iron silicates. Asbestos and erionite fibers are extremely dangerous because they split longitudinally (**C**) into long strands that remain in the lung tissue for a long time after inhalation. By contrast, artificial fibers break into shorter pieces and are therefore eliminated more easily.

About 60% of the inhaled asbestos fibers are eliminated by mucociliary action with a half-life of 1–5 h. Prolonged exposure to asbestos dust causes characteristic diseases: asbestosis, lung tumors, and mesotheliomas.

Asbestosis is the increase in connective tissue of the lungs (pulmonary fibrosis) in response to inhaled asbestos fibers. When activated alveolar macrophages attempt to eliminate the fibers by phagocytosis (**C**), they release lysozymes and mediators to stimulate T lymphocytes and fibroblasts. The deposition of precollagen in the interstitial spaces results in impaired lung function.

Lung tumors develop more frequently in asbestos-exposed smokers than in unexposed smokers (synergistic effect).

Mesotheliomas are very rare malignant tumors of the pleura and peritoneum, with a frequency of only 1–3 cases per 1 million individuals unexposed to asbestos. The occurrence of a mesothelioma is therefore a strong indication of asbestos exposure.

Although the use of asbestos has been dramatically restricted since 1980, the number of people becoming ill is currently still increasing. Since asbestos-induced tumors have a latency period of up to 30 years, the disease will probably not peak until around the year 2020 (**D**).

Asbestos fibers more than 5 µm long and less than 3 µm in diameter, and with a 3 : 1 ratio of length to diameter, are considered to be the most dangerous and carcinogenic. The fibers are very stable and remain in the body for a long time.

Detection of asbestos particles (fibers surrounded by iron-containing proteins) in the lung is a diagnostic indicator of asbestos exposure.

No mutagenic effects of mineral fibers have been documented. However, chromosomal aberrations, such as deletion of chromosome 3, have been found in human asbestos mesothelioma. Most mineral fibers have initiating and promoting properties and are therefore considered complete carcinogens.

Artificial Mineral Fibers

These consist mainly of oxides of silicon, aluminum, calcium, magnesium, sodium, potassium, and iron. They are predominantly used as insulating material. Most artificial fibers (with the exception of ceramic fibers) are less stable than natural fibers and therefore also less damaging to lung tissue. However, some artificial fibers have been found to be carcinogenic in animal experiments (**B**).

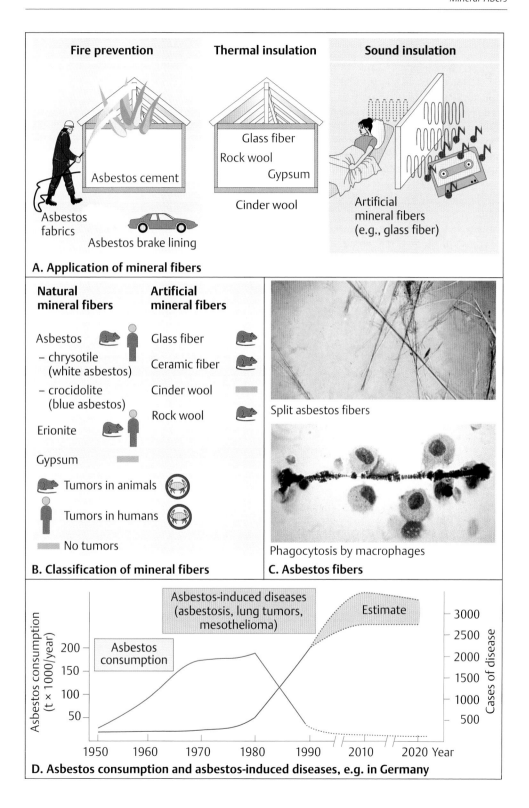

Fire prevention

Thermal insulation

Sound insulation

Asbestos cement

Glass fiber
Rock wool
Gypsum

Cinder wool

Artificial
mineral fibers
(e.g., glass fiber)

Asbestos
fabrics

Asbestos brake lining

A. Application of mineral fibers

**Natural
mineral fibers**

**Artificial
mineral fibers**

Asbestos

– chrysotile
(white asbestos)

– crocidolite
(blue asbestos)

Erionite

Gypsum

Glass fiber

Ceramic fiber

Cinder wool

Rock wool

Split asbestos fibers

Tumors in animals

Tumors in humans

No tumors

B. Classification of mineral fibers

Phagocytosis by macrophages

C. Asbestos fibers

Asbestos-induced diseases
(asbestosis, lung tumors,
mesothelioma)

Estimate

Asbestos
consumption

Asbestos consumption
(t × 1000/year)

Cases of disease

D. Asbestos consumption and asbestos-induced diseases, e.g. in Germany

■ Aluminum (Al)

Application. Aluminum is used in the automobile, aviation, and packaging industries as well as in medicine (predominantly as Al^{3+} in antacids) for treating gastritis and ulcers.

Absorption. Aluminum is absorbed in the gastrointestinal tract ($\sim 1\%$), and in the lungs (as aluminum-containing dust up to 10%) (**A**).

Distribution. After absorption, Al^{3+} is mainly bound to transferrin in the blood and then distributed in the body. The following aluminum concentrations have been measured in individuals not exposed to aluminum: 50 mg/kg in the lungs, 10 mg/kg in muscles and bones, 2 mg/kg in the brain, and 10 µg/L in the blood serum (**A**).

Elimination. Aluminum is excreted almost exclusively by the kidneys (**A**).

The uptake of aluminum after cooking or storing food in aluminum containers (e.g., camping pots) is negligible. However, very acidic foods (e.g., cola, pickles) may cause aluminum to dissolve and these foods should never be stored in such containers. In addition, aluminum is taken up by certain foods; e.g., carrots may contain up to 400 mg/kg.

In medicine, aluminum is used as a constituent of antacids. In the past, Al^{3+}-containing antacids were often used in dialysis patients with renal insufficiency to bind phosphate and thus reduce the dialysis frequency. In patients receiving Al^{3+}-containing antacids, $Al(OH)_3$ is converted by the gastric acid to $AlCl_3$ (neutralization). $AlCl_3$ reacts with phosphate to form the insoluble $AlPO_4$ (binding of phosphate) and is then eliminated in the feces (**C**). If the aluminum intake is high, the Al^{3+} ions generated in the stomach are also absorbed in the gastrointestinal tract.

Acute and chronic toxicity. When aluminum levels in the serum rise above 200 µg/L, certain disease symptoms (e.g., dialysis encephalopathy) may occur (**B**).

Such symptoms have also been observed in dialysis patients after receiving dialysis fluid prepared with water containing Al^{3+}. Dialysis patients need to exchange more than 30 000 L of blood per year with dialysis fluid. The EU standard for the maximum permissible aluminum level in dialysis fluid is 30 µg/L.

Today, aluminum-induced dialysis encephalopathy is prevented by administering calcium carbonate to bind phosphate.

Dialysis encephalopathy has been found in individuals with aluminum levels of more than 9 mg/kg in the brain. The symptoms include dementia, speech disorders, myoclonia, and seizures (**B**). Other toxic effects of aluminum include the development of pulmonary fibrosis (mainly observed in workers in the aluminum-processing industry) due to inhalation of aluminum-containing dust, mostly as bauxite ($Al_2O_3 \cdot 3 H_2O$) admixed with silicates.

Furthermore, aluminum can cause anemia and osteoporosis (**B**). Aluminum delays the formation of bones, and it may also cause disintegration of bone tissue.

Aluminum inhibits the absorption of fluoride, calcium, iron, phosphate, and cholesterol in the gastrointestinal tract. It affects intestinal motility by inhibiting acetylcholine-induced intestinal contractions. As a result, patients taking Al^{3+}-containing antacids often have obstipation (**B**). Antacid mixtures consisting of Al $(OH)_3 + Mg^{2+}$ (acting as a laxative) are therefore preferred.

Therapy. Deferoxamine is recommended as an antidote for poisoning with aluminum or aluminum compounds, and also for reducing the aluminum content of dialysis fluids (**D**).

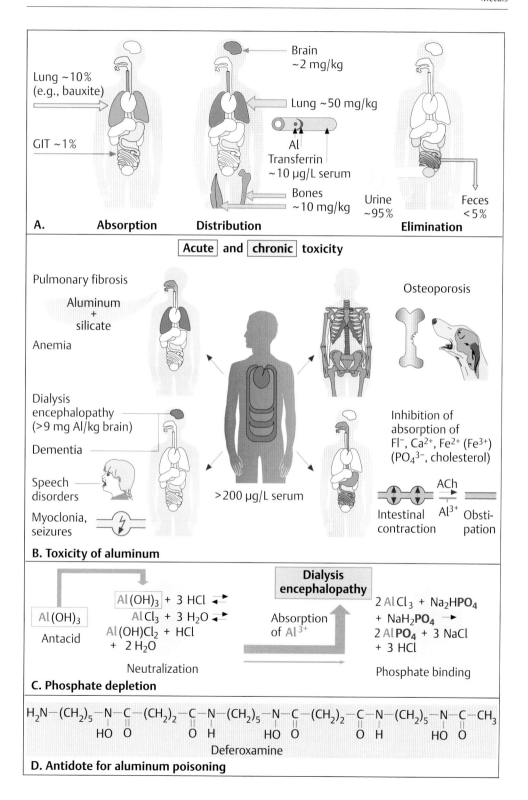

A.   **Absorption**   **Distribution**   **Elimination**

Lung ~10% (e.g., bauxite)

GIT ~1%

Brain ~2 mg/kg

Lung ~50 mg/kg

Al Transferrin ~10 µg/L serum

Bones ~10 mg/kg

Urine ~95%

Feces <5%

Acute and chronic toxicity

Pulmonary fibrosis

Aluminum + silicate

Anemia

Dialysis encephalopathy (>9 mg Al/kg brain)

Dementia

Speech disorders

Myoclonia, seizures

>200 µg/L serum

Osteoporosis

Inhibition of absorption of Fl^-, Ca^{2+}, Fe^{2+} (Fe^{3+}) (PO_4^{3-}, cholesterol)

Intestinal contraction Al^{3+} Obsti-pation

ACh

B. Toxicity of aluminum

Dialysis encephalopathy

$Al(OH)_3$

Antacid

$Al(OH)_3$ + 3 HCl ⇄
$AlCl_3$ + 3 H_2O ⇄
$Al(OH)Cl_2$ + HCl + 2 H_2O

Neutralization

Absorption of Al^{3+}

2 $AlCl_3$ + Na_2HPO_4 + NaH_2PO_4 →
2 $AlPO_4$ + 3 NaCl + 3 HCl

Phosphate binding

C. Phosphate depletion

$$H_2N-(CH_2)_5-\underset{HO}{N}-\underset{O}{C}-(CH_2)_2-\underset{O}{C}-\underset{H}{N}-(CH_2)_5-\underset{HO}{N}-\underset{O}{C}-(CH_2)_2-\underset{O}{C}-\underset{H}{N}-(CH_2)_5-\underset{HO}{N}-\underset{O}{C}-CH_3$$

Deferoxamine

D. Antidote for aluminum poisoning

■ Arsenic (As)

Application. Arsenic trioxide (As_2O_3) is tasteless, odorless, and colorless. In the past it was difficult to detect, and it was therefore used as a poison by murderers. Arsenic compounds were frequently used as medication for various diseases (e.g., syphilis, psoriasis). Today, they are still in use worldwide as biocides and wood preservatives, and in industrial manufacturing processes. Currently, increasing amounts of arsenic are required in the computer industry for the manufacture of semiconductors (gallium and indium arsenides). The toxicity of arsenic depends on the valency of the atom and the type of compound. Compounds of trivalent inorganic arsenic, As(III), are generally more toxic than those of pentavalent As(V); they have an increased tendency to react with compounds featuring adjacent sulfhydryl groups (e.g., inhibition of lipoic acid residues in the enzyme pyruvate dehydrogenase, **D 1–2**). The toxicity of organic arsenic compounds varies widely.

The gaseous compound arsane (AsH_3) and the chemical warfare agent lewisite (see p. 244) are considered extremely toxic.

Occurrence. The average arsenic content of uncontaminated soils is around 6 mg/kg. In Europe the seawater contains approximately 2 µg/L and the air 16 ng/m³. For Europeans, the average intake of arsenic with food is about 11 µg/day (**A**).

Absorption. Inorganic arsenic compounds are mainly absorbed in the gastrointestinal tract (~80%) and the lungs (~10%). The skin takes up very little arsenic (**A**).

Distribution. Following absorption, arsenic is rapidly distributed in the blood. The liver and kidneys absorb most of it, followed by the spleen and lungs. After prolonged arsenic exposure, the highest arsenic concentrations are measured in the skin and in the keratin-rich hair and nails (**A**).

Since little arsenic is excreted in the feces, despite the fact that high arsenic levels are found in the small intestine, the existence of an enterohepatic cycle for arsenic is assumed.

Elimination. Arsenic is eliminated within 24 h in the urine (30%) and feces (4%) (**A**).

Acute toxicity. Inorganic arsenic compounds have gastrointestinal, cardiovascular, and neurological effects (**B**). As_2O_3 in aqueous solution damages the gastrointestinal tract, causing clear, watery diarrhea. For humans, a dose of 0.01–0.05 g As_2O_3 is toxic, and 0.3 g is lethal.

Chronic toxicity. Prolonged uptake of arsenic by inhalation primarily damages mucosae and airways. Damage to the liver and skin (hyperkeratosis on hands and feet) is observed after oral uptake (**B**). The appearance of Mees' lines in fingernails is characteristic of arsenic poisoning (**B**).

The mutagenic and teratogenic effects of arsenic are undisputed. Studies have also indicated a carcinogenic effect.

Biotransformation. Inorganic As(III) compounds are mainly methylated to form the less toxic compounds dimethylarsinic acid (DMA) and, to a lesser extent, monomethylarsonic acid (MMA); or else they are oxidized to form inorganic As(V) which can be more efficiently excreted in the urine (**C**). The capacity for methylation is age-dependent. Children methylate As(III) faster than adults.

Therapy. The antidotes recommended are the same as for mercury poisoning (see p. 176); for example, dimercaptopropanesulfonate (DMPS) binds arsenic to form a stable five-membered ring compound (As–DMPS complex, **D 3–5**), which can be more efficiently eliminated in the urine.

As shown in animal experiments, administration of colestyramine interrupts the enterohepatic cycling of the As–DMPS complex and thus increases arsenic elimination in the feces.

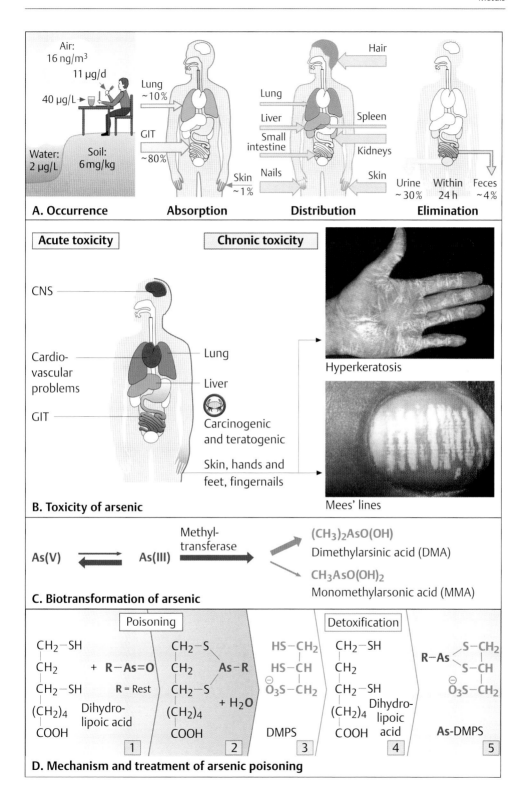

A. Occurrence   **Absorption**   **Distribution**   **Elimination**

Air:
16 ng/m^3
11 μg/d
40 μg/L
Water:
2 μg/L
Soil:
6 mg/kg

Lung
~10%
GIT
~80%
Skin
~1%

Hair
Lung
Liver
Spleen
Small
intestine
Kidneys
Nails
Skin

Urine   Within   Feces
~30%   24 h   ~4%

Acute toxicity   **Chronic toxicity**

CNS

Cardio-
vascular
problems

GIT

Lung
Liver

Carcinogenic
and teratogenic

Skin, hands and
feet, fingernails

Hyperkeratosis

Mees' lines

B. Toxicity of arsenic

$$As(V) \rightleftarrows As(III) \xrightarrow{\text{Methyl-transferase}}$$

$(CH_3)_2AsO(OH)$
Dimethylarsinic acid (DMA)

$CH_3AsO(OH)_2$
Monomethylarsonic acid (MMA)

C. Biotransformation of arsenic

Poisoning   Detoxification

CH_2-SH
CH_2
CH_2-SH
$(CH_2)_4$
COOH
Dihydro-
lipoic acid

$+$ **R$-$As$=$O**
R = Rest

CH_2-S
CH_2 **As$-$R**
CH_2-S
$(CH_2)_4$
COOH

$+ H_2O$

$HS-CH_2$
$HS-CH$
$\overset{\ominus}{O_3S}-CH_2$
DMPS

CH_2-SH
CH_2
CH_2-SH
$(CH_2)_4$
COOH
Dihydro-
lipoic
acid

R$-$As
$\begin{array}{l} S-CH_2 \\ S-CH \\ \overset{\ominus}{O_3S}-CH_2 \end{array}$
As-DMPS

1   2   3   4   5

D. Mechanism and treatment of arsenic poisoning

Lead (Pb)

History and application. Lead poisoning has been known for more than 2000 years. In the past large quantities of lead were used in the construction of pipes (plumbing). Today, about 40% of the demand for lead is for batteries; the rest is used in the manufacture of paints and bullets, as well as counterweights and balance weights. The most important lead compound in toxicology is probably tetraethyl lead, which serves as an antiknock agent in gasoline engines. To clean lead from engines, ethylene dihalides (ethylene dichloride and dibromide) are added; they react with lead to form PbBrCl, which then appears in the exhaust gas (**A**).

Occurrence. In Europe, the lead content of drinking water is 30 µg/L on average; the air contains 1 µg/m^3 and food usually not more than 0.5 mg/kg. For Europeans, the average uptake of lead is 200 µg/day (**A**).

Absorption. Lead compounds are predominantly absorbed in the lungs (as aerosols up to 70%) and in the gastrointestinal tract (8%) (**A**). Children may absorb up to 50% of the dose in the gastrointestinal tract.

Distribution. After absorption, lead is bound in the blood mainly to hemoglobin and then rapidly distributed in the body. For Europeans, the average normal lead concentrations are: blood 0.3 µg/mL, urine 0.03 µg/mL, brain 0.1 mg/kg, kidneys 0.8 mg/kg, liver 1.0 mg/kg, and bones up to 20 mg/kg (**A**). Lead combines with phosphate to form the highly insoluble lead phosphate in bones and teeth, where it is stored for a very long time (lead deposition, half-life up to 30 years).

Elimination. Lead is excreted in the urine (75%) and feces (15%). Up to 10% of the dose can be eliminated via hair, nails and sweat (**A**).

Acute toxicity. The first symptoms of lead poisoning appear when lead levels rise above 1 µg/mL blood or 0.1 µg/mL urine. Lead toxicity is characterized by severe lead colics, neurological symptoms (insomnia, apathy, stupor, aggression), lead encephalopathy (with disturbed motor and sensory functions), and lead paraly-sis of the arms (weakness of the extensor muscle) (**B**).

Chronic toxicity. This is characterized by anemia, subicteric discoloration, a lead line (gray–black discoloration along the gingiva), loss of appetite, and stomach aches. Sudden mobilization of lead from the skeleton (triggered by factors causing bone absorption, such as stress, acidosis, and infectious diseases) can also result in acute symptoms, such as lead encephalopathy ("lead crisis") (**B**).

Acute and chronic lead exposure damages the hematopoietic system (**C**). Lead inhibits the δ-aminolevulinic acid dehydratase (δ-ALA-D), an enzyme that catalyzes the conversion of δ-aminolevulinic acid (δ-ALA, provided by the succinate–glycine cycle) to porphobilinogen (**C**). The δ-ALA levels in the blood and urine then rise, which is an important diagnostic parameter; values of more than 0.3 µg δ-ALA/mL urine indicate lead poisoning. Inhibition of coprogenase and ferrochelatase lead to an increase in coproporphyrin III in the urine (the brown compound gives the skin a subicteric coloration) and protoporphyrin IX in the erythrocytes. The inhibition of iron incorporation finally leads to hypochromic anemia (**C**).

So far, studies have not confirmed mutagenic, teratogenic, or carcinogenic effects of lead in humans.

Therapy. Chelators, such as calcium disodium ethylenediaminetetraacetic acid (CaNa$_2$ EDTA), D-penicillamine, British antilewisite (BAL, see p. 176), and dimercaptosuccinic acid (DMSA, see p. 176) are considered effective antidotes for lead intoxication (**D**).

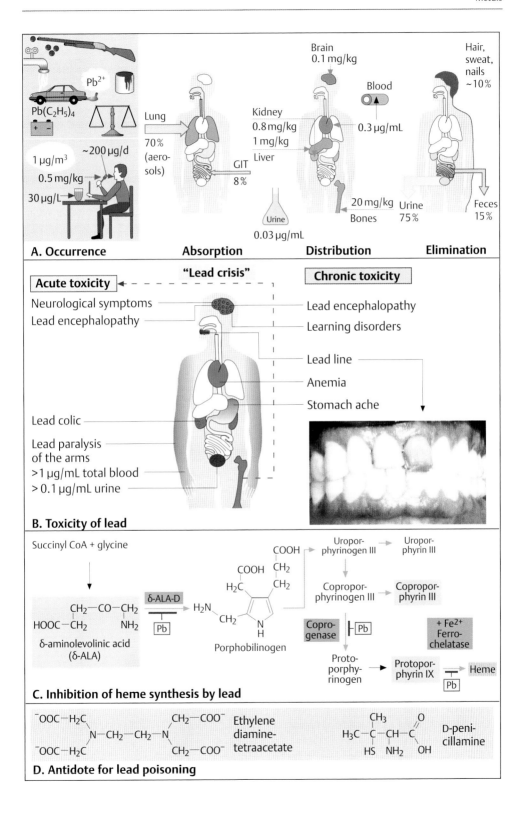

A. Occurrence · **Absorption** · **Distribution** · **Elimination**

Brain
0.1 mg/kg

Hair,
sweat,
nails
~10%

Blood
0.3 µg/mL

Pb^{2+}

$Pb(C_2H_5)_4$

Lung
70%
(aerosols)

Kidney
0.8 mg/kg
1 mg/kg

Liver

GIT
8%

$1 µg/m^3$
0.5 mg/kg
30 µg/L
~200 µg/d

20 mg/kg
Bones

Urine
75%

Feces
15%

Urine
0.03 µg/mL

B. Toxicity of lead

"Lead crisis"

Acute toxicity

Chronic toxicity

Neurological symptoms
Lead encephalopathy

Lead encephalopathy
Learning disorders

Lead line
Anemia
Stomach ache

Lead colic

Lead paralysis
of the arms
>1 µg/mL total blood
> 0.1 µg/mL urine

C. Inhibition of heme synthesis by lead

Succinyl CoA + glycine

δ-ALA-D
Pb

CH_2—CO—CH_2
HOOC—CH_2 NH_2
δ-aminolevolinic acid
(δ-ALA)

H_2N CH_2
     COOH CH_2
H_2C CH_2
       COOH

N
H
Porphobilinogen

Uropor-
phyrinogen III → Uropor-
phyrin III

Copropor-
phyrinogen III → **Coproporphyrin III**

Copro-
genase ⊢ Pb

+ Fe^{2+}
Ferro-
chelatase

Proto-
porphy-
rinogen → Protopor-
phyrin IX → Heme
Pb

D. Antidote for lead poisoning

^-OOC—H_2C CH_2—COO^-
         N—CH_2—CH_2—N
^-OOC—H_2C CH_2—COO^-

Ethylene
diamine-
tetraacetate

CH_3 O
H_3C—C—CH—C
     HS NH_2 OH

D-peni-
cillamine

165

■ Cadmium (Cd)

Application. About 60% of the current demand for cadmium is for alloys (as a corrosion protection), and the rest is for manufacturing dry batteries, cathode ray tubes, paint pigments (for luminous traffic signs, and for hard plastic toys —which are considered safe for children, since it is the bioavailability rather than the presence of cadmium that is of concern).

Occurrence. Cadmium is ubiquitous. In Europe, unpolluted air contains on average $3\,ng/m^3$, while polluted air contains up to $60\,ng/m^3$. The maximum permissible cadmium concentration in drinking water is $5\,ng/L$. For Europeans, the average uptake of cadmium with food is $50\,\mu g/$ day. Smoking 20 cigarettes/day increases the daily uptake of cadmium by around $2\,\mu g$. The highest cadmium concentrations are found in oysters and pork kidneys (up to $1\,mg/kg$), root vegetables ($0.5\,mg/kg$), and wheat ($0.1\,mg/kg$) (**A**).

Absorption. Cadmium compounds are absorbed in the lungs (as aerosols up to 50%) and in the gastrointestinal tract (up to 5% depending on the composition of the food) (**A**).

Distribution. After absorption, cadmium is bound in the blood to albumin and transported to the liver and kidneys, where it stimulates the synthesis of the metal-binding protein metallothionein (MT) (**B**). Once this is taken up into the tubular epithelium, cadmium is cleaved from the Cd–MT complex. This free form of cadmium is thought to be the toxic component that causes kidney damage when the concentration rises above $200\,mg/kg$. MT is a heat-resistant protein with a molecular weight of $5-6\,kDa$. It is characterized by the absence of aromatic amino acids and the presence of up to 20 free sulfhydryl groups (separated into two clusters) to which heavy metals can bind (e.g., seven Cd atoms create a Cd_3 and a Cd_4 cluster) (**B**). The biological role of MT seems to be the storage of essential metals (Cu, Zn) as well as the binding of heavy metals (Hg, Cd) for detoxification (**B**).

In unexposed nonsmokers, the highest cadmium concentrations are found in the renal cortex (up to $20\,mg/kg$), followed by liver and muscle (**A**). The biological half-life of cadmium in these organs is 10–35 years. Exposed smokers may have three to four times as much cadmium. A nonsmoker in Europe has an average body burden of $1\,\mu g/L$ blood (**A**).

Elimination. Intestinal absorption is marginal; around 95% of ingested cadmium is excreted in the feces. Depending on age, a small portion is eliminated by the kidneys (more in old age) (**A**).

Acute toxicity. When cadmium compounds are taken up by inhalation, the first disease symptoms are cough, headache, and fever. After a latency period of 24 h, toxic pulmonary edema and pneumonitis may develop. The lethal inhaled dose for humans is $6\,mg/m^3$ in 8 h. Vomiting and severe diarrhea are observed after ingestion of cadmium (**C**).

Chronic toxicity. This is characterized by a cadmium line around the necks of the teeth (yellow rings of CdS), degeneration of the mucosae in the nose and throat (cadmium rhinitis), destruction of olfactory epithelium (hyposmia, anosmia), obstructive airway disease, and severe kidney damage (**C**). Cadmium poisoning was observed for the first time in Japan in 1946. The individuals affected (predominately women) showed severe osteomalacia, osteoporosis, and iron-deficiency anemia after eating cadmium-contaminated foods (Itai itai disease). The poisoned individuals also had severe pain and suffered from skeletal deformation and shrinkage in body size (**C**). The cause was traced back to a disturbed metabolism of calcium, phosphate, and vitamin D_3 due to cadmium.

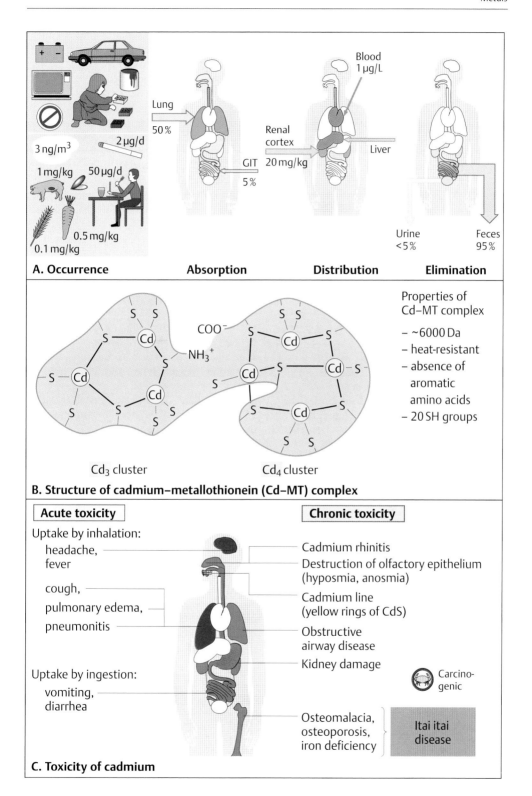

A. Occurrence

Lung 50%

3 ng/m³   2 µg/d

1 mg/kg   50 µg/d

0.5 mg/kg

0.1 mg/kg

Absorption

GIT 20 mg/kg
5%

Distribution

Blood
1 µg/L

Renal cortex

Liver

Elimination

Urine
<5%

Feces
95%

B. Structure of cadmium–metallothionein (Cd–MT) complex

COO⁻
NH₃⁺

Cd₃ cluster

Cd₄ cluster

Properties of Cd–MT complex

– ~6000 Da
– heat-resistant
– absence of aromatic amino acids
– 20 SH groups

Acute toxicity

Uptake by inhalation:
  headache, fever

  cough,
  pulmonary edema,
  pneumonitis

Uptake by ingestion:
  vomiting,
  diarrhea

Chronic toxicity

Cadmium rhinitis

Destruction of olfactory epithelium (hyposmia, anosmia)

Cadmium line (yellow rings of CdS)

Obstructive airway disease

Kidney damage

Carcinogenic

Osteomalacia, osteoporosis, iron deficiency

Itai itai disease

C. Toxicity of cadmium

167

Mechanism of toxicity. Vitamin D_3 is converted in the liver to 25-hydroxy-D_3 (25-OH-cholecalciferol, 25-OH-D_3). In the tubular epithelium of the kidney, 25-OH-D_3 is hydroxylated to 1,25-dihydroxy-D_3 (1,25-[OH]$_2$-cholecalciferol, 1,25-[OH]$_2$-D_3), the active metabolite of vitamin D_3. 1,25-(OH)$_2$-D_3 activates the release of calcium from the bones and stimulates the absorption of calcium from the small intestine into the blood plasma. Cadmium inhibits both mechanisms. Furthermore, cadmium inhibits the uptake of calcium into the tubular epithelium of the kidney by inactivating the enzyme adenylate cyclase (**D**).

So far, studies have not confirmed mutagenic and teratogenic effects of cadmium in humans, but there are indications of a carcinogenic effect.

Therapy. The treatment of poisoning by inhalation or by oral uptake of cadmium compounds is mainly symptomatic (**E**). In case of *inhalation* of cadmium vapors (e.g., CdO formed during heating, welding, and other technical applications of cadmium), it is important to keep the airways free and to apply fresh air immediately, and if necessary, artificial ventilation. After an uneventful latency period lasting for several hours, toxic pulmonary edema may develop, causing damage to the alveolar structures. Inhalation of high doses of glucocorticoid is indicated as a first aid. Acute intoxication by inhalation calls for British antilewisite (BAL; see mercury poisoning, p. 176) (**E**). In case of *ingestion* of cadmium, induction of vomiting or gastric lavage is recommended. Administration of activated charcoal is helpful (**E**).

In case of chronic intoxication following inhalation or ingestion of cadmium compounds, administration of BAL is not recommended because of redistribution of cadmium from the tissues to the kidneys (risk of kidney damage).

■ Chromium (Cr)

Application. Chromium is used for manufacturing batteries and stainless steel, for tanning, and for wood staining (as $K_2Cr_2O_7$). Some soluble chromium salts are critical. Chromium is considered an essential element in humans. The daily requirement for chromium in humans is approximately 60 µg. Chromium is a constituent of the glucose tolerance factor, which has important metabolic functions (**A**).

Absorption. Depending on the compound, chromium is absorbed in the lungs (up to 70%), in the gastrointestinal tract (up to 2%), and through the skin (**A**).

Distribution. In unexposed individuals, the highest chromium concentrations are found in the kidneys (0.6 mg/kg), liver (0.2 mg/kg), and brain (0.02 mg/kg).

Elimination. Chromium is mainly excreted by the kidneys (**A**).

Acute toxicity. Chromium inhalation of more than $2\,\mu g/m^3$ air for several hours may lead to ulceration of the nasal septum, bronchitis, pneumoconiosis, rhinorrhea, and asthma. Necrotic areas in the kidneys have been observed after ingestion of chromium (the lethal dose in humans is $2\,g\ K_2Cr_2O_7$ by mouth) (**B**).

Chronic toxicity. This is characterized by gingivitis, gastritis, gastric ulcers, and chromium enteropathy (ulcerous gastroenterocolitis) (**B**).

Hypersensitivity reactions associated with typical contact eczema are common in construction workers (chromium-containing cement).

Therapy. In case of *skin contact* with soluble chromium salts, the area should be immediately rinsed with water, and a CaNa$_2$–EDTA solution (see lead poisoning, p. 158) in polyglycol should be applied topically. After *ingestion* of chromium, the chromium should be eliminated by induction of vomiting and subsequent drinking of plenty of water (dilution therapy). Cr(VI) can be transformed into the less toxic Cr(III) by administering ascorbic acid. DMPS (see mercury poisoning, p. 176) is recommended as an antidote for chromium poisoning (**C**).

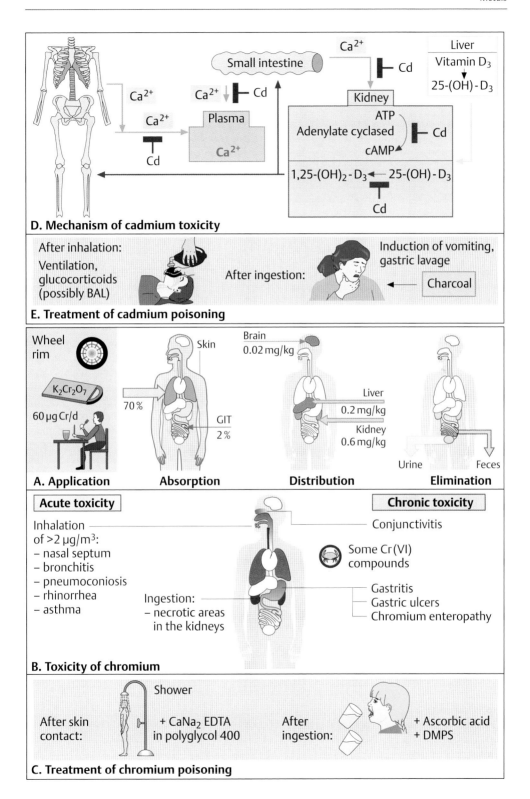

D. Mechanism of cadmium toxicity

After inhalation:
Ventilation, glucocorticoids (possibly BAL)

After ingestion:

Induction of vomiting, gastric lavage

Charcoal

E. Treatment of cadmium poisoning

Wheel rim

$K_2Cr_2O_7$

$60\,\mu g\,Cr/d$

Skin

70%

GIT 2%

Brain 0.02 mg/kg

Liver 0.2 mg/kg

Kidney 0.6 mg/kg

Urine   Feces

A. Application   **Absorption**   **Distribution**   **Elimination**

Acute toxicity

Chronic toxicity

Inhalation of >2 µg/m³:
– nasal septum
– bronchitis
– pneumoconiosis
– rhinorrhea
– asthma

Conjunctivitis

Some Cr(VI) compounds

Ingestion:
– necrotic areas in the kidneys

Gastritis
Gastric ulcers
Chromium enteropathy

B. Toxicity of chromium

Shower

After skin contact:

+ CaNa₂ EDTA in polyglycol 400

After ingestion:

+ Ascorbic acid
+ DMPS

C. Treatment of chromium poisoning

▪ Precious Metals

Silver (Ag)

Application. Silver is used for manufacturing jewelry, coins and tableware, and also in photography and medicine. Silver nitrate ($AgNO_3$) is still used for cauterization of wound granulations; it is also applied to the conjunctiva of newborns for gonorrhea prophylaxis. In the past, organic silver compounds were often used for treating gastric ulcers. The above-mentioned applications frequently caused severe cauterization in the eyes and the gastrointestinal tract.

Intoxication. This is characterized by a gray discoloration of the skin (argyria) due to deposition of tiny granules of silver sulfide (AgS). A characteristic argyric line may also form along the gums (**A**).

Therapy. Induction of vomiting, followed by administration of 0.9% NaCl solution to convert $AgNO_3$ to insoluble AgCl, which is then excreted in the feces. In case of chronic silver intoxication, administration of DMPS (see mercury poisoning, p. 176) is recommended.

Gold (Au)

Application. Gold is used in the form of organic compounds (e.g., aurothioglucose, aurothiopolypeptide) for treating rheumatoid arthritis.

Toxicity. Toxic side effects are common (up to 25% of the patients treated). Stomatitis, dermatitis, kidney damage, hemorrhagic diathesis, and bronchitis may develop. Allergic reactions accompanied by thrombocytopenia have been observed (**B**).

Therapy. Administration of chelators (e.g., BAL or DMPS, see mercury poisoning, p. 176) is recommended. In the presence of allergic symptoms, administration of glucocorticoids should be considered.

Platinum (Pt)

Application. The group of platinum elements includes the closely related metals ruthenium (Ru), rhodium (Rh), palladium (Pd), osmium (Os), iridium (Ir), and platinum (Pt). Platinum is predominantly used in the jewelry and electronics industries, and in the production of catalytic converters for car exhaust systems. Platinum complexes (e.g., *cis*-diamminedichloroplatinum(II), *cis*-DDP) are used for cancer treatment (**C**).

Distribution. Studies with animal experiments have shown that, after administration of chloroplatinum compounds, up to 90% of the platinum binds to plasma proteins. The highest platinum concentrations are found in the kidneys, followed by liver and spleen.

Elimination. Platinum compounds are eliminated within 24 h by the kidney (up to 50%) and, in smaller amounts, in the feces (**C**).

Acute and chronic toxicity. The application of platinum compounds in cancer treatment is limited by their toxicity. Nausea and vomiting are characteristic mainly for acute toxicity. After prolonged therapeutic use of platinum compounds, hypersensitivity reactions (eczema, dermatitis) as well as severe nephrotic and ototoxic symptoms have been observed, and above all, an increase in platinum allergy (type I, platinosis) accompanied by conjunctivitis, rhinitis, and bronchial asthma (**D**).

The platinum metals Rh, Pd, and Pt are emitted mainly as elements from the catalytic converters of cars; they increasingly pollute the atmosphere. In Europe, the platinum concentration in the air is currently about 10^{-10} mg/m^3. The toxicological role of the increased atmospheric platinum concentration is controversial. In animal experiments, *cis*-platinum compounds proved carcinogenic, leading to the development of pulmonary adenomas in mice. Complex formation with the heterocyclic bases of the DNA is assumed to be the cause. In cultured human cells (HeLa cells), an increase in DNA breaks has been observed after adding *cis*-platinum.

Therapy. The treatment of intoxication with platinum compounds is symptomatic.

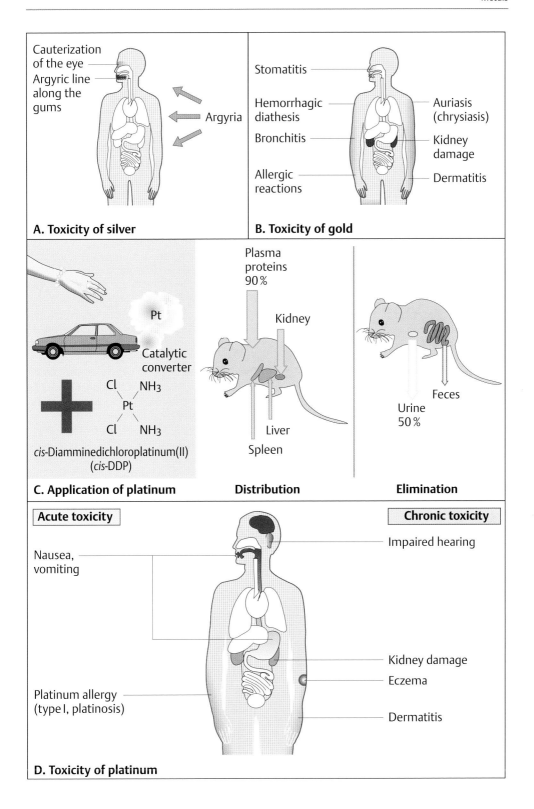

A. Toxicity of silver

Cauterization of the eye
Argyric line along the gums

Argyria

B. Toxicity of gold

Stomatitis
Hemorrhagic diathesis
Bronchitis
Allergic reactions
Auriasis (chrysiasis)
Kidney damage
Dermatitis

C. Application of platinum

Catalytic converter

cis-Diamminedichloroplatinum(II) (cis-DDP)

Distribution

Plasma proteins 90%
Kidney
Liver
Spleen

Elimination

Feces
Urine 50%

D. Toxicity of platinum

Acute toxicity

Chronic toxicity

Nausea, vomiting

Impaired hearing

Platinum allergy (type I, platinosis)

Kidney damage
Eczema
Dermatitis

▪ Copper (Cu)

Application. More than 50% of the demand for copper today is for manufacturing electric cables; the rest is for coins, alloys (e.g., bronze), cookware, and herbicides (especially for treating grape vines) (**A**).

Occurrence. In Europe, the average copper content of drinking water is less than 0.01 mg/L (the EU guide value is 0.1 mg/L) (**A**). Copper is an essential trace element for humans: the copper requirement of adults in Europe is specified as 2 mg/day. Copper is a constituent of many metalloenzymes (e.g., cytochrome oxidase, superoxide dismutase, uricase, tyrosinase). Both copper deficiency and copper overload cause characteristic disease symptoms in humans.

Absorption. Depending on the composition of the food, up to 40% of the ingested copper is absorbed in the gastrointestinal tract, about 15% of it in the stomach (**A**).

Distribution. After absorption, copper is bound in the blood mainly to albumin. It is then transported to the liver where it is bound to metallothionein, which in turn transfers the copper to ceruloplasmin. Finally, ceruloplasmin distributes the copper with the plasma to the tissues (**A**). For Europeans, the average normal copper concentrations are: plasma 0.13 µg/mL, kidney 2 mg/kg, heart 3 mg/kg, liver 5 mg/kg, and brain 6 mg/kg (**A**). Copper concentrations in the liver and spleen of children unexposed to copper are 3–4 times higher than for adults.

Elimination. Within 72 h, only up to 1% of copper is excreted in the urine and up to 10% in the feces. Up to 3% can be eliminated in the sweat (**A**).

Deficiency. This is characterized by dyshemopoiesis (hypochromic anemia). A rare disorder of copper metabolism is the genetically based Menke's disease (kinky hair syndrome) with X-linked recessive inheritance. This disease shows characteristic anomalies of hair, blood vessels, and brain (**B**) and the life expectancy of children with this condition is less than 4 years.

Acute toxicity. Uptake of more than 10 g copper may cause symptoms of poisoning (**C**). Copper toxicity is characterized by lethargy, vomiting, and icterus. Contact allergy is rare (~1%) (**C**).

Chronic toxicity. Indian/German childhood cirrhosis (ICC/GCC) is a disease pattern observed in children in India and Germany after drinking water or eating food that has been stored in copper pots. These children showed severe damage to the liver (cirrhosis) and a weakened immune system. Irritation of the gastrointestinal tract is almost always observed with chronic copper poisoning (**C**).

A genetically based disturbance in the synthesis of ceruloplasmin leads to hepatolenticular degeneration as a result of copper overload (Wilson's disease, frequency 1:100 000) (**C**). Copper also affects iron metabolism.

Copper is cytotoxic (hepatic cirrhosis), but there are currently no indications of teratogenic, mutagenic, or carcinogenic effects.

Therapy. *Copper deficiency* is treated by administration of copper orotate or copper gluconate and/or food rich in copper, such as chocolate, cacao, or mushrooms (**D**).

As an antidote for *copper poisoning*, administration of D-penicillamine is recommended (see lead poisoning, p. 164). In case of intolerance to D-penicillamine (frequency ~5%), triethylene tetramine dihydrochloride (TRIEN-2HCl) should be administered (**E**).

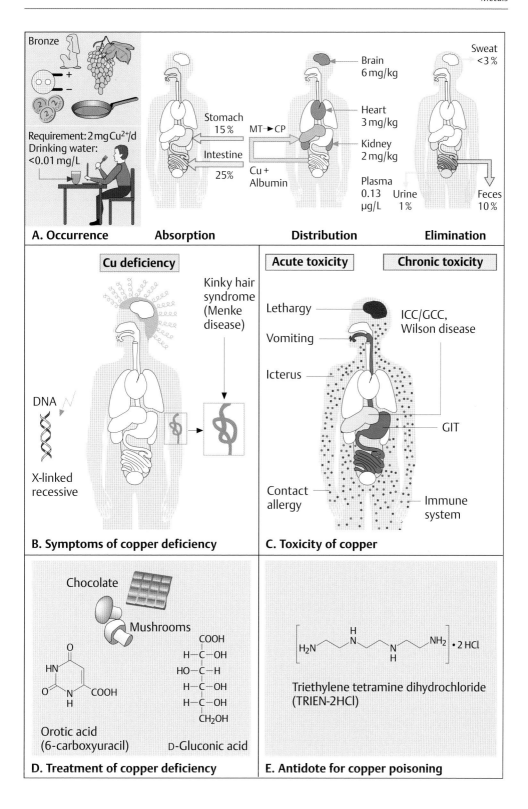

A. Occurrence **Absorption** **Distribution** **Elimination**

Bronze

Requirement: 2 mg Cu²⁺/d
Drinking water:
<0.01 mg/L

Stomach 15% MT → CP
Intestine 25% Cu + Albumin

Brain 6 mg/kg
Heart 3 mg/kg
Kidney 2 mg/kg
Plasma 0.13 µg/L

Sweat <3%
Urine 1%
Feces 10%

B. Symptoms of copper deficiency

Cu deficiency

Kinky hair syndrome (Menke disease)

DNA

X-linked recessive

C. Toxicity of copper

Acute toxicity   Chronic toxicity

Lethargy
Vomiting
Icterus
Contact allergy

ICC/GCC, Wilson disease
GIT
Immune system

D. Treatment of copper deficiency

Chocolate
Mushrooms

Orotic acid
(6-carboxyuracil)

D-Gluconic acid

E. Antidote for copper poisoning

Triethylene tetramine dihydrochloride
(TRIEN-2HCl)

173

Nickel (Ni)

Application. Nickel is used mainly in the steel industry. A smaller quantity is used for manufacturing cookware, dry batteries, jewelry, spectacle frames, coins, buttons, belt buckles, and textile fasteners.

Occurrence. The nickel content of food usually does not exceed 2 mg/kg. In Europe, the air contains on average $10 \, ng/m^3$ and a cigarette around 2 ng. For Europeans, the average uptake of nickel is 500 µg/day (**A**).

Absorption. Depending on the nickel compound, up to 35% of nickel inhaled as dust is absorbed in the lungs. Water-soluble nickel compounds taken in by mouth are absorbed up to 10%, and water-insoluble nickel compounds are phagocytosed in the gastrointestinal tract. Nickel is also taken up by human skin (**A**).

Distribution. After absorption, nickel is bound in the blood mainly to albumin and rapidly distributed in the body. For Europeans, the normal nickel content of the serum is about 2 µg/L. The highest nickel concentrations are found in the kidneys, liver, and lungs (**A**).

Elimination. Nickel taken up by ingestion is mainly excreted in the urine (90%). A small portion is eliminated in the feces, saliva, and sweat (**A**).

Acute and chronic toxicity (B). In individuals exposed to nickel (primarily in the steel industry), continuous inhalation of nickel aerosols may cause epithelial dysplasia of the nasal mucosa, asthmatic symptoms, and pneumoconiosis. Early symptoms of nickel poisoning are observed when nickel concentrations of the urine rise above 100 µg/L.

In a small proportion of the population (~10%, mainly women), nickel toxicity is characterized by allergic symptoms. Since nickel is often a constituent of jewelry and other personal items, as mentioned above, direct skin contact may lead to cellular hypersensitivity. The result is nickel dermatitis. The classic picture of a hypersensitivity reaction to nickel is contact eczema.

The most poisonous nickel compound is nickel tetracarbonyl, $Ni(CO)_4$, which is a liquid at 25 °C. It is used for manufacturing pure nickel. Since $Ni(CO)_4$ is lipophilic, it can easily penetrate the blood–brain barrier. In the blood, carbon monoxide is cleaved from $Ni(CO)_4$. In a person poisoned with this substance, the highest nickel contents are therefore found in the blood; the released carbon monoxide is immediately bound to hemoglobin. The toxicity of this substance in humans is characterized by cough, nausea, headache, dyspnea, and toxic pulmonary edema. Hemorrhages and edema in the human brain have also been described.

Teratogenic effects of nickel have not been documented in humans, but its mutagenic and carcinogenic effects are undisputed.

Nickel is a constituent of metalloenzymes (e.g., lactate dehydrogenase, malate dehydrogenase, alcohol dehydrogenase). Nickel deficiency causes retardation of growth and wound healing, and it leads to dyshemopoiesis.

Therapy. An effective antidote for nickel intoxication is triethylene tetramine (TRIEN, see copper poisoning, p. 172). The calcium salt of cyclohexylsulfamic acid (calcium cyclamate) (**C**) promotes the elimination of nickel.

In case of poisoning with nickel tetracarbonyl, sodium diethyldithiocarbamate trihydrate (DDTC) is effective (**C**).

For individuals with nickel hypersensitivity, a nickel-deficient diet may alleviate the symptoms. The following foods are considered rich in nickel: cereals, legumes, tomatoes, asparagus, mushrooms, pears, tea, and cacao.

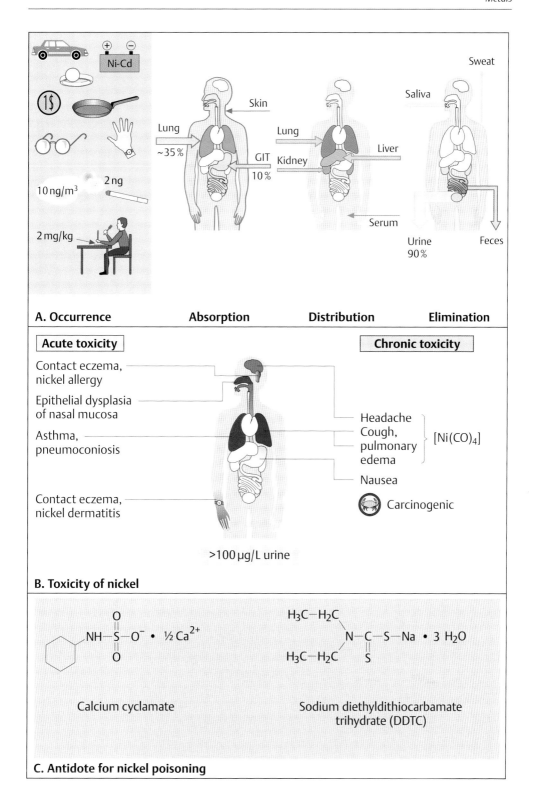

A. Occurrence **Absorption** **Distribution** **Elimination**

Acute toxicity **Chronic toxicity**

Contact eczema, nickel allergy

Epithelial dysplasia of nasal mucosa

Asthma, pneumoconiosis

Headache
Cough, pulmonary edema $[Ni(CO)_4]$

Nausea

Contact eczema, nickel dermatitis

Carcinogenic

>100 µg/L urine

B. Toxicity of nickel

Calcium cyclamate

Sodium diethyldithiocarbamate trihydrate (DDTC)

C. Antidote for nickel poisoning

■ Mercury (Hg)

History and application. Pliny the Elder described the application of mercury for separating gold and silver in AD 59. Today, mercury and mercury compounds are used in electrical engineering, as catalysts in the production of chlorine and lye, and in many countries as a crop protection agent. Mercury is also used in medicine as an antiseptic agent and in dentistry as a component of amalgam. Mercury from dental amalgam is released into the air by crematoria. Mercury occurs in the oxidation states 0, +1, and +2.

Mercury Vapor (Hg⁰)

Up to 80% of mercury vapor is retained in the lungs, where it is oxidized by catalases to Hg^{2+}. Hg^0 crosses the cell membranes faster than Hg^{2+}, which explains the high central nervous system toxicity of mercury vapor. It is eliminated in the feces (42%) and urine (52%). Mercury may persist in some tissues over a considerable period of time.

Acute toxicity. Short-term exposure (1–3 h) to high concentrations of Hg^0 (1–3 mg/m³) causes acute signs of poisoning, which manifest themselves as symptoms of pneumonia.

Chronic toxicity. Repeated long-term exposure to Hg^0 (0.1–0.2 mg/m³) causes tremor, erethism, periodontosis, increased salivation, and a metallic taste in the mouth (**A**).

Inorganic Mercury Compounds (Hg⁺ and Hg²⁺)

These are distributed between plasma and erythrocytes in a 1:1 ratio. After ingestion, only about 10% of Hg^{2+} and less than 2% of Hg^+ are absorbed in the intestine. Hg^+ and Hg^{2+} compounds penetrate the blood–brain barrier and the placental membrane only under certain conditions. Their uptake and elimination by various organs varies considerably. Enzymes with sulfhydryl groups are inactivated by Hg^{2+} (mercaptide formation) (**B**). Inorganic mercury compounds are eliminated in the urine (60%) and feces (40%).

Acute toxicity. After ingestion, Hg^{2+} salts cause cauterization of the oral cavity, throat, and esophagus, accompanied by nausea and vomiting.

Chronic toxicity. The target organ of poisoning with Hg^{2+} is the kidney (polyuria to anuria). Acrodynia (Feer's disease, pink disease, infantile mercury poisoning,) is caused by uptake of Hg^+ or Hg^{2+}; it is associated with irritability, insomnia, sensitivity to light, and generalized exanthem (**A**).

Organic Mercury Compounds

Because methylmercury is biosynthesized by aquatic microorganisms and subsequently bioaccumulates in fish, high consumption of fish may lead to high mercury uptake in humans (e.g., Minamata disease) (**C**). About 90% of methylmercury is absorbed in the gastrointestinal tract. It penetrates the blood–brain barrier and the placental membrane; hence, the portion of the total load is higher in the brain and fetus, but lower in the kidneys, than after exposure to Hg^{2+} salts. The ratio of methylmercury distribution in erythrocytes and plasma is ~20:1 in humans. Methylmercury is eliminated in the feces (90%) and urine (10%).

Acute and chronic toxicity. The target organ in primates is the brain. Here, the reaction with sulfhydryl groups and nucleic acids (DNA, RNA) interferes with protein synthesis, membrane structure, and oxygen consumption and may lead to cell death. Methylmercury mainly interferes with the sensory areas in the brain. The first clinical symptoms include paresthesia, followed by ataxia, auditory and visual defects (**A**).

Therapy. Administration of British antilewisite (BAL, dimercaptopropanol) is recommended as an antidote for poisoning with inorganic mercury compounds. In poisoning with Hg^0 and organic mercury compounds, BAL application is not indicated because the mercury accumulates in the central nervous system. Recent derivatives, such as dimercaptosuccinic acid (DMSA) and dimercaptopropanesulfonate (DMPS) have proved to be suitable antidotes in humans for poisonings with Hg^0, Hg^+, and Hg^{2+} (**D**).

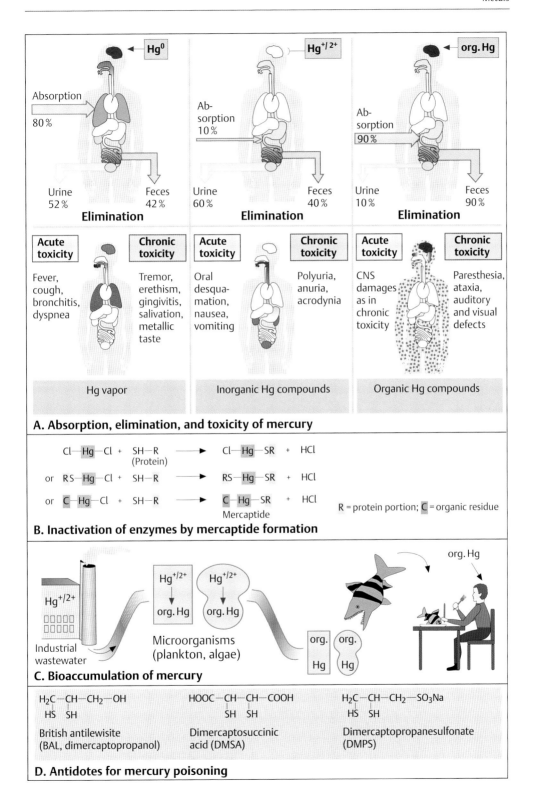

A. Absorption, elimination, and toxicity of mercury

| Hg⁰ | Hg⁺/²⁺ | org. Hg |

Absorption 80%

Ab-sorption 10%

Ab-sorption 90%

Urine 52% | Feces 42%
Elimination

Urine 60% | Feces 40%
Elimination

Urine 10% | Feces 90%
Elimination

Acute toxicity — Fever, cough, bronchitis, dyspnea

Chronic toxicity — Tremor, erethism, gingivitis, salivation, metallic taste

Acute toxicity — Oral desquamation, nausea, vomiting

Chronic toxicity — Polyuria, anuria, acrodynia

Acute toxicity — CNS damages as in chronic toxicity

Chronic toxicity — Paresthesia, ataxia, auditory and visual defects

Hg vapor

Inorganic Hg compounds

Organic Hg compounds

B. Inactivation of enzymes by mercaptide formation

Cl—Hg—Cl + SH—R (Protein) ⟶ Cl—Hg—SR + HCl

or RS—Hg—Cl + SH—R ⟶ RS—Hg—SR + HCl

or C—Hg—Cl + SH—R ⟶ C—Hg—SR + HCl
Mercaptide

R = protein portion; C = organic residue

C. Bioaccumulation of mercury

Hg⁺/²⁺
Industrial wastewater

Hg⁺/²⁺ ↓ org. Hg   Hg⁺/²⁺ ↓ org. Hg
Microorganisms (plankton, algae)

org. Hg   org. Hg

org. Hg

$H_2C—CH—CH_2—OH$
   HS   SH

British antilewisite (BAL, dimercaptopropanol)

$HOOC—CH—CH—COOH$
         SH   SH

Dimercaptosuccinic acid (DMSA)

$H_2C—CH—CH_2—SO_3Na$
   HS   SH

Dimercaptopropanesulfonate (DMPS)

D. Antidotes for mercury poisoning

■ Thallium (Tl)

Application. Thallium is mainly used in the electronics industry. It is also used in smaller amounts in the chemical industry as a catalyst and, because of its low melting point, in thermometers for measuring low temperatures. Thallium glows green in a flame and is therefore favored for manufacturing fireworks. The tasteless, odorless Tl_2SO_4 has been used for more than 50 years as a rodenticide for controlling animal pests (e.g., rats, mice) (**A**). Despite restrictions on its sale, reports of murder and suicide by means of this "rat poison" are not uncommon. The lethal dose of Tl_2SO_4 for adults is 1 g.

Occurrence. The thallium content of food derived from animals and plants is usually less than 0.1 mg/kg, but mushrooms and some types of cabbage may accumulate thallium up to 1 mg/kg (**A**).

Absorption. Up to 80% of ingested thallium is absorbed in the gastrointestinal tract. Small amounts are taken up through the skin (**A**).

Distribution. Following absorption, thallium is rapidly distributed in the body by the blood. The highest thallium concentrations are found in the kidney, liver, bones, cartilage, epididymis, and above all in hair (**A**).

Elimination. Thallium is excreted very slowly. Only 20% of the ingested dose has been found in the urine of poisoned individuals 2 months after intoxication (**A**). Furthermore, thallium is excreted with the bile into the intestinal lumen, from where it is largely reabsorbed (enterohepatic cycle). Thallium is eliminated in small amounts with sweat, saliva, milk, hair, and skin (**A**). It has been shown in animal experiments that Tl^+ can also be actively transported from the blood directly into the intestinal lumen.

Acute toxicity. Early symptoms of poisoning usually appear after a latency period of one or two symptom-free days. They are followed by disturbances of the gastrointestinal tract (e.g., nausea, diarrhea) and the nervous system (e.g., polyneuropathy) (**B**). During the first 14 days, emotional disturbances and disturbed sensations are common (e.g., a penny resting on the forearm may suddenly cause severe pain). Disturbed vision, hypertension, and encephalopathy develop later on. Severe loss of hair occurs after about 3 weeks (alopecia areata) (**B**).

Chronic toxicity. This is similar to acute toxicity and primarily characterized by polyneuropathy with severely disturbed vision. A typical sign of chronic thallium poisoning is the appearance of white transverse lines in the fingernails (Mees' lines, see also arsenic poisoning, p. 162) (**B**).

No teratogenic, mutagenic, or carcinogenic effects of thallium have been confirmed for humans.

Mechanism of action. Tl^+ behaves like K^+ because of its similar ionic radius. Hence, Tl^+ ions can replace K^+ ions in all cellular systems (e.g., in the Na^+,K^+-ATPase system), thus causing changes in the intracellular and extracellular ion balance (**C**). Biological changes may result, e.g., in biosynthesis, metabolism, and membrane potentials.

Therapy. Colloidal, nonabsorbable Fe(III) hexacyanoferrate(II) (Prussian blue) is administered by mouth to bind Tl^+ in the intestine, thus interrupting the enterohepatic cycle and promoting elimination of thallium from the body (**D**). Forced diuresis further increases the elimination of thallium.

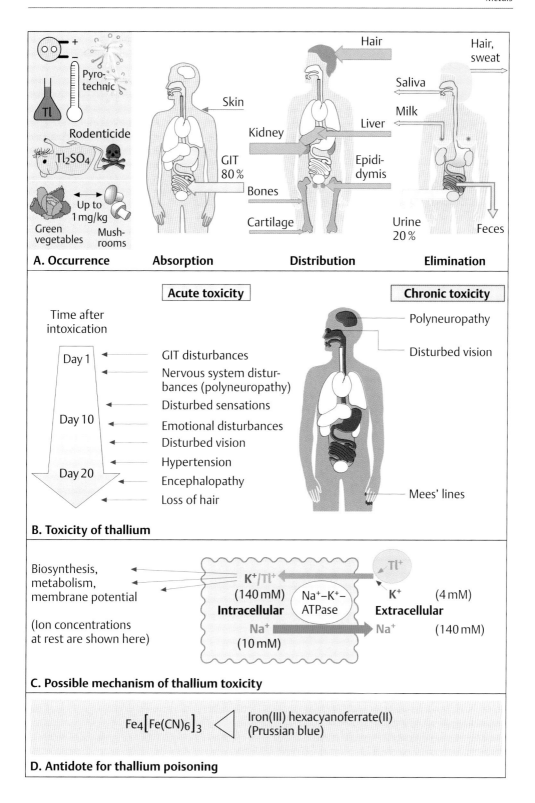

A. Occurrence **Absorption** **Distribution** **Elimination**

Hair

Hair, sweat

Saliva

Milk

Skin

Liver

Kidney

GIT 80%

Epididymis

Bones

Cartilage

Urine 20%

Feces

Pyrotechnic

Tl

Rodenticide

Tl_2SO_4

Up to 1 mg/kg

Green vegetables Mushrooms

Acute toxicity

Chronic toxicity

Time after intoxication

Day 1

Day 10

Day 20

GIT disturbances

Nervous system disturbances (polyneuropathy)

Disturbed sensations

Emotional disturbances

Disturbed vision

Hypertension

Encephalopathy

Loss of hair

Polyneuropathy

Disturbed vision

Mees' lines

B. Toxicity of thallium

Biosynthesis, metabolism, membrane potential

(Ion concentrations at rest are shown here)

Tl^+

K^+/Tl^+ (140 mM) **Intracellular**

Na^+-K^+- ATPase

K^+ (4 mM) **Extracellular**

Na^+ (10 mM)

Na^+ (140 mM)

C. Possible mechanism of thallium toxicity

$Fe_4\left[Fe(CN)_6\right]_3$ Iron(III) hexacyanoferrate(II) (Prussian blue)

D. Antidote for thallium poisoning

▪ Tin (Sn)

Application. Tin is used primarily in the manufacture of iron products such as weapons, cans, tin lids, etc. It is also a constituent of bronze alloys. Tin compounds are used in smaller amounts in the chemical industry as catalysts and in the plastics industry as stabilizers. Organotin compounds are frequently used as biocides (e.g., fungicides, insecticides) and as algicides and molluscicides in antifouling paints for vessels over 25 m in length (**A**).

Inorganic tin compounds play a minor role in toxicology.

Absorption. Inorganic tin compounds are absorbed only under certain conditions. Depending on the compound, the gastrointestinal tract can absorb up to 100% of tin from organotin compounds (e.g., triethyltin). A small portion of tin from organotin compounds is also taken up by the skin (**A**).

Distribution. Organotin compounds show different patterns of distribution. After uptake of trimethyltin and triethyltin, the highest tin content is found in the blood, followed by liver, kidney, and brain (**A**).

Elimination. This varies depending on the tin compounds. Monoethyltin is predominantly eliminated in the urine, while diethyltin and dibutyltin are excreted almost exclusively in the feces (**A**).

Acute and chronic toxicity. The toxicities of individual tin compounds differ widely. Signs of intoxication have been observed in individuals after drinking orange juice containing tin (2 g Sn/L). The orange juice in this case had been stored in tin cans for 24 h. Only uptake of large amounts of inorganic tin—more than 2 g of Sn(II)—leads to inhibition of enzymes in humans (e.g., succinate dehydrogenase or acid phosphatase). However, no late toxic effect or lethal damage has been observed (**B**).

In 1954, during a mass poisoning episode in France, around 100 individuals died after taking medication contaminated with triethyltin. The poisoned individuals were found to have developed brain edema (**B**).

Ingestion of trimethyltin causes insomnia, hyperactivity, loss of appetite, and severe seizures (**B**).

Studies have found evidence that triethyltin inhibits oxidative phosphorylation, glucose oxidation, and the synthesis of phospholipids in the central nervous system (**B**). Teratogenic and carcinogenic effects of inorganic and organic tin compounds in humans have not been confirmed. There are indications for a genotoxic effect of organotin compounds.

Mechanism of action. Tetraethyltin is rapidly dealkylated in the liver to the more toxic triethyltin (toxin generation). Subsequent slow dealkylation leads to diethyltin, which is about 20 times more toxic than tetraethyltin. Diethyltin is then very rapidly dealkylated to the nontoxic monoethyltin, which is then excreted in the urine (**C**).

Therapy. After ingestion of inorganic tin compounds (e.g., from contaminated tin cans), the treatment is symptomatic.

If lesions in the mouth, esophagus, and stomach are suspected to be caused by uptake of organic tin compounds, drinking plenty of lukewarm water (500 mL = 2 cups) immediately after intoxication is essential (dilution therapy).

To prevent formation of edema or stricture, the use of glucocorticoids should be considered (**D**).

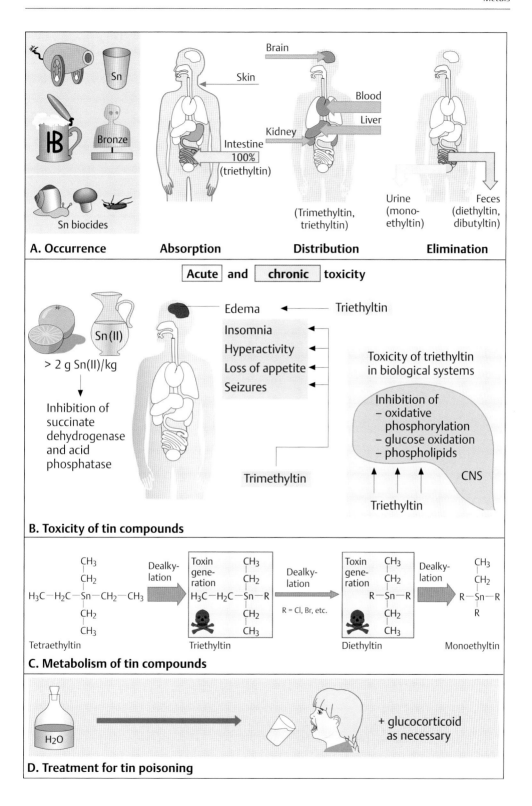

A. Occurrence **Absorption** **Distribution** **Elimination**

Acute and chronic toxicity

B. Toxicity of tin compounds

C. Metabolism of tin compounds

Tetraethyltin   Triethyltin   Diethyltin   Monoethyltin

R = Cl, Br, etc.

D. Treatment for tin poisoning

◾ Radioactive Metals

The harmfulness of radioactive metals is primarily based on tissue damage due to radiation (α- and β-rays, see chapter on radiation, p. 294). It is assumed that a single radiation hit can alter the cell structure and induce formation of a tumor under certain conditions (see p. 298).

Radium (Ra)

The isotope ^{226}Ra behaves similarly to calcium in the body and is therefore incorporated into the bones. Because of its long physical and biological half-life, tiny amounts (20 μg) suffice to induce damage to the bone marrow (hematopoiesis) and to the bones (osteosarcoma) (**A**). Radium disintegrates into the noble gas radon (Rn, an α-emitter), which occurs in underground mines and is used in several spas for treating rheumatism, gout, and other diseases (the air in the mines of Bad Gastein, Germany, contains up to 150 Bq/L). Radium is used in the manufacture of luminous paint for clock faces. An increased rate of leukopenia, gastrointestinal complaints, osteosarcoma, and bronchial carcinoma has been observed in workers at radium-processing plants (**A**).

Thorium (Th)

In the past, thorium in the form of ^{232}ThO$_2$ was used for diagnostic radiology. Thorium is mainly stored in the spleen, liver, and bone marrow. As a result, hemangioma in the liver and osteosarcoma may develop with a latency period of up to 20 years (**A**).

Strontium (Sr)

The isotope ^{90}Sr is closely related to calcium; it is therefore incorporated into osseous tissues. Children require a lot of calcium and are therefore especially prone to incorporate ^{90}Sr (development of osteosarcoma) (**A**).

Cesium (Cs)

The isotope ^{137}Cs behaves in the body like potassium (electrolyte replacement). ^{137}Cs is excreted mainly by the kidneys; hence, its main toxic effect is the development of kidney tumors. ^{137}Cs is easily taken up from the soil by edible mushrooms, and these are a favorite food for wild animals. The radioactivity in mushrooms and venison may be 100 times that in other foods (see also p. 284) (**A**).

Uranium (U)

The isotope ^{235}U is used as a nuclear fuel. Uranium was used as the explosive in the Hiroshima bomb. The most common and toxicologically most important isotope is ^{238}U. The uranyl(VI) ion (UO$_2$$^{2+}$) causes damage to the kidneys in humans (uranium nephritis), and uranium hexafluoride (UF$_6$) causes damage to the lungs (toxic pulmonary edema) (**A**).

Plutonium (Pu)

The isotope ^{239}Pu was used in the plutonium bomb dropped on Nagasaki (August 9, 1945). Up to 1% of plutonium is absorbed in the lungs and gastrointestinal tract, and 99% is excreted in the feces. Plutonium is bound in the blood to transferrin (in competition with iron) and stored primarily in the bone marrow (hematopoiesis) and in the liver. Its toxicity is characterized by the development of tumors (**B**).

Nuclear explosions. The following fission products, among others, are generated as fall-out by nuclear explosions: ^{90}Sr, ^{239}Pu, ^{137}Cs, ^{131}I. After uptake of a lethal dose (> 6 Sv), the symptoms listed in **C** have been observed in radiation-damaged individuals about 2 days after the explosion. Death typically occurs around day 10. After uptake of a dose of less than 6 Sv, symptoms of radiation sickness occurred around 60 days after the explosion. Even decades after the explosion, there have been reports of the development of tumors (e.g., thyroid tumors) (**C**).

Therapy. In case of skin contamination, rinse immediately with warm water (shower). For poisoning by strontium or radium, administration of NaSO$_4$+BaSO$_4$ (adsorbents) is recommended. For plutonium poisoning, administration of zinc diethylenetriaminepentaacetic acid (DTPA), or hydroxypyridinone derivatives, or more recent antidotes of the LICAM group are recommended (**D**).

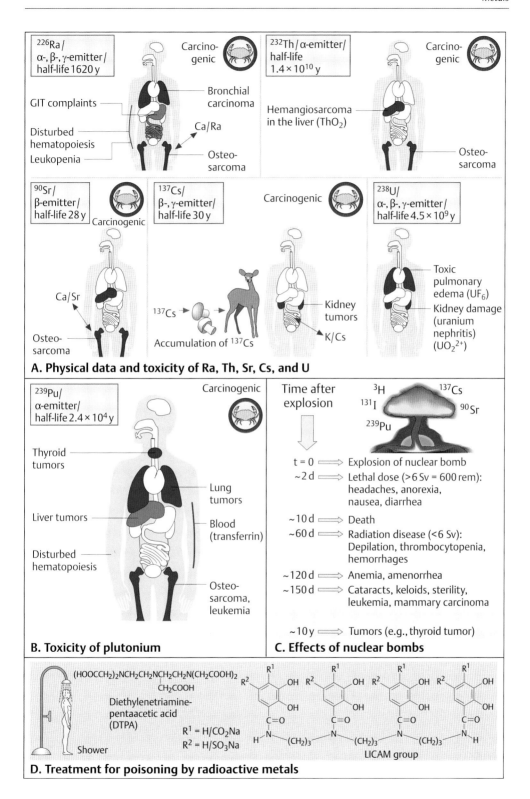

A. Physical data and toxicity of Ra, Th, Sr, Cs, and U

226Ra/
α-, β-, γ-emitter/
half-life 1620 y

Carcino-
genic

Bronchial
carcinoma

GIT complaints

Disturbed
hematopoiesis

Leukopenia

Ca/Ra

Osteo-
sarcoma

232Th / α-emitter/
half-life
1.4×10^{10} y

Carcino-
genic

Hemangiosarcoma
in the liver (ThO$_2$)

Osteo-
sarcoma

90Sr/
β-emitter/
half-life 28 y

Carcinogenic

Ca/Sr

Osteo-
sarcoma

137Cs/
β-, γ-emitter/
half-life 30 y

Carcinogenic

137Cs

Accumulation of 137Cs

238U/
α-, β-, γ-emitter/
half-life 4.5×10^9 y

Toxic
pulmonary
edema (UF$_6$)

Kidney damage
(uranium
nephritis)
(UO$_2{}^{2+}$)

Kidney
tumors

K/Cs

B. Toxicity of plutonium

239Pu/
α-emitter/
half-life 2.4×10^4 y

Carcinogenic

Thyroid
tumors

Lung
tumors

Liver tumors

Blood
(transferrin)

Disturbed
hematopoiesis

Osteo-
sarcoma,
leukemia

C. Effects of nuclear bombs

Time after
explosion

3H   137Cs
131I   90Sr
239Pu

t = 0 ⟹ Explosion of nuclear bomb

~2 d ⟹ Lethal dose (>6 Sv = 600 rem):
headaches, anorexia,
nausea, diarrhea

~10 d ⟹ Death

~60 d ⟹ Radiation disease (<6 Sv):
Depilation, thrombocytopenia,
hemorrhages

~120 d ⟹ Anemia, amenorrhea

~150 d ⟹ Cataracts, keloids, sterility,
leukemia, mammary carcinoma

~10 y ⟹ Tumors (e.g., thyroid tumor)

D. Treatment for poisoning by radioactive metals

(HOOCCH$_2$)$_2$NCH$_2$CH$_2$NCH$_2$CH$_2$N(CH$_2$COOH)$_2$
CH$_2$COOH

Diethylenetriamine-
pentaacetic acid
(DTPA)

R^1 = H/CO$_2$Na
R^2 = H/SO$_3$Na

Shower

LICAM group

■ Plastics

Basics

Application and importance. The use of products made of plastics is commonplace today (**A, B**). Properties such as outdoor durability, flame resistance, high elasticity, and impact strength explain their wide range of applications. About a fourth of plastic products are used in construction. Of special importance to the consumer are essential commodities (e.g., food packaging material), consumer goods (e. g., toys), and medical products.

Chemical structure. Plastics are *polymers* consisting of many identical or similar chemical building blocks (*monomers*). The properties of plastics are determined by the type and quantity of monomers, and also by auxiliaries and additives. Depending on their different properties, plastics are classified as *thermoplastics* (linear and branched chains, thermally deformable), *duroplastics* (highly cross-linked, thermally not deformable), and *elastomers* (loosely cross-linked, partly thermally deformable) (**C**).

Monomers are reactive products made of hydrocarbons. They contain either unsaturated bonds (polymerization) or reactive end groups (polyadduct formation or polycondensation) (**D**).

Toxicity of monomers and polymers. Unlike the situation for reactive monomers, neither severe irritation nor carcinogenic effects have been identified for polymers.

It has been known for many years that the monomer vinyl chloride (see p. 108) is carcinogenic in experimental animals as well as humans, but as yet there is no evidence for carcinogenic effects of polyvinyl chloride (PVC). In Germany, for example, in the period from 1978 to 1990, only 14 cases of cancer were traced back to exposure to vinyl chloride (for comparison, there were 2445 cases relating to asbestos and 99 cases relating to dusts from oak and beech wood), and they have been recognized as an occupational disease. The small number of cancer cases linked to exposure to vinyl chloride is due, at least in part, to closed industrial systems that limit occupational exposures.

The international threshold values for PVC dust are about $5\,mg/m^3$; they correspond to the values of other dusts, such as flour and wood dust, and are not based on any special toxicity of PVC. Unlike PVC, which is predominantly processed as a powder, other thermoplastics are processed as granulates; exposure to dust during manufacturing is therefore negligible, although it may occur as a result of abrasion.

Auxiliaries

Auxiliaries (initiators, blowing agents, cross-linking agents) are used during the manufacturing process.

Initiators enable the polymerization, polycondensation, or adduct formation of the monomers. Azo compounds (e.g., azodicarbonamide) and hydrazine derivatives are used as *blowing agents* (sensitization is possible). Organic peroxides are used as *cross-linking agents*. These may have irritating, sensitizing, or carcinogenic effects.

Since the auxiliaries, like the monomers, become firmly integrated into the polymer matrix, only the free residual constituents are of toxicological importance for the consumer or user. Improved manufacturing techniques (e.g., intensive degassing) have reduced the free constituents by a factor of up to 1000.

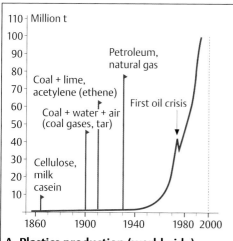

A. Plastics production (worldwide)

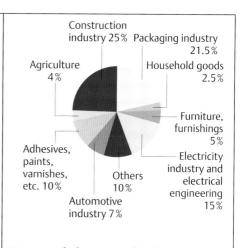

Construction industry 25% Packaging industry 21.5%
Agriculture 4%
Household goods 2.5%
Coal + lime, acetylene (ethene)
Petroleum, natural gas
First oil crisis
Coal + water + air (coal gases, tar)
Cellulose, milk casein
Furniture, furnishings 5%
Adhesives, paints, varnishes, etc. 10%
Others 10%
Electricity industry and electrical engineering 15%
Automotive industry 7%

B. Areas of plastics application

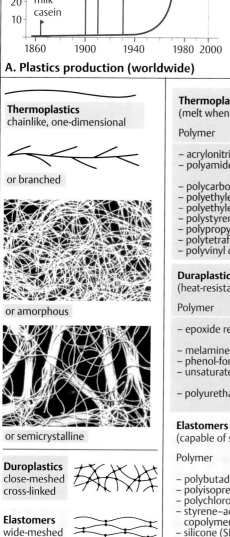

Thermoplastics
chainlike, one-dimensional

or branched

or amorphous

or semicrystalline

Duroplastics
close-meshed cross-linked

Elastomers
wide-meshed cross-linked

C. Structure of polymers

Thermoplastics
(melt when heated)

Polymer	Monomer
– acrylonitrile-butadiene-styrene (ABS)	acrylonitrile, styrene, butadiene
– polyamide (PA)	lactam derivatives, diamines, dicarboxylic acids
– polycarbonate (PC)	e.g., bisphenol A
– polyethylene (PE)	ethylene
– polyethylene terephthalate (PET)	dimethyl terephthalate
– polystyrene (PS)	styrene
– polypropylene (PP)	propylene
– polytetrafluorethylene (PTFE)	tetrafluorethylene
– polyvinyl chloride (PVC)	vinyl chloride

Duraplastics
(heat-resistant)

Polymer	Monomer
– epoxide resin (EP)	e.g., bisphenol A, epichlorohydrin
– melamine resin	melamine, formaldehyde
– phenol-formaldehyde resin (PF)	phenol, formaldehyde
– unsaturated polyester (UP)	hydroxycarboxylic or dicarboxylic acid, alcohols
– polyurethanes (PUR)	isocyanate, dicarboxylic acids, polyol compounds

Elastomers
(capable of swelling, rubber-elastic)

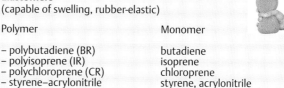

Polymer	Monomer
– polybutadiene (BR)	butadiene
– polyisoprene (IR)	isoprene
– polychloroprene (CR)	chloroprene
– styrene–acrylonitrile copolymer (SAN)	styrene, acrylonitrile
– silicone (SI)	e.g., methylchlorosilane
– styrene–butadiene copolymer (SB)	styrene, butadiene

D. Polymers and monomers

Additives

Once the polymerization is complete, additives are admixed to improve the properties of the plastic. Additives act as *stabilizers, plasticizers, lubricants,* or *flame retardants.* Also used are *fillers, reinforcing agents,* and *dyes* (**A**).

Unlike auxiliaries, which are added during polymerization, additives are incorporated subsequently and may be released from the polymer by diffusion. Exposure of consumers to additives is therefore possible, in principle.

Stabilizers

Thermal stabilizers. These include cadmium stearate (for cadmium, see pp. 166–169) and organotin compounds (heavy metal soaps; for tin, see p. 180). When *cadmium stearate* is heated, cadmium-containing compounds are released, e.g., cadmium oxide which is a strong irritant and induces toxic pulmonary edema; it also leads to renal dysfunction when absorbed in large quantities. These heat-generated cadmium compounds are considered potential carcinogens (**B**). Cadmium compounds are no longer used in PVC manufacturing, and their role as dyes in other polymers manufactured at high temperatures is diminishing. *Organotin compounds* are highly poisonous and act as local irritants.

Antioxidants (e.g., butylhydroxytoluene). The irritating action and toxicity of these are low. In contrast to their use as food additives, they are toxicologically insignificant when used as stabilizers (of polypropylene or polyethylene) in a largely closed system.

Light stabilizers. These include aliphatic amino compounds, nickel compounds, hydroxybenzophenone, and hydroxyphenylbenzotriazole.

Plasticizers

The esters of phthalic acid and adipic acid, as well as phosphates, are used as plasticizers.

Di-(2-ethylhexyl) phthalate (DEHP). Damage to the testes has been observed in rodents exposed to high doses of DEHP, and at more than 500 mg/kg, teratogenic effects also. The European Commission (EEC, 1990) has not classified DEHP as a carcinogen or irritant.

Diphenylcresyl phosphate. After conversion to the active metabolite saligenin phosphate, it acts as a neurotoxin because of its *o*-cresyl content.

Di-(2-ethylhexyl) adipate (DEHA). So far, carcinogenic effects (liver carcinoma) have been observed exclusively in rodents after long-term exposure to DEHA or DEHP. The acute toxicity of these compounds is very low. The "no observed effect level" (NOEL) is ~40 mg/kg per day for DEHA and DEHP, and the daily exposure is probably much lower (by a factor of 500).

Lubricants

Lubricants facilitate further processing of the polymer. Primarily used are paraffins (nontoxic, if not contaminated), and also alcohols (cetyl alcohol), stearates and fatty acid esters (low toxicity).

Flame Retardants

Five different classes of substances are used as flame retardants (**A**). Apart from tri-*o*-cresyl phosphate, the acute toxicity of these compounds is low.

Tricresyl phosphate. Depending on the production procedure, this mixture of isomers contains various amounts of esterified *o*-cresol, which is neurotoxic when metabolized to saligenin cyclic *o*-tolyl phosphate (SCOTP) (**C, D**). There is no evidence for mutagenic, teratogenic, or carcinogenic effects.

Fillers and Reinforcing Agents

These include metals and metal oxides, quartz, talcum, chalk, and glass fibers.

Dyes

The following substances are used as dyes: soot, iron oxide (black pigments), titan dioxide, zinc oxide (white pigments), and various colored pigments (compounds containing metals, such as cadmium, iron, manganese, chromium, zinc, molybdenum, and organic dyes).

A. Plastic additives

Stabilizers

– thermal stabilizers
– antioxidants
– photo-stabilizers

Softeners

– phthalates
– adipates
– phosphates

Lubricants

– paraffins
– alcohols
– stearates
– fatty acid esters

Dyes

– black pigments
  (soot, iron oxide)
– white pigments
  (titanium oxide, zinc oxide)
– colored pigments
  (metal compounds,
  organic dyes)

Plastic

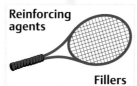

Reinforcing agents

Fillers

Flame retardants

– inorganic compounds
– halog. org. compounds
– org. phosphorus compounds
– halog. org. phosphorus compounds
– high-nitrogen compounds

B. Toxicity of cadmium stearate

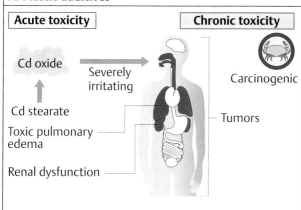

| Acute toxicity | | Chronic toxicity |

Cd oxide

Cd stearate

Severely irritating

Carcinogenic

Tumors

Toxic pulmonary edema

Renal dysfunction

C. Toxicity of saligenin cyclic *o*-tolyl phosphate

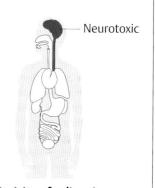

Neurotoxic

D. Toxin generation from the flame retardant tri-*o*-cresyl phosphate

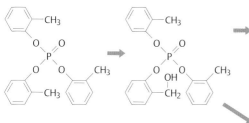

Tri-*o*-cresyl phosphate

2'-Hydroxy-tri-*o*-cresyl phosphate

2,2'-Dihydroxy-tri-*o*-cresyl phosphate

Saligenin cyclic *o*-tolyl phosphate (SCOTP)

Saligenin cyclic *o*-hydroxytolyl phosphate

Saligenin cyclic *o*-hydroxy-benzyl phosphate

■ Carcinogenic Effect of Plastic Implants

Plastics implanted under the skin have caused sarcomas in experimental animals (rodents) after long-term retention. It appears that the carcinogenic effect depends not on the chemical composition of the plastic but rather on its physical properties (solid-state carcinogenesis). Thin implants with a smooth surface were more likely to cause malignant tumors than compact, perforated implants with a rough surface (**A**). The pathological mechanism of this phenomenon is unclear. Epidemiological studies are still pending.

■ Allergic Reactions

Monomers. Monomers are highly reactive agents; they combine with the amino groups of proteins and thus become immunogenic (haptenization). A classic example of a highly reactive monomer is *formaldehyde* (see p. 94); it easily binds to proteins and acts as an immunogen. Formaldehyde can induce contact dermatitis and various other allergic conditions. Some individuals with an existing formaldehyde allergy may be so sensitive to this allergen that even traces of formaldehyde in the printing ink of a newspaper can trigger an allergy attack (**B**). This example highlights the great importance of protecting consumers from sensitizing substances.

On the other hand, plastic products made of soft PVC are recommended for individuals who are allergic to natural rubber.

Nonsensitized users of plastic products are virtually unaffected by the very low concentrations of residual monomers (free formaldehyde rapidly evaporates or is removed by washing). The workers involved in manufacturing the polymer, however, must be protected from acute exposure in the workplace.

Severe allergic diseases (asthma, contact dermatitis) have been observed in workers after handling *toluylene diisocyanates*. The allergic effects caused by these compounds have been confirmed in experimental animals after exposure to above-threshold concentrations both on the skin and by inhalation.

After sensitization by toluylene diisocyanates, some patients developed cross-reactivity to other diisocyanates which they had never been in contact with before. Patients sensitized by toluylene diisocyanates experienced asthma attacks even years after the last contact with this allergen. It is therefore hypothesized that this allergen sensitizes the airways, and other air pollutants (see smog, p. 134) later trigger an asthma attack.

Animal experiments have also shown that dermal exposure to diisocyanates may lead to systemic sensitization, and subsequent exposures of the lungs will trigger immediate asthma attacks.

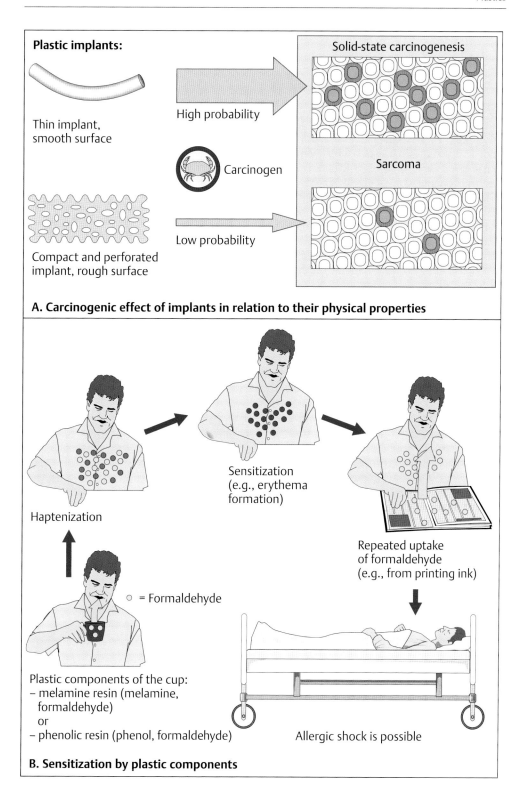

Plastic implants:

Thin implant, smooth surface

High probability

Solid-state carcinogenesis

Carcinogen

Sarcoma

Compact and perforated implant, rough surface

Low probability

A. Carcinogenic effect of implants in relation to their physical properties

Haptenization

Sensitization (e.g., erythema formation)

Repeated uptake of formaldehyde (e.g., from printing ink)

○ = Formaldehyde

Plastic components of the cup:
– melamine resin (melamine, formaldehyde)
  or
– phenolic resin (phenol, formaldehyde)

Allergic shock is possible

B. Sensitization by plastic components

■ Consumer Protection

Studies examining the health effects of plastics and the auxiliaries and additives used in their production began in the 1950s. Numerous laws and regulations are currently in place for the protection of consumers, for example, the EU guidelines: "Plastic materials and articles intended to come into contact with foodstuff" (Commission Directive 90/128 EEC in connection with Commission Directive 89/109 EEC). These specify the specific monomer migration limits and the maximum residual concentration for individual compounds; the maximum value for total migration is 60 mg/kg food simulant, or 10 mg/100 cm^2 plastic contact surface. Limits for compounds used in medical products are regulated separately.

■ Recycling

Many plastics used in homes and businesses are currently sorted by type and then recycled. The portion of post-consumer products recycled in industrial quantities is now increasing as well (e.g., recycling of PE or PVC pipes into new pipes; PVC window recycling). Plastics not sorted by type or unsuitable for remelting can be separated by means of solvolysis/hydrolysis, pyrolysis, or hydration (**A**) into monomers and low-molecular raw material. In the case of PVC, chlorine is recovered for producing new PVC. In many cases, however, plastic waste is still disposed of together with the domestic garbage (in Germany, for example, the plastic portion of garbage is ~6–7% w/w); it is then burnt in waste incinerators under the stringent conditions for waste gas purification specified by varying national legislation in different countries. Some of the energy consumed for manufacturing plastics is recovered in this way (**B**). Some polymers can be enzymatically degraded by bacteria into CO_2, H_2O, and humus (biological destruction); others are first photochemically cleaved into smaller molecules (degradation by UV irradiation).

■ Toxicity of Combustion Products; Treatment of Poisoning

Incomplete combustion of plastics (smoldering fire) releases poisonous products. The combustion gases *carbon monoxide* (CO, see p. 138) and *hydrogen cyanide* (HCN, see p. 140) and also *HCl vapors* (damage to the mucosa) are acutely dangerous for exposed individuals, and for their rescuers (**C**).

Treatment of severe poisoning by combustion gases includes oxygen supply to antagonize CO poisoning (if necessary, 100% O_2 under hyperbaric pressure, 3 atmospheres) and IV injection of hydroxocobalamin (vitamin B_{12}; 5 mg/70 kg BW) (**D**). Hydroxocobalamin rapidly combines with cyanide to form a nonpoisonous complex, but large volumes (~1 L) must be administered for galenic reasons. This costly therapeutic principle ensures that the oxygen transport capacity, which is already weakened by CO poisoning, is not further reduced by therapeutic methemoglobin formation (e.g., by 4-DMAP, see p. 140).

Depending on their composition, burning plastics may also release small amounts of polychlorinated dibenzodioxins (PCDDs, see pp. 116–120; the term dioxin includes about 75 different halogenated dibenzodioxins), polychlorinated dibenzofurans (PCDFs, see pp. 116–120; over 100 different compounds), as well as benzene, aromatic hydrocarbons, phenols, metals, and acids. However, no increased levels of PCDDs/PCDFs have been detected in the blood of firefighters.

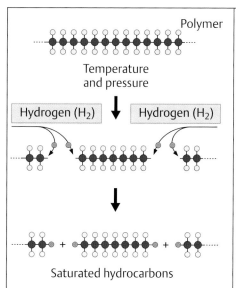

Polymer

Temperature
and pressure

Hydrogen (H₂) ↓ Hydrogen (H₂)

Saturated hydrocarbons

A. Hydration of plastic waste

Calorific values of various plastics in
comparison to other materials (kJ/kg)

Polystyrene	46 000
Polyethylene	46 000
Polypropylene	44 000
Heating oil	44 000
Fats	37 800
Natural gas	34 000
Hard coal	29 000
Brown coal briquettes	20 000
Leather	18 900
PVC	18 900
Paper	16 800
Wood	16 000
Household waste	8 000

B. Calorific values

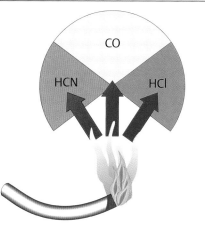

**C. Acutely dangerous products from
plastics in a smoldering fire**

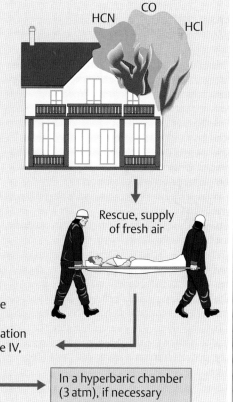

Rescue, supply
of fresh air

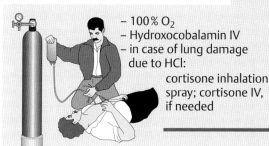

– 100% O₂
– Hydroxocobalamin IV
– in case of lung damage
  due to HCl:

  cortisone inhalation
  spray; cortisone IV,
  if needed

In a hyperbaric chamber
(3 atm), if necessary

D. Treatment of acute poisoning from plastics in a smoldering fire

▓ Biocides

Basics

Biocides are used to control pests attacking food or other essential goods (building materials, clothing, leather), transmitting diseases, or causing diseases themselves. In some regions of the world (Africa, Asia), more than 50% of the harvest is destroyed by plant diseases, insects, and rodents (**A**). The occurrence of diseases transmitted by insects, such as malaria (**B**) which is still one of the most important diseases worldwide, has been dramatically reduced by the use of biocides (mainly DDT).

Biocides are classified according to their target organisms (**C**):

Insecticides are used against hygiene pests (e.g., cockroaches, bugs, fleas, lice), plant pests (e.g., potato beetles, fruit flies, aphids), forest pests (e.g., bark beetles), and pests of stored food (e.g., mealworm, moths).

Acaricides (miticides) are used against mites (mostly spider mites) in the cultivation of fruits, grapevines, hops, and ornamental plants.

Fungicides are used against fungi or their spores for crop protection, in foods, textiles, walls, paper, and wood, and in medicinal preparations (antimycotics).

Herbicides kill undesired wild plants ("weeds") and wild grasses.

Nematicides are mainly used against pathogenic nematodes in plants and pathogenic parasites in humans (anthelmintics).

Rodenticides are used for controlling rodents (mice, rats).

Molluscicides are used against mollusks (snails).

The activity spectrum of *insecticides* includes essentially one or more of the following components: knockout, repellent, expulsion, and killing effects, and these effects may be specific for certain developmental stages (adulticides, larvicides, pupicides, ovicides). Depending on the way of uptake by the pest organism, they are classified as respiratory, contact, and stomach insecticides.

Currently, there are around 1000 biocide preparations based on approximately 200 active agents (although this number is tending to decline).

The problems with biocide application relate to the selection and resistance development of the pest organisms, the contamination of the environment, and the exposure of the general public (residue problems). The goals of modern "integrated pest control" include a targeted use of the most selective and environmentally safe systems possible and a reduction in biocide use by combining it with biological and physical/mechanical procedures, such as the promotion of natural pest controls (beneficial organisms) and pheromone traps (using insect hormones that attract the opposite sex).

Guide values. The maximum tolerable levels of pesticide active ingredients and their degradation products in food, in consideration of their toxicity and application conditions, have been established by most national regulatory authorities and are further supplemented by recommendations of the Joint FAO/WHO Meeting on Pesticide Residues (see http://www.codexalimentarius.net/web/jmpr.jsp). In Europe, regulations limit the presence of any given pesticide active ingredient to no more than 0.1 µg/L, and no more than 0.5 µg/L for the sum of all pesticides. The aim is to make drinking-water practically free of pesticides. Most of the active ingredients have *ADI values* recommended by FAO/WHO.

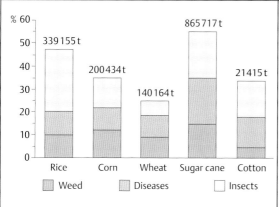

% 60

50 — 339 155 t

40 — 200 434 t

30 — 140 164 t — 865 717 t

20 — 21 415 t

10

0

Rice   Corn   Wheat   Sugar cane   Cotton

☐ Weed   ☐ Diseases   ☐ Insects

A. Harvest losses in five important crops

Number of disease cases before and after treatment, mainly with DDT		
Bulgaria	1946	144 631
	1969	10
Italy	1945	411 602
	1868	37
Romania	1948	338 198
	1969	4
Turkey	1950	1 188 969
	1969	2 173
India	1935	>1 000 000
	1969	286 962
Ceylon (now Sri Lanka)	1946	2 800 000
	1961	110
	1968/69 (4 y without DDT)	2 500 000

B. Malaria morbidity

Insecticides

Acaricides

Chlorinated cyclic hydrocarbons, organophosphates, carbamates, pyrethroids, hydrogen cyanide, methyl bromide, phosphine-generating compounds, carbon monoxide, nitrogen, boric acid, triazines, etc.

Fungicides

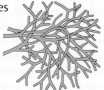

Material protection (e.g., wood, paints):
– formaldehyde-producing compounds, phenols, metal salts, copper and chromium compounds, etc.
Plant protection:
– carbamates, dithiocarbamates, triazoles, triazines, imidazoles, etc.

Herbicides

Chlorinated phenoxycarboxylic acids, carbamates, bipyridilium compounds, ureas, triazoles, triazines, simazines, etc.

Nematicides

Organophosphates, carbamate, soil fumigates (e.g., D-D mixture: 1,2-dichloropropane and 1,3-dichloropropane), methyl bromide, etc.

Rodenticides

Cumarins, sulfonamides, vitamins D_2 and D_3, thallium sulfate, zinc phosphide, hydrogen cyanide, etc.

Molluscicides

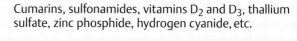

Metaldehyde (a cyclic oligomer of acetaldehyde), carbamates, desiccating agents (e.g., CaO), etc.

C. Classification of biocides with selected active ingredients

■ Chlorinated Cyclic Hydrocarbons

Cyclic organochlorine compounds (**A**) (see p. 112) act on insects as contact poisons. They penetrate into the arthropods through the chitinous exoskeleton and paralyze their nervous system.

Dichlorodiphenyltrichloroethane (DDT). DDT (see p. 219) is the best-known representative of this group of substances. It was discovered by the chemist P. Müller, who received the Nobel Prize in 1948. DDT is an extremely effective insecticide with a comparatively low toxicity for warm-blooded animals. Millions of tonnes of DDT were used in the 1950s and 1960s for the control of epidemics (malaria, yellow fever, typhus, etc.) and for pest control (in agriculture, forestry, and horticulture). The sale and use of DDT is now prohibited in many countries worldwide.

Aldrin, dieldrin, and heptachlor. These chlorinated cyclodienes were applied mainly in the fruit and vegetable growing sector and in forestry for controlling soil pests and ants.

Hexachlorocyclohexane (HCH). HCH includes a group of eight isomers, of which only the γ-isomer (lindane) acts as an insecticide. Lindane is still approved; apart from its application in agriculture and forestry, it has been—and still is—used also as a wood preservative, as a household and garden insecticide (ants, cockroaches, lice), as a textile preservative (e.g., for controlling moths in wardrobes), in veterinary medicine, and for topical treatment in humans.

Hexachlorobenzene (HCB). This was used as a pesticide for crop seeds until 1974 when its application was prohibited. It is generated as a by-product in various industrial processes (e.g., production of tri- and tetrachloroethene, chlorination of hydrocarbons, and manufacture of other biocides, such as pentachlorophenol and HCH).

Absorption and basic exposure. DDT and related substances are completely absorbed in the gastrointestinal tract and through the skin. The ubiquitous occurrence of these substances has led to exposure of entire populations worldwide (see p. 112). Exposure predominantly results from ingestion with food (> 90 %), especially lipid-rich foods (milk and dairy products, meat, fish, and eggs) (**B**).

Distribution and metabolism. DDT and related substances are lipophilic. They are therefore predominantly distributed in fatty tissues (**C**), from which they are mobilized very slowly. Their elimination half-lives are usually very long (~ 1 year in the case of DDT). Certain metabolites, such as dichlorodiphenyldichloroethylene (DDE) from DDT or heptachloroepoxide from heptachlor, are stored in fatty tissue like their parent substances. When fat depots are rapidly broken down because of hunger or disease (e.g., cancer), concentrations rapidly rise in all tissues. Fat depots are also broken down during breastfeeding, so that the substances may appear in the milk. Hence, breast milk may serve as a bioindicator of a population's exposure to these compounds. The individual isomers of HCH behave differently: whereas γ-HCH (lindane) is eliminated from the blood with a half-life of several days, the β-isomer (a contaminant of technical HCH) accumulates more extensively in the environment than lindane and metabolizes more slowly in humans.

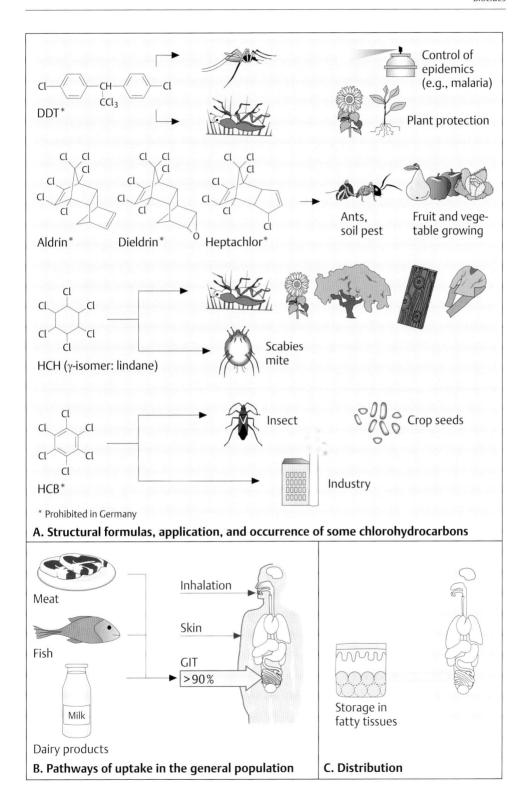

DDT*

Aldrin*   Dieldrin*   Heptachlor*

HCH (γ-isomer: lindane)

HCB*

* Prohibited in Germany

Control of epidemics (e.g., malaria)

Plant protection

Ants, soil pest   Fruit and vege-table growing

Scabies mite

Insect   Crop seeds

Industry

A. Structural formulas, application, and occurrence of some chlorohydrocarbons

Meat

Fish

Milk

Dairy products

Inhalation

Skin

GIT
>90%

Storage in fatty tissues

B. Pathways of uptake in the general population

C. Distribution

Acute toxicity. Cyclic organochlorine compounds are neurotoxic when taken up in larger quantities. They all have similar poisoning symptoms (**A**): paresthesia in the tongue, lips, face, and in the skin of limbs; vertigo, dizziness, and headache. The following symptoms occur after very high doses: agitation, seizures (> 16 mg DDT/kg BW), vomiting, mydriasis, and unconsciousness (after several hours). The clinical picture of poisoning may be complicated by contaminants in technical products and by additives in commercial products (e.g., solvents). The acute human toxicity of dienes (LD_{oral} 0.03–0.07 g/kg BW) is higher than that of HCH (LD_{oral} 0.15–0.9 g/kg BW) and DDT (LD_{oral} 0.1–1 g/kg BW). The acute toxicity of HCB is very low ($LD_{50\ oral}$ 1–10 g/kg BW). Controlled studies in humans are not available.

Therapy. No specific treatment is known. Treatment consists of gastric lavage and administration of activated charcoal and Na_2SO_4. Diazepam is administered in case of seizures, and atropine in case of bradycardia. Catecholamines (risk of atrial fibrillation), alcohol, and fatty or oily substances must be avoided because they increase absorption.

Chronic toxicity. Induction of microsomal liver enzymes and acceleration of the oxidative metabolism of xenobiotics have been observed after intense occupational handling of DDT (> 0.25 mg/kg BW over years) (**A**). Epidemic HCB poisoning due to bread made with treated crop seeds in Turkey (1954–56) manifested itself as porphyria cutanea tarda and photosensitization (~ 4000 people were affected, with a daily uptake of 50–200 mg/person for several months). Reproductive toxicity (DDT) and tumor-promoting properties (HCH) were observed in experimental animals, but epidemiological studies did not confirm these effects in humans (not even for persons with occupational exposure).

The international threshold values are in the range of: DDT, 1 mg/m³; aldrin and dieldrin, 0.25 mg/m³; HCH, 0.5 mg/m³, HCH, 20 µg/L blood and 25 µg/L plasma/serum.

Ecological importance. DDT and related substances are lipophilic and very stable in the environment (*persistence*) because their abiotic degradation (e.g., photolysis) and microbial degradation are very slow. Circulation in the ecosystem (air, soil, water) has resulted in a uniform global distribution (**B**); DDT is found today even in the polar surface ice. These compounds enter the aquatic and terrestrial food chains, in which they are very stable and are degraded only slowly, as they are in the abiotic world. This leads to *accumulation* of the substances in individual members of the food chain, and humans are especially affected as an end point of the chain. Significantly higher concentrations are therefore found in breast milk than in cow's milk. In the 1960s it became known that these substances are stored in fatty tissue of animals and humans, and their application in Germany and other Western industrialized countries has been largely prohibited since the early 1970s (with the exception of lindane). In tropical countries, however, DDT is currently still essential as an inexpensive insecticide and also as one of the most effective agents in controlling malaria.

In Germany, the *basic exposure* of the general public to these substances has been declining for years because of prohibition or restriction of their use.

Daily uptake: lindane, < 0.001 µg/kg BW; HCB, ~ 1 µg/kg BW.

Breast milk: β-HCH, 0.02 mg/kg fat; HCB, 0.02–0.2 mg/kg fat.

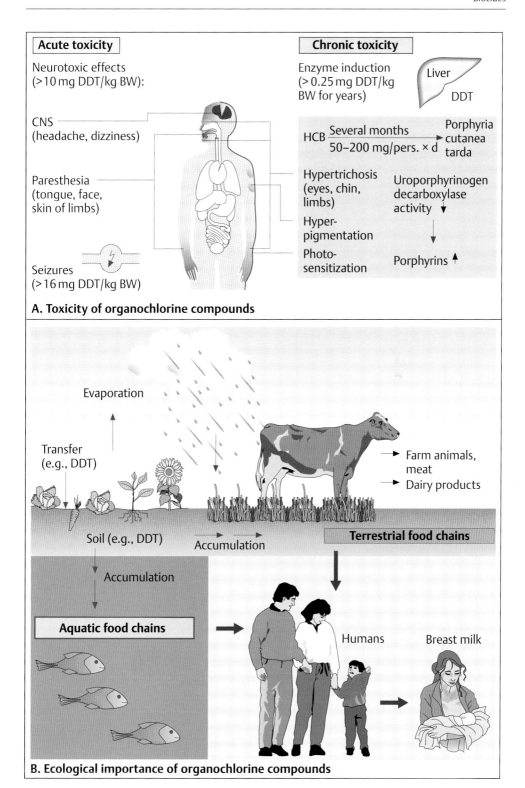

Acute toxicity

Neurotoxic effects
(>10 mg DDT/kg BW):

CNS
(headache, dizziness)

Paresthesia
(tongue, face,
skin of limbs)

Seizures
(>16 mg DDT/kg BW)

Chronic toxicity

Enzyme induction
(>0.25 mg DDT/kg
BW for years)

Liver

DDT

HCB $\dfrac{\text{Several months}}{\text{50–200 mg/pers.} \times \text{d}}$ → Porphyria cutanea tarda

Hypertrichosis
(eyes, chin,
limbs)

Hyper-
pigmentation

Photo-
sensitization

Uroporphyrinogen
decarboxylase
activity ↓

Porphyrins ↑

A. Toxicity of organochlorine compounds

Evaporation

Transfer
(e.g., DDT)

Farm animals,
meat

Dairy products

Soil (e.g., DDT)   Accumulation

Terrestrial food chains

Accumulation

Aquatic food chains

Humans

Breast milk

B. Ecological importance of organochlorine compounds

Pentachlorophenol

Pentachlorophenol (PCP) was widely used as a fungicide in wood preservatives until the end of the 1970s. Because of its persistence, considerable concentrations of PCP can be detected in treated materials even many years later. Basic exposure of the general public to PCP is caused primarily by ingestion with food ($0.1-6\,\mu g$/day). Other residues in food, particularly HCB, are degraded to PCP in the body and thus contribute to the exposure. Exposure has been declining in recent years because of the worldwide decrease in PCP use.

Toxicokinetics. Unlike other persistent organochlorine compounds, PCP does not tend to accumulate in fatty tissues because of its polar hydroxyl groups and its strong binding to plasma proteins ($> 90\%$). It is excreted (either unchanged or as glucuronide) mainly in the urine; the elimination half-life is around 20 days (**B**).

Acute toxicokinetics. Extremely high doses of PCP inhibit the energy metabolism of cells (uncoupling of oxidative phosphorylation) and lead to tachypnea, tachycardia, sweating, thirst, and muscular weakness. The oral LD_{50} is > 30 mg/kg BW (**C**).

Therapy. Symptomatic treatment. Alkalization of the urine ($NaHCO_3$) accelerates elimination.

Chronic toxicity. Long-term occupational exposure causes irritation of skin and mucosae, neuralgia, toxic myocarditis, dysfunction of liver and kidney, and changes in blood counts (leukocytosis, eosinophilia). Various symptoms (e.g., chloracne) are attributed to contamination of technical PCP with PCDDs/PCDFs (see p. 116).

The *wood preservative syndrome* is a clinical presentation thought to be associated with chronic exposure to PCP and other active ingredients of wood preservatives (e.g., lindane) (**C**). The clinical picture includes an extraordinary variety of symptoms. The main complaint is malaise, but many other symptoms are reported that indicate problems relevant to internal medicine, dermatology, neurology, and otolaryngology. A causal relationship with exposure to PCP and other constituents of wood preservatives has not yet been confirmed scientifically, despite extensive studies including groups of particularly sensitive individuals, such as children in schools and kindergarten.

Reference values (A). *Wood:* untreated, less than 5 mg PCP/kg; slightly treated, more than 5 mg/kg; heavily treated, > 100 mg/kg.

Dust: uncontaminated dwelling, less than 5 mg PCP/kg; slightly contaminated, 5–10 mg/kg; heavily contaminated, more than 10 mg/kg.

Air: uncontaminated dwelling, less than $0.1\,\mu g/m^3$; the value of intervention is $1\,\mu g/m^3$.

Carcinogenicity. PCP has been shown to have carcinogenic effects in experimental animals, prompting a lively debate about corresponding effects in humans. So far, however, no such effects have been confirmed beyond those in the animal studies.

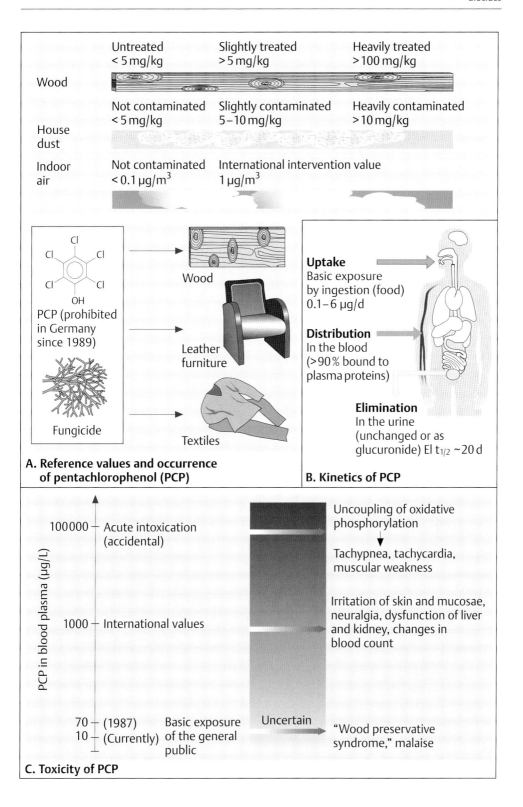

A. Reference values and occurrence of pentachlorophenol (PCP)

B. Kinetics of PCP

C. Toxicity of PCP

199

Organophosphates

Organophosphates are esters, amides, and thiol derivatives of orthophosphoric acid, phosphonic acid, thiophosphoric acid, and thiophosphonic acid (**A**). Parathion (E 605) is the best known (**B**). Organophosphates are used as contact and systemic insecticides (stomach poisons; present in all plant parts after uptake through the root system); they are applied for plant protection and malaria control, as fungicides, against ecto- and endoparasites in veterinary medicine, and as miotics in human medicine (glaucoma therapy). Unlike chlorinated hydrocarbons, organophosphates are biodegradable and are not stored externally or internally by organisms. However, their acute toxicity is high. Some highly toxic and volatile representatives (sarin, soman, tabun) have been tested as chemical warfare agents (see p. 240).

Toxicokinetics. Organophosphates are well absorbed after uptake by ingestion and inhalation (maximum blood levels ~1 h after ingestion), and also through the skin. They are rapidly distributed into all organs and tissues. Some of these compounds (e.g., parathion) are converted in the body to more active metabolites. Degradation is mostly by oxidation (cytochrome P450-dependent monooxygenases of the liver) and by hydrolytic cleavage of the ester bonds (esterases).

Mechanism of action. Organophosphates (like carbamates) are neurotoxic for insects and warm-blooded animals. They inhibit acetylcholine esterase (AChE) in the nervous system (**C**). The organophosphate, like acetylcholine (ACh), is covalently bound to the active center of the enzyme while giving off the substituent X. Cleavage of this bond (spontaneous or enzymatic) occurs very slowly (days or weeks) and is incomplete, unlike the release of ACh (where there is rapid reactivation of the enzyme). At this stage, certain oxime antidotes are still able to cleave the bond. However, removal of another substituent from the organophosphate results in a very stable complex (aging of the enzyme). The enzyme is then irreversibly inhibited, i. e., it cannot be reactivated either spontaneously or by oximes.

Acute toxicity (D). *Muscarinic effects* (on parasympathetic nerve endings) predominate initially, but these are rarely life-threatening; they include nausea (without vomiting), anorexia, abdominal cramps, sweating, salivation, and lacrimation. Exposure to higher doses causes diarrhea, tenesmus, uncontrolled defecation and urination, pale skin, miosis, blurred vision, pronounced bronchial secretion, asthma-like dyspnea, pulmonary edema with cyanosis.

Subsequently, *nicotinic effects* (on autonomic ganglia, neuromuscular end plates) predominate; they include fibrillar twitching initially in the eyelids and the tongue, later in the muscles of face, neck, and eyes (sudden movements of eyeballs), and finally generalized twitches and muscle weakness (respiratory muscles).

Initial effects on the central nervous system: malaise, restlessness, anxiety, and vertigo; then headache and insomnia. In case of more severe poisoning: ataxia, tremor, poor concentration, and confusion; in extreme cases: coma, areflexia, and generalized cramps.

Main risks: life-threatening respiratory dysfunction because of the restriction of alveolar gas exchange (due to increased bronchial secretion), risk of bronchoconstriction, peripheral and central respiratory paralysis. The course is usually fulminant after uptake by ingestion (possibly death within a few minutes), while symptoms are slowly increasing after dermal uptake. In case of inhalation, respiratory symptoms are very pronounced.

Laboratory tests. An important diagnostic parameter is AChE activity, which can be measured in erythrocytes (**C**). However, only at the initial stage of poisoning does the extent of inhibition correlate with the manifestation of symptoms (first symptoms at inhibition by 50%; severe poisoning at < 30% of the initial activity). Activity of (pseudo)cholinesterase in the serum is a less specific parameter.

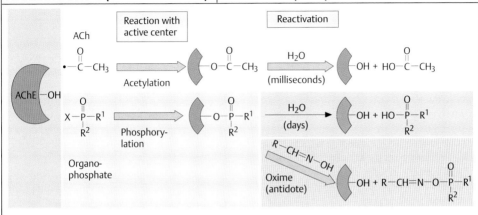

A. Basic structure (Schrader formula)

$X = $ phenoxy, alkoxy, halogen, pseudohalogen, etc.
$R^1 = $ alkoxy
$R^2 = $ alkoxy, alkyl, dialkylamino, etc.

B. Parathion (E605)

Insecticide

C. Mechanism of action of organophosphates

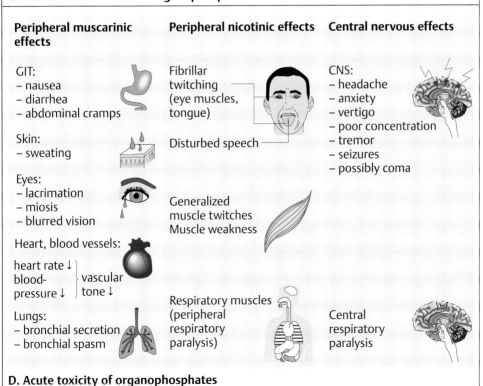

D. Acute toxicity of organophosphates

Peripheral muscarinic effects

GIT:
– nausea
– diarrhea
– abdominal cramps

Skin:
– sweating

Eyes:
– lacrimation
– miosis
– blurred vision

Heart, blood vessels:
heart rate ↓
blood-pressure ↓ } vascular tone ↓

Lungs:
– bronchial secretion
– bronchial spasm

Peripheral nicotinic effects

Fibrillar twitching (eye muscles, tongue)

Disturbed speech

Generalized muscle twitches
Muscle weakness

Respiratory muscles (peripheral respiratory paralysis)

Central nervous effects

CNS:
– headache
– anxiety
– vertigo
– poor concentration
– tremor
– seizures
– possibly coma

Central respiratory paralysis

Chronic toxicity. Additive effects, but also adjustment, have been observed after repeated uptake of small quantities. The international threshold values (also valid for carbamates, e.g., carbaryl) are in the range of 5 mg/m^3: reduction of the erythrocyte AChE activity to 70% of the individual activity prior to exposure.

Delayed neuropathy (A). Some organophosphates (e.g., dichlorvos) lead to neuropathy with a latency period of 1–4 weeks (acute symptoms may be absent). After initial paresthesia, ascending pareses develop slowly (within weeks or months), being flaccid at first, then spastic, and occurring first in the legs but later in the arms also. Trunk, cranial nerves, and sensory nerves are less affected. The symptoms are most likely caused by irreversible inhibition of neurotoxic esterase (neuropathy target esterase, NTE), a carboxyesterase in nerve tissue which is phosphorylated in the same way as AChE. Symptoms disappear very slowly and often incompletely.

Therapy. Treatment of organophosphate poisonings with *oximes* (**B**): in case of some organophosphates (e.g., parathion), reactivation of choline esterase may be attempted within the first 24–48 h (prior to aging of the enzyme) by administering obidoxime (250 mg, IV or IM), but this should never be done without atropine protection.

Order of therapeutic measures (**D**):

1. *Maintaining respiration* (intubation, bellows respiration during transport, no mouth-to-mouth ventilation, possibly artificial ventilation for days, aspiration of the airways) *and circulation*.

2. *Atropine* in high doses (2–5 mg IV every 10 min) to antagonize the effects of ACh (if possible, only after correction of severe hypoxia because there is a risk of atrial fibrillation; the cardinal symptom for dosing is bronchial hypersecretion).

3. *Detoxification:* in case of ingestion, gastric lavage and administration of activated charcoal and Na$_2$SO$_4$; in case of dermal contact, cleaning of the skin with water and soap, but preferably with 5–10% NaHCO$_3$ solution.

Carbamates

Esters of carbamic acid (**C**) are used as insecticides, fungicides, herbicides, and nematicides in agriculture, for malaria control and indoor pest control, and as a topical miotic agent (neostigmine). The consumption worldwide is 20 000–30 000 t/year. Like organophosphates and ACh, carbamates bind to the active center of AChE. The difference is in the speed with which the original enzyme structure is restored: ACh, rapidly; carbamate, slowly but completely (reversible inhibition); organophosphates, very slowly and incompletely (irreversible inhibition).

Kinetics. Carbamates are absorbed after uptake by ingestion (>90%), inhalation (spray or dust), and through the skin. They are rapidly metabolized and completely eliminated.

Toxicity. The symptoms are, in principle, the same as in organophosphate poisoning. They disappear much faster, and fatalities are very rare.

Therapy (D). High doses of atropine and symptomatic treatment as with organophosphate poisoning. Oximes are contraindicated (increase of carbamate activity and damage due to its own toxicity).

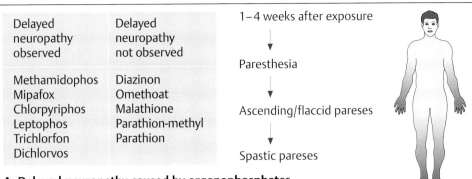

Delayed neuropathy observed	Delayed neuropathy not observed
Methamidophos	Diazinon
Mipafox	Omethoat
Chlorpyriphos	Malathione
Leptophos	Parathion-methyl
Trichlorfon	Parathion
Dichlorvos	

1–4 weeks after exposure
↓
Paresthesia
↓
Ascending/flaccid pareses
↓
Spastic pareses

A. Delayed neuropathy caused by organophosphates

Only in case of organo-phosphate poisoning: possibly obidoxime

Obidoxime

B. Treatment of poisoning with organophosphates

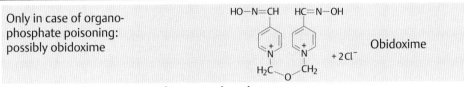

– methyl → Insecticide → Carbaril

$R^2O-\overset{\overset{O}{\|}}{C}-NHR^1$

R^2 = aliphatic or aromatic group

– aromatic → Herbicide

– benzimi-dazole → Fungicide → Carbendazim

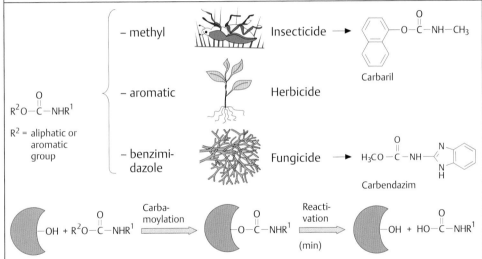

$-OH + R^2O-\overset{\overset{O}{\|}}{C}-NHR^1$ →(Carba-moylation)→ $-O-\overset{\overset{O}{\|}}{C}-NHR^1$ ⇌(Reacti-vation) (min)→ $-OH + HO-\overset{\overset{O}{\|}}{C}-NHR^1$

C. Structural formulas and mechanism of action of carbamates

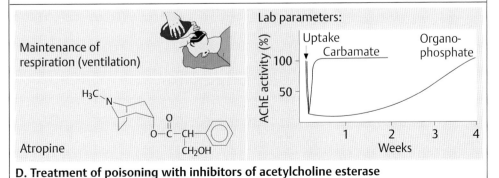

Maintenance of respiration (ventilation)

Atropine

Lab parameters:

Uptake — Carbamate — Organo-phosphate

AChE activity (%): 100, 50

Weeks: 1 2 3 4

D. Treatment of poisoning with inhibitors of acetylcholine esterase

Pyrethroids

Pyrethroids are synthetic compounds, similar to the pyrethrins in certain pyrethrum (*Chrysanthemum*) species; they are esters of chrysanthemic acid, pyrethric acid, and various ketoalcohols (**A**). They are more effective and last longer than their natural counterparts. Since their development in the 1970s, pyrethroids have been increasingly used as insecticides for textile preservation (clothes, carpets) and wood preservation (as supplements to PCP and lindane), in households (for indoor pest control), in horticulture, forestry, and agriculture, and also in veterinary and human medicine.

Based on their characteristic action, pyrethroids are divided into two types that differ in the absence (type I) or presence (type II) of an α-cyano group (**A**). Their relatively low toxicity for warm-blooded animals (**B**) and their low persistence in the environment are advantageous. They are rapidly degraded (within a few days) by hydrolysis, photolysis, and microorganisms. However, they are relatively stable in dry, heated rooms (photodegradation is slow because window glass acts as a filter).

Toxicokinetics. Pyrethroids are only partly absorbed by ingestion and hardly at all through the skin. They are completely metabolized (mainly by esterase-mediated cleavage and monooxygenase-catalyzed hydroxylation). They are largely eliminated (80–100%) after conjugation of their metabolites, usually within a few hours or days.

Acute toxicity. The target organ is the nervous system (effects on sodium channels). In animal experiments, type I pyrethroids cause "T symptoms" (tremor, etc.), while type II pyrethroids cause "CS symptoms" (choreoathetosis, salivation, etc.) (**C**). Acute poisoning in humans has been observed only in a few cases of improper handling. After *ingestion* (accidentally through contaminated food or in the workplace) (**D**), gastrointestinal symptoms (nausea, vomiting, diarrhea) occurred within 10–60 min. In severe cases, absorption was followed by slowly developing central nervous symptoms (clouded consciousness, seizures). The symptoms usually disappeared after a few days; no persistent nerve damage was noticed. After *direct skin contact* (undiluted preparation, heavily contaminated surfaces) (**D**), local paresthesia (tingling, burning, itching) may occur after a latency period of a few minutes to several hours. These symptoms are explained by local irritation of sensory nerve endings in the skin; they persist for about 24 h and are reversible. Apart from these, irritation of the mucosae, airways, and eyes, as well as dizziness and headache, have also been observed. Distinct individual differences exist; children are at greater risk from dermal exposure than adults because their skin is more sensitive.

Chronic toxicity. The question of whether bioaccumulation of pyrethroids in nerve tissue will lead to irreversible neurotoxic effects is still controversial, as experimental studies in animals have been inconclusive. So far, no chronic organic damage has been observed in individuals with long-term exposure.

In animal experiments, pyrethroids have shown no reproductive, embryotoxic, or teratogenic effects. Experimental results regarding their mutagenic, carcinogenic, and immunotoxic potency were inconsistent, and there is no evidence for such effects in humans.

Pyrethrins: ingredients of extracts from pyrethrum (*Chrysanthemum*) flowers

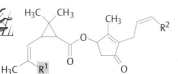

Chrysanthemum

	R^1	R^2
Pyrethrin I	—CH$_3$	—CH=CH$_2$
Pyrethrin II	—COOCH$_3$	—CH=CH$_2$
Cinerin I	—CH$_3$	—CH$_3$
Cinerin II	—COOCH$_3$	—CH$_3$
Jasmolin I	—CH$_3$	—C$_2$H$_5$
Jasmolin II	—COOCH$_3$	—C$_2$H$_5$

Pyrethroids: synthetic derivatives

Type I ("soft" pyrethroids)

Permethrin

Type II (cyanopyrethroids, "hard" pyrethroids)

Cypermethrin

A. Pyrethrins, pyrethroids

Compounds	LD$_{50}$ in insects (mg/kg)	LD$_{50}$ in rats (mg/kg)	Selection factor (LD$_{50}$ rats/LD$_{50}$ insects)
Carbamates	2.8	45	16
Organophosphates	2.0	67	34
Chlorinated hydrocarbons	2.6	230	90
Pyrethroids	0.45	2000	4400

B. Comparison of insecticide toxicities

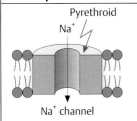

Pyrethroid
Na$^+$
Na$^+$ channel

Experimental animal

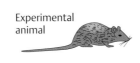

Type I ⟶ "T syndrome"

Tremor, ataxia, increased agitation, hypersensitivity to external stimuli

Type II ⟶ "CS syndrome"

Choreoathetosis, **s**alivation, coarse tremor, clonic seizures

C. Pathomechanism, toxicity in animal experiments

Ingestion:

(2–250 mg Deltamethrin/kg BW)

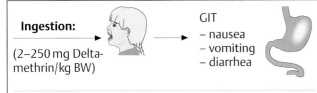

GIT
– nausea
– vomiting
– diarrhea

Severe poisoning with deltamethrin (100–200 mg/kg BW)

After absorption, increase in CNS symptoms
– clouded consciousness
– seizures

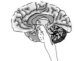

Skin contact:

Local reactions:
– paresthesia (burning, itching, tingling)

Reversibility of symptoms within one to several days

D. Toxicity of pyrethroids in humans

205

Dithiocarbamates

Dithiocarbamates are esters and salts of dithio-carbamic acid (**A**). They are classified as dialkyl derivatives (thiram, ziram, disulfiram) and alky-lene bisthio derivatives (maneb, zineb). They are mainly used in agriculture as fungicides, herbi-cides, and insecticides. In addition, they are used in the rubber industry (vulcanization), pa-permaking, and wastewater treatment, and also in human medicine for treating parasitic skin diseases and alcoholism (disulfiram). Dithiocar-bamates are not very persistent in the environ-ment. They are degraded in water and soil with-in hours or days.

Toxicokinetics. Absorption, primarily that of the alkylene bisthio derivates, is poor after uptake by ingestion or dermal contact (~30%). Ab-sorbed dithiocarbamates are largely eliminated unchanged or after being metabolized (mainly in the liver) within 24–72 h. Dialkyl derivates are converted into dialkylthiocarbamic acid, carbon disulfide (CS_2), dialkylamine, sulfate, and formaldehyde. Alkylene bisthio derivatives are degraded to ethylene thiourea, ethylene di-amine, CS_2, H_2S, and CO_2.

Acute toxicity. The potential toxicity of dithio-carbamates in humans is well described in the scientific literature, although acute systemic poisoning hardly ever occurs. Local irritations of the skin and mucosae, as well as allergic con-tact dermatitis, have been observed after use for pest control and, above all, in the rubber indus-try (**B**). Dialkyl derivatives lead to delayed etha-nol degradation and alcohol intolerance (Anta-buse effect) by inhibiting alcohol dehydrogen-ase and, particularly, acetaldehyde dehydrogen-ase. Immediately after alcohol consumption, they trigger the following symptoms: nausea, vomiting, an increase in both respiratory rate and heart rate, and a rise or drop in blood pres-sure leading to life-threatening circulatory col-lapse.

Chronic toxicity. Chronic toxic effects in persons with long-term occupational exposure have not been established, and most mutagenicity tests have been negative. In animal experiments, high doses of the metabolite ethylene thiourea (> 60 mg/kg food) have lead to thyroid carcino-

ma, but no increased risk of carcinoma has been observed in exposed individuals.

Therapy. Treatment is symptomatic.

Chlorinated Phenoxycarbonic Acids

Herbicides based on chlorinated phenoxycar-bonic acids (**C**) inhibit the growth of plants be-cause they are chemically similar to the natural growth hormone auxin (3-indolylacetic acid). 2,4-Dichlorophenoxyacetic acid (2,4-D) and 2,4,5-trichlorophenoxyacetic acid (2,4,5-T) are, perhaps, the best known of this class. Since the mid 1980s, 2,4,5-T is no longer used in Germany because 2,3,7,8-TCDD (see p. 120) is generated as a by-product during its synthesis.

Toxicokinetics. These compounds are well ab-sorbed (> 90%) after uptake by ingestion and through the skin. They are poorly metabolized and are rapidly and completely eliminated in the urine (within hours or days). They are not stored in tissues because they are hydrophilic.

Toxicity (D). Acute poisonings occur after acci-dental or suicidal uptake of high doses. The symptoms are not characteristic. They include autonomic disturbances (headache, gastrointes-tinal symptoms), muscle dysfunction (stiffness of trunk and limb muscles, most likely because glycolysis is inhibited), and neural symptoms (peripheral neuropathies). Extremely high doses may lead to clouded consciousness, car-diovascular failure, respiratory paralysis, and possibly death.

Therapy. Treatment is symptomatic.

Dialkyl derivatives

Dithiocarbamate

$$R^1 \quad S$$
$$N-C-S-Metal$$
$$R^2$$

R^1, R^2 = alkyl groups
Metal = Na, Mn, Zn, etc.

Thiram

$$R^1 \quad S \qquad S \quad R^1$$
$$N-C-S-S-C-N$$
$$R^2 \quad R^1, R^2 = CH_3 \quad R^2$$

Ethylene bisthio derivatives

Cyclic form

Metal

Polymeric form

$$\left[-CH_2-CH_2-NH-C-S-C-NH- \right]_x$$
$$\qquad\qquad\qquad S \quad S$$

Insecti-cide

Herbicide

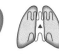
Fungi-cide

A. Structural formulas and biocidal effects of dithiocarbamates

Local effects:
Skin, mucosae
– irritation
– contact eczema

Epi-dermis  Mucosa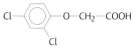

After ingestion:
Alcohol intolerance (Antabuse effect)
immediately after alcohol uptake

 Heart rate ↑
Blood pressure ↑

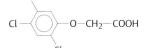

Vomiting

Respiratory rate ↑

B. Toxicity of dithiocarbamates

$$Cl-\text{⬡}-O-CH_2-COOH$$
$$\qquad Cl$$

2,4-Dichlorophenoxyacetic acid (2,4-D)

$$Cl-\text{⬡}-O-CH_2-COOH$$
$$\qquad Cl \qquad\qquad Cl$$

2,4,5-Trichlorophenoxyacetic acid (2,4,5-T)

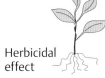
Herbicidal effect

C. Chlorinated phenoxycarbonic acids

NOAEL for humans: 5–36 mg 2,4-D/kg BW
Lethal oral dose: 80–1000 mg 2,4-D/kg BW

Muscles
– myotonia
– painful rigidity of trunk
  and limb muscles
  (peripheral respiratory paralysis)

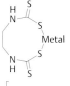

GIT
– irritation
– nausea
– vomiting
– diarrhea

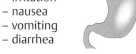

CNS
– sedative effect,
  headache

High doses:
– unconsciousness
– central respiratory paralysis

PNS
– neuropathy
  (paresthesia, paresis,
  loss of reflexes)

D. Acute toxicity of chlorinated phenoxycarbonic acids

Bipyridinium Compounds

The bipyridinium compounds *paraquat* and *diquat* are highly effective herbicides (**A**). The phytotoxic effect is based on the inhibition of photosynthesis by the formation of radicals, thus blocking NADP reduction and energy transfer. They undergo rapid photolysis in the environment, although this may be slowed down by their adsorption to soil particles; the annual degradation rate is 5–10%.

Toxicokinetics (B). Absorption after ingestion is minor (5–10% in case of paraquat). Absorption of paraquat in toxicologically relevant amounts is possible after uptake through previously injured skin. Absorbed paraquat (but not diquat) accumulates in the lungs; a sixfold rise in plasma levels is observed 30 h after ingestion. Reactive oxygen species (radicals) are generated during metabolism, and these are responsible for the damaging effects on cells.

Acute and chronic toxicity. Accidents and suicide attempts have led to many fatalities. *Topical contact* (**C**) leads, after a characteristic latency period of a few hours to 2 days, to painful reactions of the skin (erythema, ulcers, changes of the nails) or the outer portion of the eyes (possibly deep ulcers with long-lasting scarring defective healing). In case of inhalation, irritation and inflammation of the airways up to the toxic pulmonary edema are possible. The course of *oral poisoning* (**D**) is divided into three typical phases:

Phase 1: After immediate vomiting and a symptom-free latency period of several hours, the mucosa of the gastrointestinal tract is attacked (gastroenteritis, ulcers).

Phase 2: This is followed by toxic nephritis associated with renal dysfunction (including anuria) that disappears after 5–10 days. This may be accompanied by liver dysfunction (liver cell necrosis with cholestasis, icterus) and central nervous symptoms (headache, vertigo, rarely seizures and coma), and also by rapidly progressing normochromic anemia (rarely also arrhythmias).

Phase 3: After about 10 days, rapidly progressing pulmonary fibrosis follows. Severe alveolitis and bronchiolitis obliterans causes rapidly increasing dyspnea and finally death from suffocation.

The LD_{50} for paraquat is 40–60 mg/kg BW. The *ADI values* for paraquat and diquat are 0.001 and 0.008 mg/kg BW, respectively.

Therapy. Because of the high mortality, all possible means of primary detoxification (gastric and intestinal lavage, activated charcoal, saline laxatives) and secondary detoxification (forced diuresis, possibly hemodialysis or, preferably, hemoperfusion with application of charcoal filters) should be employed. Lowering the pH of the urine (e.g., arginine–HCl infusion) increases elimination of the poison by inhibiting renal reabsorption (paraquat and diquat are powerful bases). Renal insufficiency and hepatolysis are treated as required. Lowering the partial pressure of oxygen in the respiratory air is supposed to alleviate damage to the lungs (oxygen administration increases fibrosis by forming toxic peroxides). The benefit of high doses of glucocorticoids and immunosuppressive agents is controversial.

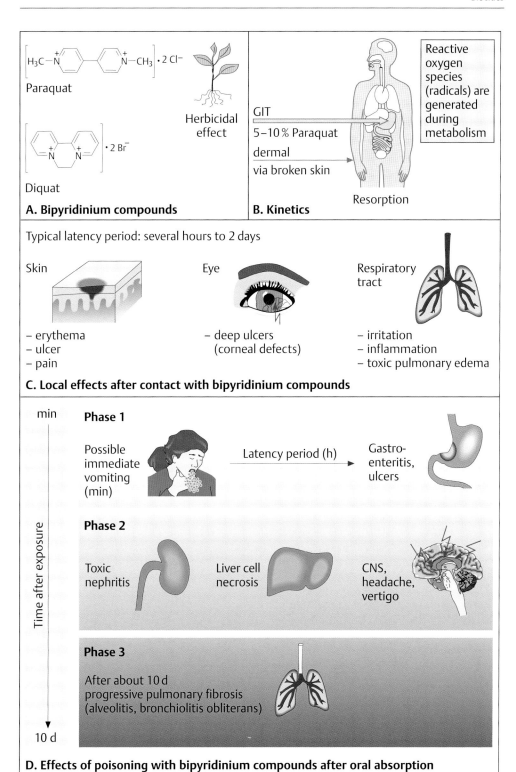

A. Bipyridinium compounds

Paraquat

Diquat

Herbicidal effect

B. Kinetics

GIT

5–10% Paraquat

dermal

via broken skin

Resorption

Reactive oxygen species (radicals) are generated during metabolism

Typical latency period: several hours to 2 days

Skin
– erythema
– ulcer
– pain

Eye
– deep ulcers
(corneal defects)

Respiratory tract
– irritation
– inflammation
– toxic pulmonary edema

C. Local effects after contact with bipyridinium compounds

min

Phase 1

Possible immediate vomiting (min)

Latency period (h)

Gastro-enteritis, ulcers

Phase 2

Toxic nephritis

Liver cell necrosis

CNS, headache, vertigo

Phase 3

After about 10 d progressive pulmonary fibrosis (alveolitis, bronchiolitis obliterans)

Time after exposure

10 d

D. Effects of poisoning with bipyridinium compounds after oral absorption

■ Toxins in Foods

Almost 90% of all food poisonings are due to toxins produced by bacteria.

Exotoxins. These are synthesized inside the bacterial cell and then excreted (see also bacterial poisons, p. 286). *Staphylococcus aureus* grows on cooked, protein-rich foods where it releases its exotoxins (e.g., staphylococcus α-toxin). To inhibit bacterial multiplication, foods should be stored below 4 °C or above 65 °C. However, the toxins are heat resistant. In humans, the ingestion of tainted, toxin-containing food leads to vomiting and diarrhea. Treatment with antibiotics is ineffective because the symptoms are caused by the ingested exotoxins. *Bacillus cereus* grows on cereal products, egg dishes, and meat dishes that have been kept warm, where it releases a toxin that also causes diarrhea and vomiting when ingested by humans. *Clostridium perfringens* grows preferentially in reheated meat dishes and desserts. Ingestion of its toxin leads to loss of appetite, abdominal cramps, and diarrhea. Heating the foods destroys the toxin. The exotoxin of *Clostridium botulinum* (botulinum toxin) rarely induces food poisonings these days; the bacterium is inactivated by the commonly used food processing methods (e.g., heating to 80 °C for 30 min). Since the spoilage of foods (e.g., homemade preserves) is not recognized by the senses, bulged cans and food jars must be discarded. Ingestion of this extremely poisonous toxin (the lethal dose for humans is 2 μg) inhibits the release of acetylcholine and thus results in paralysis (see bacterial poisons, p. 292).

Endotoxins. These originate from dead Gram-negative bacteria. Endotoxins are largely lipopolysaccharides and act without an incubation period; for example, the characteristic symptoms of septicemia and enteritis (salmonellosis) occur in humans 6–8 h after ingestion of salmonella endotoxin. The main sources of contamination are insufficiently heated eggs and egg products, ground meat, poultry meat, sausages, and clams (salmonella toxin is destroyed by heating at 70 °C for 10 min). In addition to the widely distributed *Salmonella typhimurium*, *Salmonella enteritidis* has become common since 1987; it occurs primarily in poultry farms where it infects the eggs prior to shell formation. In humans, ingestion of the toxin results in severe fever with vomiting and diarrhea (**A**).

Mycotoxins. Ergot alkaloids (see p. 72) are produced by the fungus *Claviceps purpurea*, which often grows in wet years on rye plants and forms the purplish-black ergot resembling a grain of corn (**B**). Its alkaloids (e.g., ergometrine) (**C**) are heat resistant. Uptake of even a few milligrams of these toxins is toxic for humans. A single ergot grain (e.g., in bread) triggers headaches and cramps. Aflatoxins (**C**) are produced by molds (e.g., *Aspergillus flavus*) that grow on nuts, spices, and cereals stored in humid conditions. After ingestion of toxin-contaminated foods, a mother may transfer aflatoxins to her baby in the breast milk. Aflatoxins are considered hepatotoxic and carcinogenic. The epoxide generated during aflatoxin metabolism is extremely toxic for trout and birds. Islanditoxin and patulin are produced by *Penicillium islandicum* and *P. expansum*, while ochratoxin A is formed by *Aspergillus ochraceus* (**C**). These fungi grow on rotting fruits, vegetables, and nuts. Consumption of toxin-contaminated foods may damage the liver and kidneys in humans. There is evidence for carcinogenic effects of patulin and ochratoxin on humans.

EU regulations on aflatoxin (since 1990) permit up to 2 μg aflatoxin B_1 per kg of food.

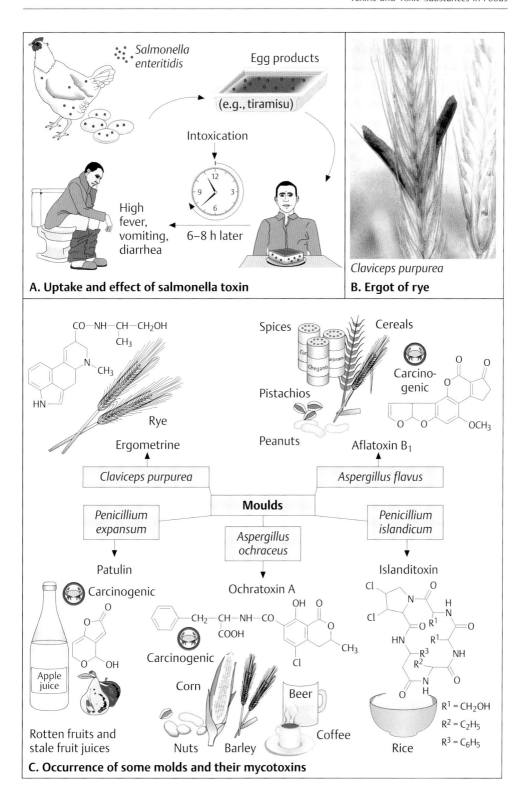

A. Uptake and effect of salmonella toxin

Salmonella enteritidis

Egg products
(e.g., tiramisu)

Intoxication

6–8 h later

High fever, vomiting, diarrhea

B. Ergot of rye

Claviceps purpurea

CO—NH—CH—CH₂OH

Rye

Ergometrine

Claviceps purpurea

Penicillium expansum

Patulin

Carcinogenic

Apple juice

Rotten fruits and stale fruit juices

Spices

Pistachios

Peanuts

Cereals

Carcinogenic

Aflatoxin B₁

Aspergillus flavus

Moulds

Aspergillus ochraceus

Ochratoxin A

Carcinogenic

Corn

Nuts   Barley

Beer

Coffee

Penicillium islandicum

Islanditoxin

R¹ = CH₂OH
R² = C₂H₅
R³ = C₆H₅

Rice

C. Occurrence of some molds and their mycotoxins

Toxic Substances Generated in Foods or in the Human Digestive System

Biogenic amines. These are generated in microorganisms by enzymatic decarboxylation (**A**). Foods produced by microbial methods (e.g., cheese, beer) are therefore rich in biogenic amines. Their concentrations rise dramatically in spoiled foods as a result of the multiplication of microbes. A high uptake of amines in food may lead to hypertension when certain medications are taken simultaneously. For example, *tyramine* is normally degraded in the intestinal wall by monoaminoxidase (MAO). However, this enzyme may be inhibited by antihypertensives, antidepressives, or tuberculostatics, thus leading to increased tyramine levels in the intestine. Increased tyramine absorption then triggers the release of norepinephrine from sympathetic nerve endings, resulting in a rise in blood pressure (**B**). Tyramine is present in cheese, beer, wine (especially Chianti), chocolate, and sauerkraut. The tyramine level in foods is usually around 50 μg/g, but mature cheese may contain up to 900 μg/g and yeast extract even more than 2000 μg/g. Patients with high blood pressure are therefore particularly at risk if they consume these foods frequently. The biogenic amine *serotonin* (e.g., in bananas, walnuts, tomatoes) also raises blood pressure. *Histamine* in connection with ethanol seems to induce intolerance to certain wines that may contain up to 25 mg histamine/L (normally only ~2 mg/L). Acute histamine intoxication in humans occurs only after uptake of more than 1000 mg; it is associated with severe headaches and spasms.

The level of biogenic amines in foods can be reduced, e.g., by discarding the cooking water or preserving liquid into which the biogenic amines are released (**C**).

Nitrosamines, nitrosamides. These are generated by the chemical reaction of secondary amines in the body and are to some extent already present in food (e.g., sausages, meat, cheese; see pp. 124–129) (**D**). Humans take in about 1 μg/day nitrosamines. In addition to this exogenous exposure, there may be an endogenous burden due to amines and nitrates that can be nitrosated (see also nitrates and nitrosamines, p. 214).

Food Allergies

Allergies are primarily triggered by certain proteins in the food. The most common allergens include *α-lactalbumin, β-lactoglobulin, casein,* and *lipoproteins* of cow's milk. Of the proteins contained in wheat, *albumin* has the most allergenic effect. Also common are allergies to nuts, citrus fruits, stone fruits, various vegetables (e. g., legumes, tomatoes), chicken and fish proteins, and chemical food additives (see additives, p. 220). In 90% of individuals with an existing food allergy, irritation of skin and airways are observed. The mucosae of lips, eyes, and tongue are most frequently affected. The following symptoms may also occur: nausea, headache, seizures, and cardiovascular complaints, although reactions of the gastrointestinal tract (diarrhea) are particularly common. Irritant foods, such as onions, radishes, hot spices, alcohol, and caffeine, or an imbalance in the intestinal flora (e.g., due to fungal infection) promote allergic reactions. The allergen content of a plant may vary significantly depending which part of the plant is used and its different stages of maturity. Some allergens are easily denatured (e.g., those in cow's milk and wheat by heating to 120 °C, and those in apples by air oxidation). By contrast, the allergens in hen's eggs, fish, nuts, and beans are very resistant to denaturation. Some of the triggers of food allergies are very difficult to identify. If in doubt, the only protection from allergic reactions is to avoid the suspected foods.

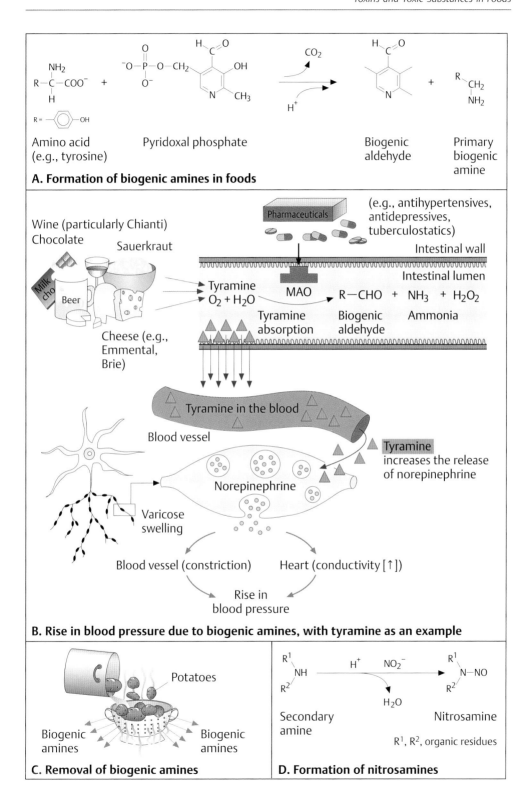

A. Formation of biogenic amines in foods

Amino acid (e.g., tyrosine) Pyridoxal phosphate Biogenic aldehyde Primary biogenic amine

B. Rise in blood pressure due to biogenic amines, with tyramine as an example

Wine (particularly Chianti)
Chocolate
Sauerkraut
Beer
Cheese (e.g., Emmental, Brie)

Pharmaceuticals
(e.g., antihypertensives, antidepressives, tuberculostatics)

Intestinal wall
Intestinal lumen

Tyramine
$O_2 + H_2O$
MAO
$R-CHO + NH_3 + H_2O_2$

Tyramine absorption
Biogenic aldehyde
Ammonia

Tyramine in the blood
Blood vessel

Tyramine increases the release of norepinephrine

Norepinephrine
Varicose swelling

Blood vessel (constriction)   Heart (conductivity [↑])

Rise in blood pressure

C. Removal of biogenic amines

Potatoes
Biogenic amines
Biogenic amines

D. Formation of nitrosamines

Secondary amine   Nitrosamine

R^1, R^2, organic residues

213

■ Naturally Occurring Toxic Substances in Foods

Naturally occurring toxic substances are of little toxicological importance, since they are usually destroyed by the traditional methods of food preparation (see Environmental Toxicology, p. 62). The following substances are exceptions:

Nitrate. Some plants can accumulate up to 7000 mg nitrate per kg (**A**). In addition, nitrate is added as a preservative to cheese and meat (see additives, p. 220). It may also be present in the drinking water. Exposure by infants is particularly dangerous during the first 3 months, since nitrate is reduced to nitrite in the small intestine (**A**).

Nitrite. Nitrite leads to the formation of methemoglobin and may thus inhibit oxygen transport in the erythrocytes. Intake of around 6 mg nitrate/kg BW may lead to cyanosis in infants (**B**). Nitrate is reduced to nitrite by bacteria during the storage of vegetables at temperatures above 8 °C, and also in the saliva of adults (**A**). Exposure to nitrate-containing foods may also result in the formation of carcinogenic nitrosamines or nitrosamides from secondary amines (e.g., dimethylamine contained primarily in fish, cheese, and vegetables) due to the acidic environment of the stomach (see pp. 124–129). Some nitrosamines and nitrosamides may be present in some foods. Ascorbic acid and tocopherols inhibit nitrosation in the human body, whereas chlorogenic acid derived from coffee stimulates nitrosation (**A**).

Hydrocyanic acid. Present in the stones of fruits and in bitter almonds, HCN inhibits cellular respiration by forming a complex with Fe^{3+} in the cytochrome of the respiratory chain (see p. 140). The amount present in 5–10 bitter almonds may be enough to be lethal for children.

Several naturally occurring toxic substances in foods inhibit mineral uptake:

Oxalic acid. This occurs in spinach and black tea, among other foods, and inhibits calcium metabolism. By forming calcium oxalate, it may result in kidney stones in humans.

Tannins. These are found in coffee and tea. They inhibit iron uptake and increase the elimination of calcium and magnesium.

Hemagglutinins, protease inhibitors. Hemagglutinins (e.g., lectins) and protease inhibitors (e.g., in wheat, beans) reduce the uptake of iron, zinc, and calcium.

■ Novel Foods

These include:

1. *Products manufactured by using genetic technology to create foods that last longer, are larger, and look more appetizing.* Nutritional concerns for humans may arise when these genetically modified (GM) foods (e.g., milk, tomatoes, meat) contain less vitamins and minerals, or more fat or salt, than traditional foods. When ingested with foods, genetically modified microorganisms may release foreign proteins that trigger allergic reactions in humans.

2. *Foods not easily available on the international market.* These include mycoprotein-based products as meat analogues for vegetarians (e.g., Quorn) and artificial compounds, such as indigestible fat substitutes that taste like fat but have no calories (e.g., Olestra) (**C**). During the digestion of normal fat (triglycerides), up to three fatty acids are cleaved off by enzymes and are absorbed in the intestinal tract; the physiological calorific value of fat is 39 kJ/g (= 9 kcal/g). By contrast, fat substitutes contain sucrose as a central molecule, to which 6–8 fatty acids bind in a radial arrangement. This renders the fatty acids inaccessible to enzymes so that they cannot be cleaved off and absorbed in the intestinal tract; the calorific value of fat substitutes is 0 kJ/g (**C**). Eating fat substitutes is thought to lead to reduced uptake of lipophilic vitamins (A, D, E, and K); it can also cause increased defecation (anal leakage) due to forced lubrication in the intestinal tract. Fat substitutes are not yet biologically degradable and are therefore still considered special waste.

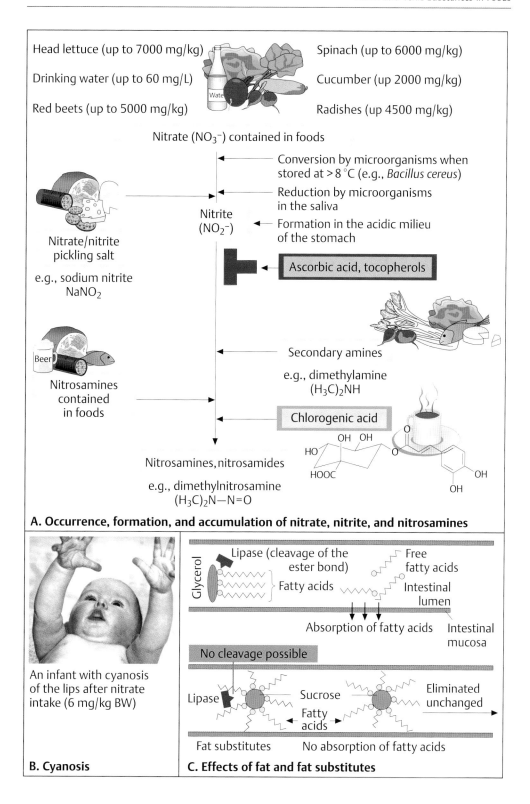

Head lettuce (up to 7000 mg/kg)

Spinach (up to 6000 mg/kg)

Drinking water (up to 60 mg/L)

Cucumber (up 2000 mg/kg)

Red beets (up to 5000 mg/kg)

Radishes (up 4500 mg/kg)

Nitrate (NO_3^-) contained in foods

Conversion by microorganisms when stored at $> 8\,°C$ (e.g., *Bacillus cereus*)

Reduction by microorganisms in the saliva

Nitrite (NO_2^-)

Formation in the acidic milieu of the stomach

Ascorbic acid, tocopherols

Nitrate/nitrite pickling salt

e.g., sodium nitrite $NaNO_2$

Secondary amines

e.g., dimethylamine ($H_3C)_2NH$

Nitrosamines contained in foods

Chlorogenic acid

Nitrosamines, nitrosamides

e.g., dimethylnitrosamine ($H_3C)_2N-N=O$

A. Occurrence, formation, and accumulation of nitrate, nitrite, and nitrosamines

An infant with cyanosis of the lips after nitrate intake (6 mg/kg BW)

Glycerol

Lipase (cleavage of the ester bond)

Free fatty acids

Fatty acids

Intestinal lumen

Absorption of fatty acids

Intestinal mucosa

No cleavage possible

Lipase

Sucrose

Eliminated unchanged

Fatty acids

Fat substitutes

No absorption of fatty acids

B. Cyanosis

C. Effects of fat and fat substitutes

215

■ Irradiation of Foods

The treatment of foods with ionizing radiation is currently considered the most advanced method of preservation. There is no evidence that the ingestion of irradiated foods poses any danger to animals or humans. When properly applied, irradiation does not generate radioactive isotopes in foods.

Advantages of food irradiation. Irradiation prolongs the ripening period of fruits and vegetables and thus increases shelf life (e.g., bananas). It kills pests (e.g., beetles in cereals). Vegetables no longer sprout (e.g., potatoes, onions), and many molds and bacteria are destroyed (e.g., salmonellae on chicken). The yield of food processing increases (e.g., more fruit juice from irradiated fruits) (**A**).

Disadvantages of food irradiation. Certain vitamins (e.g., A, B$_1$, E, C) and amino acids (e.g., tyrosine, phenylalanine) are sensitive to radiation (**B**). Unsaturated fatty acids may lose their protective effect when irradiated. Furthermore, free radicals may form (see p. 146). A contentious issue is the effect of irradiation on veterinary drug residues in meat (e.g., hormones) or pesticides in vegetables. Irradiation does not kill all microbes. Resistant species, such as the spore-forming bacterium *Clostridium botulinum*, may survive. Signs of perishability, such as the growth of molds (e.g., on strawberries) or the opening of mushroom caps, are suppressed. Irradiated foods also simulate freshness despite the fact that some of the vitamins have been degraded by irradiation and subsequent long-term storage (**C**).

European law permits certain contaminated foods (e.g., liquefied eggs) to re-enter the market after irradiation although these foods may already be spoiled.

Food irradiation is preferentially done with γ-radiation (e.g., up to 10 kGy) using cobalt-60 (^{60}Co) as a source of radiation. The penetrating power of γ-rays is high, and their production is inexpensive. Because of the formation of easily identifiable, radiation-specific metabolites, it is possible in the case of most foods to detect unambiguously if they have been treated by ionizing radiation. Food irradiation is still prohibited in Germany, but it is used in more than 30 countries around the world for about 50 different foods (see also p. 62).

■ Residues from Packaging Materials, Cleaning Agents, and Disinfectants

The following substances are used in polymerization processes for manufacturing the plastics used in food packaging (e.g., plastic films). These substances partly remain in the packaging material and may therefore migrate into the packaged foods (migration).

Polychlorinated biphenyls (PCBs). Until the early 1990s, these were used as plastic softeners in food packaging materials. They can migrate into the packaged foods and are highly toxic (see p. 114). Their application is now prohibited.

Monomers. These include molecules (e.g., vinyl chloride) that are combined to macromolecules (e.g., polyvinyl chloride) for the manufacture of packaging materials (see pp. 108 and 184). For technical reasons, traces of monomers remain in the plastic material and may then migrate into packaged foods. The vinyl chloride monomer is hepatotoxic for humans and is classified as a carcinogen. In Germany, for example, the technical guideline concentration (*TRK value*, see Glossary) for vinyl chloride is 5–8 mg/m^3, depending on its application (see also p. 184).

Cleaning agents and disinfectants. These include tensides, sulfuric acid, phosphoric acid, and nitric acid (used in the brewing and dairy industries for lime removal) and perchloroethylene (a solvent used in oil production). They should not be present in foods. Nevertheless, accidents and negligence can lead to the contamination of foods. Tensides increase the permeability of the intestinal wall, thus enhancing the entrance of allergenic substances into the blood.

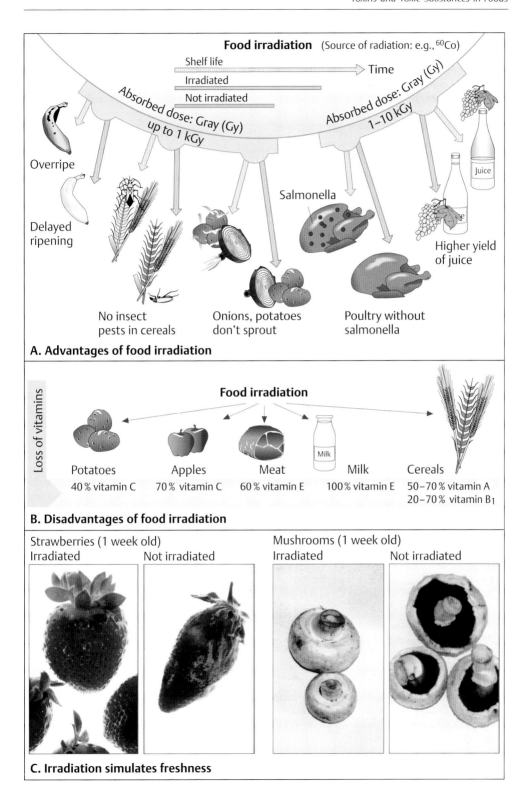

Food irradiation (Source of radiation: e.g., ^{60}Co)

Shelf life → Time

Irradiated

Not irradiated

Absorbed dose: Gray (Gy) up to 1 kGy

Absorbed dose: Gray (Gy) 1–10 kGy

Overripe

Delayed ripening

No insect pests in cereals

Onions, potatoes don't sprout

Salmonella

Poultry without salmonella

Juice

Higher yield of juice

A. Advantages of food irradiation

Loss of vitamins

Food irradiation

Potatoes	Apples	Meat	Milk	Cereals
40% vitamin C	70% vitamin C	60% vitamin E	100% vitamin E	50–70% vitamin A 20–70% vitamin B$_1$

B. Disadvantages of food irradiation

Strawberries (1 week old)
Irradiated   Not irradiated

Mushrooms (1 week old)
Irradiated   Not irradiated

C. Irradiation simulates freshness

Toxic Substances Generated during Food Preparation

Hydroperoxides and peroxides. These are formed from unsaturated fatty acids in heated oils in the presence of oxygen. Antioxidants, such as α-tocopherol (vitamin E; see free radicals, p. 146), protect foods from oxidation. However, they are partly destroyed during heating and storage, or by oxidative bleaching of flour.

Products of the Maillard reaction (A). These are generated when the carbonyl groups of reducing sugars react with the amino groups of amines, peptides, and proteins. The formation of these products during food preparation is considered desirable because they add flavor and color (browning reaction, caramelization). Also important are newly formed heterocyclic compounds, like pyridosine. Several of these substances are known to have numerous undesirable effects. There is evidence for the formation of antinutritive, toxic, and mutagenic secondary products.

Polycyclic aromatic hydrocarbons (PAHs) (B). These substances enter foods during the smoking process and also during barbecuing when fat drips on to red-hot charcoal. The concentration of *benzo[a]pyrene* in smoked ham may be up to 3 µg/kg, and in barbecued meat up to 50 µg/kg. Generally, the maximum level of benzo[a]pyrene for meat products is 1 µg/kg. When such foods are consumed in excess, dangerous health effects cannot be excluded. Grapeseed oil also contains benzo[a]pyrene up to 25 µg/kg. Vegetables and cereals may accumulate PAHs from the soil and air up to 20 µg/kg. The daily human uptake of total PAHs from a normal diet is less than about 3 µg. For certain PAHs, such as benzo[a]pyrene, there is evidence of mutagenic and carcinogenic effects in animals and humans (see PAHs, p. 100).

Residues from Substances Used in Agriculture and Animal Husbandry

Biocides (C). These include *DDT* (see p. 195), *PCBs* (see p. 114), and *dieldrin* (see p. 195). Pesticides were frequently applied in the past and have accumulated in the food chain. Foods are still contaminated today, but typically by no more than about 12 µg/kg, depending on the compound. Breast milk is considered to still be heavily contaminated with PCBs. There is evidence of carcinogenic, teratogenic, and immunosuppressive effects with some PCBs in humans (see also p. 114). Environmental lipophilic substances such as *dioxins* (see pp. 116–121) can accumulate in breast milk to a level of 2 µg/kg milk fat. Nevertheless, studies have shown that the exposure of infants to dioxins is not high enough to discourage breastfeeding.

Veterinary drugs and feed additives (D). Veterinary *antibiotics* are used both as therapeutics and as fattening supplements. When taken up by humans through the food chain, they may cause antibiotic resistance or induce allergies. *Sex hormones* (e.g., estradiol, testosterone) are also used as therapeutics and fattening supplements. *Thyreostatics* are administered to help animals gain weight; however, they are metabolized to thiourea which is carcinogenic. *Glucocorticoids* (e.g., cortisone), β-blockers, and psychopharmaceuticals (e.g., diazepam) are given to pigs as sedatives in case of stress and then may get also into humans through the food chain. *Vitamins* are used as therapeutics and fattening supplements; they accumulate in the liver of the animals (e.g., vitamin A) and induce headache and vomiting in humans who consume excessive amounts of such food.

Heavy metals. These may contaminate foods and then result in human exposure by means of canned foods and metal kitchenware (e.g., tin, copper), drinking-water (e.g., arsenic, lead), and car exhaust (e.g., platinum, lead). They have various deleterious effects (see metals, p. 160 ff.).

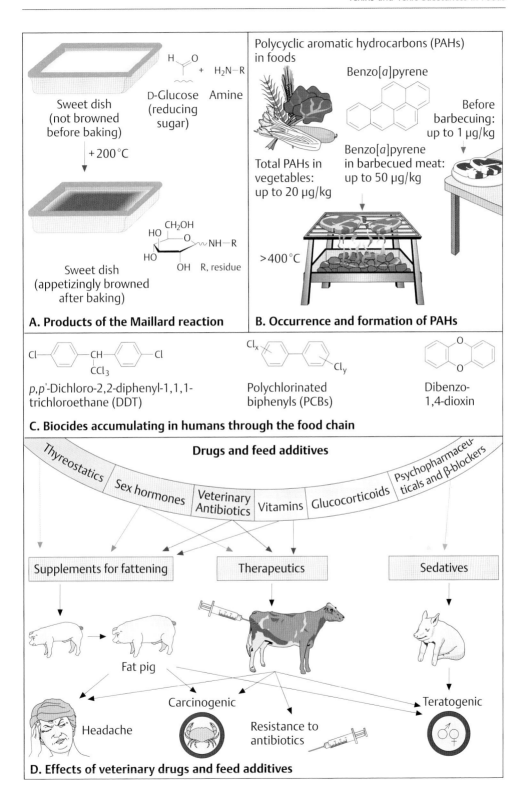

H $\diagdown$ O
$+$ H$_2$N$-$R

D-Glucose   Amine
(reducing
sugar)

Sweet dish
(not browned
before baking)

$+200\,°C$

CH$_2$OH
HO $\diagup$ O
$\diagdown$NH$-$R
HO
OH   R, residue

Sweet dish
(appetizingly browned
after baking)

A. Products of the Maillard reaction

Polycyclic aromatic hydrocarbons (PAHs)
in foods

Benzo[*a*]pyrene

Before
barbecuing:
up to 1 µg/kg

Benzo[*a*]pyrene
in barbecued meat:
up to 50 µg/kg

Total PAHs in
vegetables:
up to 20 µg/kg

$>400\,°C$

B. Occurrence and formation of PAHs

Cl$-$CH$-$Cl
CCl$_3$

p,p'-Dichloro-2,2-diphenyl-1,1,1-
trichloroethane (DDT)

Cl$_x$
Cl$_y$

Polychlorinated
biphenyls (PCBs)

O
O

Dibenzo-
1,4-dioxin

C. Biocides accumulating in humans through the food chain

Thyreostatics   Sex hormones   Veterinary Antibiotics   Vitamins   Glucocorticoids   Psychopharmaceuticals and β-blockers

Drugs and feed additives

Supplements for fattening   Therapeutics   Sedatives

Fat pig

Headache

Carcinogenic

Resistance to
antibiotics

Teratogenic

D. Effects of veterinary drugs and feed additives

■ Colors and Additives in Drugs and Foods

Basics. Colors and additives for drugs and foods are subject to stringent approval procedures and must not cause any health problems in humans. Additives are identified by reference numbers (E numbers) that are in effect throughout the European Union (**A**).

Colors. *Food colors (E100–180)* are added to make foods look more appetizing and to promote sales. Colors often simulate better quality (e.g., fruit content in ice cream). They may be natural (e.g., red carotene from carrots) or synthetic. Some synthetic colors (e.g., orange yellow and tartrazine yellow) may trigger allergies in humans. The pink-red erythrosine as well as β-naphthylamine and degradation products of azo dyes (e.g., from the red azorubin) have even been shown to initiate tumors in animals.

Acidifiers. *Orthophosphoric acid (E338)* is added to cola drinks (up to 600 mg/L). In baking powder, phosphoric acid causes leavening of the dough by releasing CO_2. Excessive uptake of phosphoric acid inhibits calcium absorption in humans. Many baking powders also contain dihydrogen phosphate as an acid-forming agent.

Thickening agents. *Alginates (E400–406)* bind water in foods (e.g., jams, sausages). They may also bind cobalt, manganese, iron, or zinc, thus leading to reduced uptake of these essential elements in humans. *Carrageenan (E407)* is obtained from red algae; it is added to foods (e. g., desserts) as a gelling agent to increase consistency. Because of its immunosuppressive effect in humans, it may promote the development of tumors.

Preservatives. *Sulfur compounds (E220–227)* are used in the form of sulfur dioxide (SO_2) for the preservation of wine (20–50 mg/L), potato products, and dried fruits. Sensitive individuals may react with nausea, headache, and diarrhea after uptake of as little as 20 mg. *Nitrate and nitrite (E250–252)* protect meat products from spoilage by bacteria. Addition of nitrite intensifies the red color of meat through the formation of nitrosohemoglobin and nitrosohemochromogen. In humans, the uptake of 0.5 g sodium nitrite leads to mild intoxication, uptake of 1–2 g causes severe intoxication, and uptake of 4 g is lethal (see nitrate, nitrite, p. 214). *Benzoic acid and benzoates (E210–213)* have antimycotic and bacteriostatic effects already at a concentration of 0.5 %. They penetrate cell membranes, inhibit the enzymes of citrate cycle and oxidative phosphorylation, and induce allergies in humans when ingested. They are primarily added to acidic foods (e.g., pickled cucumbers, mayonnaise). *Esters of p-hydroxybenzoic acid (pHB esters, E214–219)* have primarily an antimycotic effect and are used in the fillings of baked goods and in canned foods. When these foods are consumed in excess, pHB esters have a vasodilating effect in humans and may also trigger allergies.

Flavor enhancers. *Glutamates (E620–625)* intensify the taste of foods. In meat products, where glutamates develop a particularly strong effect, no more than 1 g/kg may be used. In sensitive individuals, the uptake of less than 120 mg glutamate can trigger numbness, palpitation, and headache (Chinese restaurant syndrome).

Stabilizers. *Polyphosphates (E450 a–c)* are added to certain sausages (e.g., wieners, frankfurters) to increase the binding of water. Used as melting salts in cheese, they prevent the coagulation of protein during sterilization. Polyphosphates in condensed milk prevent gelling of the thickened milk. Excessive consumption of polyphosphate-containing foods may inhibit calcium uptake in humans and trigger hyperactivity in children.

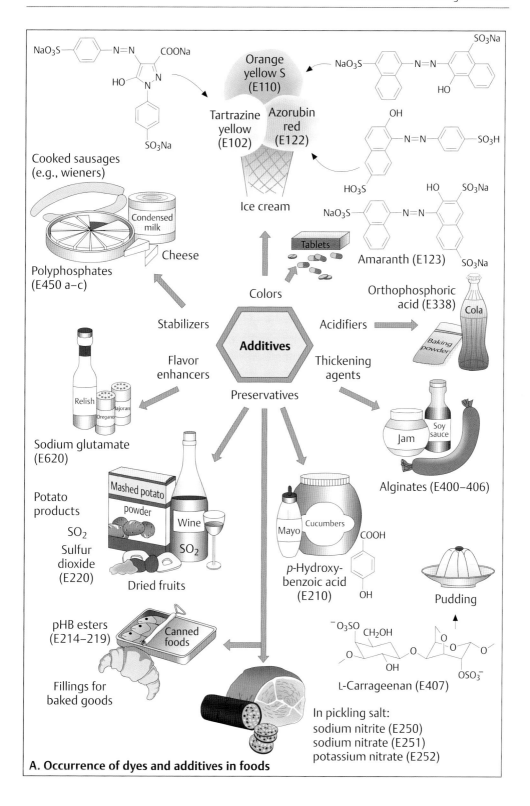

A. Occurrence of dyes and additives in foods

Orange
yellow S
(E110)

Tartrazine
yellow
(E102)

Azorubin
red
(E122)

Ice cream

Cooked sausages
(e.g., wieners)

Condensed
milk

Cheese

Tablets

Amaranth (E123)

Polyphosphates
(E450 a–c)

Colors

Orthophosphoric
acid (E338)

Cola

Stabilizers

Acidifiers

Baking
powder

Additives

Flavor
enhancers

Thickening
agents

Preservatives

Relish

Oregano

Majoram

Soy
sauce

Jam

Sodium glutamate
(E620)

Alginates (E400–406)

Potato
products

Mashed potato
powder

Wine

SO_2

Mayo

Cucumbers

COOH

SO_2
Sulfur
dioxide
(E220)

Dried fruits

p-Hydroxy-
benzoic acid
(E210)

OH

Pudding

pHB esters
(E214–219)

Canned
foods

^-O_3SO CH_2OH

OH

OSO_3^-

Fillings for
baked goods

L-Carrageenan (E407)

In pickling salt:
sodium nitrite (E250)
sodium nitrate (E251)
potassium nitrate (E252)

Cosmetics and Their Application

For thousands of years, humans have been using chemicals to improve their appearance. Today, these preparations are called *cosmetics*. They clean, protect, and beautify the skin, nails, teeth, and hair, or stimulate the olfactory senses. Cosmetics also have a high economic value. In the United States alone, more than 15 billion dollars were spent on cosmetics in 2004.

Classification of cosmetics. Cosmetics are classified primarily according to their applications (**A**). They must be manufactured and marketed in such a way that they do no harm to human health (Article 1.2 of the European Cosmetics Directive adopted in 1976).

Classes of active ingredients. In the *Blue List of Cosmetic Ingredients*, active ingredients are divided into four classes (**B**) and evaluated according to chemical, allergological, and toxicological aspects. Of the 198 substances approved, coloring agents make up the largest group.

All regulated substances mentioned in this list and in the cosmetics directive have undergone the European Union (EU) approval procedure. The scope of testing cosmetic ingredients for health and safety purposes is outlined in the EU guidelines for toxicity testing of cosmetic ingredients (started in 1983) and numerous amendments.

These guidelines include in-vitro and in-vivo toxicological tests, such as tests for acute and chronic toxicity, embryotoxicity, mutagenicity, and carcinogenicity. On the basis of the approval procedure it may be assumed that, in general, these cosmetic products are considered safe when used in the specified concentration and for the approved purpose.

Undesired reactions. Despite applying cosmetics properly, 5–10% of users report undesired reactions. These mainly include skin irritation (itching), allergic contact dermatitis, changes in skin pigmentation, phototoxic reactions, damage to nails and hair, and general paresthesia. Studies have demonstrated that such reactions predominantly occur in women after using soaps and deodorants, while in men they occur more often after using shaving preparations and soaps (**C**).

Allergic contact dermatitis. Other studies have shown that about 2–5% of the users of cosmetics develop allergic contact dermatitis, which is induced in most cases by preservatives and scents contained in cosmetic preparations (**D**). For the major groups of active substances and other ingredients of cosmetics, see p. 224.

Contact allergens. Hairdressers are particularly exposed to contact allergens. The most potent allergens are *p*-phenylenediamine (see p. 130) and thioglycolic acid glyceryl ester (**E**), which are predominantly contained in hair care products (e.g., shampoos, hair dyes).

Ingestion of the following approved ingredients can lead to severe poisoning:

Organic mercury compounds (e.g., phenylmercuric chloride/nitrate) are approved only for use as eye mascara and mascara removers. The maximum concentration must not exceed 0.007% (measured as Hg). At higher concentrations, these compounds irritate skin and mucosae. For treatment in case of ingestion, see mercury poisoning, p. 176.

Silver nitrate is approved only as a 4% solution for dyeing eyelashes and eyebrows. If it gets into the eyes, the eyes should be rinsed immediately.

Tin fluoride is only approved for oral care (mouthwash).

All other cosmetic ingredients that are approved but not listed here are toxicologically irrelevant, even if ingested as pure substances.

Application		Examples	
Skin care	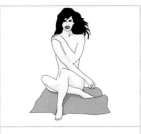	– Skin cleansers – Skin care lotions – Skin protection creams – Bath additives – Deodorants – Antiperspirants	– Hair removal creams – Shaving preparations – Make-up – Nail care products – Astringents
Dental and oral care		– Toothpastes – Dental adhesives – Mouthwashes	
Hair care		– Shampoos – Conditioners – Hair sprays – Hair dyes	
Perfumery		– Fragrances – Perfumes – Scents (compositions)	
Light and heat protection		– Suntan lotions – Sunscreen agents – Depigmentation agents – Heat protection agents	

A. Classification of cosmetics according to their application

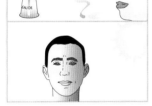

B. Classes of active ingredients

Number of substances — Coloring agents, Preservatives, Other substances, UV filter

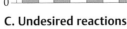

C. Undesired reactions

In women: Soaps, Deodorants, Creams, Perfumes
In men: Shaving preparations, Soaps, Deodorants, Shampoos

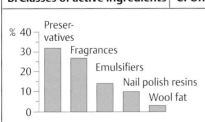

D. Allergic contact dermatitis

Preservatives, Fragrances, Emulsifiers, Nail polish resins, Wool fat

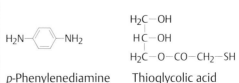

$H_2N\!-\!\langle\ \rangle\!-\!NH_2$

p-Phenylenediamine
(1,4-diaminobenzene)

$H_2C\!-\!OH$
$HC\!-\!OH$
$H_2C\!-\!O\!-\!CO\!-\!CH_2\!-\!SH$

Thioglycolic acid
glyceryl ester

E. Contact allergens

Important Groups of Cosmetic Ingredients (A)

Antioxidants. These prevent the autoxidation of fats and flavoring agents (e.g., tocopherols, butylhydroxytoluene, ascorbic acid).

Antiperspirants. These reduce the production of sweat (e.g., astringents, tannins, aluminum hydroxychloride).

Antiseptics. These kill pathogenic microbes (e. g., alcohols, salicylic acid, benzoic acid).

Antistatics. These prevent the electrostatic charging of hair (e.g., polyglycol ether, fatty acids, alkylphenols).

Astringents. These cause protein precipitation and coagulation, thus making the skin more dense on the surface and therefore protecting it (e.g., tannic acid, alum, and bismuth compounds).

Bleaching creams. These act against hyperpigmentation, such as freckles, chloasma, lentigo (e.g., H_2O_2, zinc peroxide, urea peroxide, lactic acid).

Coloring agents. These are natural colors (e.g., betaine, carotene, chlorophyll, anthraquinone).

Degreasing agents. These regulate secretion of the sebaceous glands (e.g., organic sulfur compounds).

Demulsifiers. These break up emulsions, i. e., the dispersion of immiscible liquids (e.g., salts of sulfonic acids).

Deodorants. These inhibit the growth of sweat-fermenting bacteria and thus prevent the formation of odor (e.g., triclosan, p-chloro-m-xylenol).

Depilatories. These remove unwanted body hair (e.g., strontium compounds, calcium thioglycolate).

Disinfectants. These are active against microorganisms (e.g., alcohols, phenol derivatives, usnic acid).

Emulgators. These are used for manufacturing and stabilizing emulsions (e.g., tensides, fatty acid esters, alkylphenol polyglycolether).

Fragrances. These are substances with a pleasant odor; they are either natural, derived from animals and plants (e.g., musk, rose oil), or of synthetic origin, (e.g., octanol).

Hemostatics. These stop bleeding (e.g., astringents, alum, tannin).

Moisturizers. These prevent the drying out of cosmetic preparations and make the skin softer (e.g., sorbitol, glycerol, glycols, lactic acid).

Preservatives. These prevent unwanted changes in cosmetic preparations (e.g., of odor, appearance, or consistency) caused by microorganisms (e.g., benzoate, propionate, salicylate, sorbate, formaldehyde, chlorobutanol, thiomersal).

Repellents. These are insect repellents (e.g., essential oils, such as carnation oil, lavender oil, citronella oil, or cinnamon oil; caprylic acid diethylamide, N,N-diethyl-m-toluamide, phthalic acid ester, 2-cyclohexylcyclohexanol).

Sequestration agents. These convert metal ions into an inactive but soluble form (complex formation; e.g., ethylenediaminetetraacetic acid, nitrilotriacetic acid).

Solubilizers. These dissolve water-insoluble substances (e.g., tensides, diethylene glycolether, glycerol monoaliphatic esters).

Stabilizers. These prevent undesired changes in cosmetic preparations (e.g., antioxidants, emulsifiers, preservatives).

Thickening agents. These absorb liquids and form viscous, homogenous, and colloidal solutions (e.g., tensides, fatty acid alkanolamides, waxes).

Thixotropic agents. These reversibly change from the solid to the liquid state after mechanical stress (shaking, stirring, pressure) without changing the water content (e.g., certain tenside solutions in emulsions or gels, such as massage lotions and lipsticks).

Wetting agents. Reduce the surface tension of liquids and improve wettability.

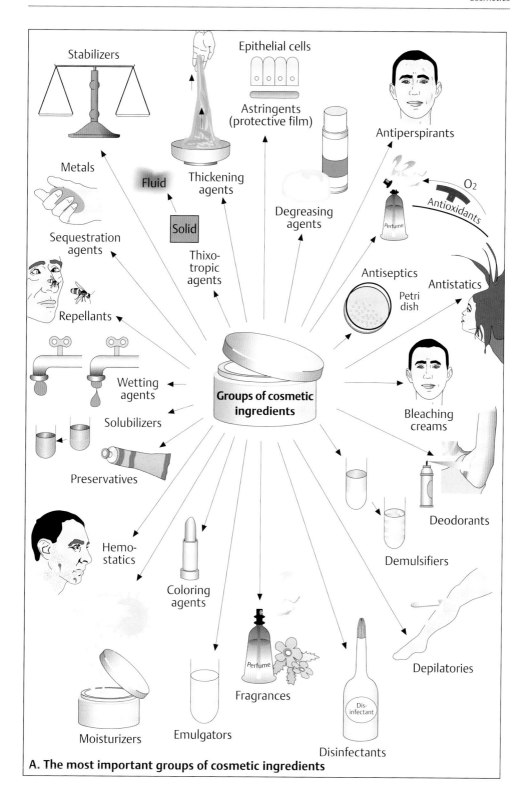

A. The most important groups of cosmetic ingredients

■ Cosmetic Changes in Color and Shape

Hair Coloring

Humans normally possess 80 000–120 000 hairs on their head. The hair shaft consists of the cortex (90 % keratin, a water-insoluble fibrous protein made of 18 amino acids with a high portion of cystine and proline) and the cuticle (keratinized dead cells) (**A1**). A hair grows 0.1–0.5 mm/day, reaching a total length of about 70 cm on average, and is shed every 4–6 years. A daily loss of 30–100 hairs is normal.

Temporary colors. These are water-soluble synthetic dyes (e.g., triarylmethane, acridine, cyanine) that adhere only loosely to the cuticle of the hair shaft. They are washed out within only one or two shampooing cycles (**A2**).

Semipermanent colors. Because of their small molecular size, they penetrate into the cortex of the hair shaft. They include *intrinsic* dyes, such as 2-nitro-p-phenylenediamine (red), 2-amino-4-nitrophenol (yellow), disperse blue 1 (blue), and *vegetable* dyes, such as henna, indigo, and extracts of chamomile or walnut. Semipermanent dyes take approximately 10 shampooing cycles to wash out, so the hair color lasts longer (**A3**).

Permanent colors. These require the following three components: a dye (e.g., p-phenylenediamine) that can penetrate easily into the hair shaft, a developer (oxidizer, e.g., hydrogen peroxide), and a coupler (e.g., resorcinol, p-amino-o-cresol). The large dye molecule forming inside the cortex becomes trapped in the hair shaft and cannot be washed out. Hence, the hair color is permanent (**A4**). Recoloring and decoloring are nevertheless possible (e.g., reductive decoloring with sodium dithionite or sodium thiosulfate). Improper handling of the substances (e.g., concentration, time of duration, temperature) or frequent dyeing (e.g., every month) may lead to hair damage (**B**) and skin irritation. Hence, permanent dyes should be allowed to grow out with the hair. Almost every desired shade of color is possible by combining hair dyes with different oxidation. Individuals with hypersensitivities or allergies to dyes (e.g.,

p-phenylenediamine or toluylenediamine) should use the less allergenic vegetable dyes.

Permanent Hair Waves

The shape, elasticity, and tensile strength of hairs depend on the structure and arrangement of the keratin molecules in the cortex (**A1**). Between the keratin molecules there are hydrogen bonds and salt links. These can be broken by water, thus making the hair stretchable. However, the original condition is regained after drying and renewed absorption of moisture. Permanent deformation of hairs (a permanent wave, or "perm") is only possible by breaking the disulfide bonds in the keratin (reduction) and subsequently forming new bonds (oxidation) (**C**). Reduction may be performed either by heat (steam), or hot alkaline solution (hot wave), or—as preferred today—with 12 % thioglycolic acid solution. Penetration into the hair shaft is facilitated by a swelling agent (e.g., urea). Acid perms (pH 5–6) are kinder to the skin than alkaline perms and are therefore preferred today. Hydrogen peroxide or sodium bromate is used for the subsequent oxidation. The newly formed disulfide bonds maintain the desired hairstyle for some time (**C**). As with hair dyeing, improper handling of perm preparations or insufficient protective measures may lead to damage to the hair (**B**), skin, or eyes.

Heat Protection and Sunscreen Agents

Heat protection agents. Firefighters and stokers are exposed to intense heat radiation. The newly developed heat protection agents contain admixed solids (e.g., titanium(IV) oxide) to reduce the heat by reflection (**D1**).

Sunscreen agents. These include fatty acid glycerides and antioxidants. They protect the skin from the harmful effects of ultraviolet (UV) radiation (**D2**) (see radiation, p. 294).

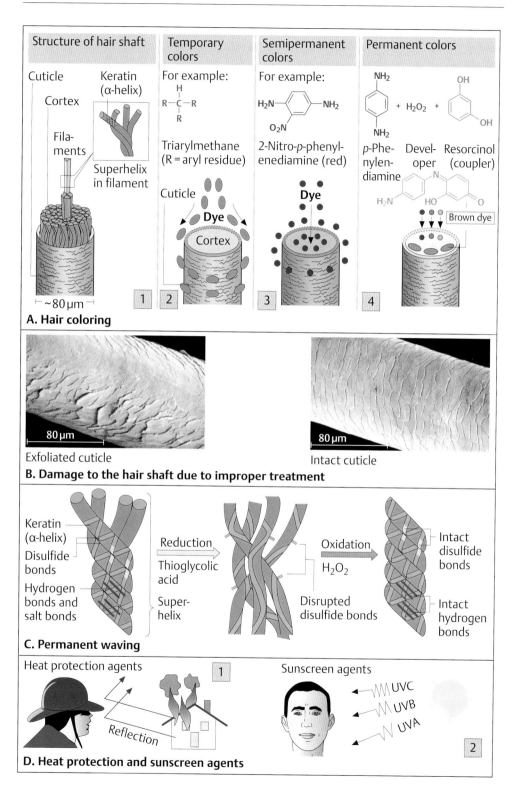

A. Hair coloring

Structure of hair shaft	Temporary colors	Semipermanent colors	Permanent colors

Structure of hair shaft:
Cuticle
Cortex
Keratin (α-helix)
Fila-ments
Superhelix in filament
~80 μm

Temporary colors:
For example:
$$R-\underset{\underset{R}{|}}{\overset{\overset{H}{|}}{C}}-R$$
Triarylmethane (R = aryl residue)
Cuticle
Dye
Cortex
1
2

Semipermanent colors:
For example:
2-Nitro-p-phenyl-enediamine (red)
Dye
3

Permanent colors:
$NH_2 + H_2O_2 +$
p-Phe-nylen-diamine
Devel-oper
Resorcinol (coupler)
Brown dye
4

B. Damage to the hair shaft due to improper treatment

80 μm
Exfoliated cuticle

80 μm
Intact cuticle

C. Permanent waving

Keratin (α-helix)
Disulfide bonds
Hydrogen bonds and salt bonds
Super-helix

Reduction
Thioglycolic acid

Oxidation
H_2O_2

Intact disulfide bonds
Disrupted disulfide bonds
Intact hydrogen bonds

D. Heat protection and sunscreen agents

Heat protection agents
Reflection
1

Sunscreen agents
UVC
UVB
UVA
2

■ Household Poisons

Basics. Earlier generations had to make do with only coarse soap, sand, and soda for the physically demanding task of keeping the house clean and well maintained, but now we have a huge arsenal of cleaning products to choose from. With the increasing use of synthetic surface-active agents (surfactants) since the late 1940s, the consumption of chemical products for household cleaning and maintenance has risen dramatically. According to estimates of the German Cosmetic, Toiletry, Perfumery and Detergent Association (IKW, *Industrieverband Körperpflege und Waschmittel e. V.*), the consumption of laundry detergents in industrialized countries amounts to about 10 kg per consumer per year.

Household chemicals are predominantly classified according to their applications (**A**).

Laws and Regulations

Unlike cosmetic ingredients, the ingredients of household cleaning products are not subject to an approval process. Cleaning products used in the household are controlled by national regulations for washing and cleansing agents. They specify the requirements for pollution control (e.g., biological degradability of surfactants) and the labeling of products.

The marketing of cleaning agents is also controlled by national regulations. These generally prohibit the marketing of any products that are dangerous to health when used according to their specification or foreseeable application. Nevertheless, household chemicals represent a potential danger, especially for small children, despite all precautions taken during selection of ingredients, labeling, and packaging. The specifications of regulations for dangerous substances therefore apply to those substances in household products that are classified as being potentially dangerous to health. These regulations are based, for example, on the 1996 EU guidelines for hazardous materials and formulations. The regulations for dangerous substances regulate the type and implementation of proper labeling (display of the relevant hazard symbols, warnings of special dangers, as well as safety recommendations) (**B, C**).

In the US, antimicrobial substances are regulated by the EPA only if pesticide claims of efficacy are made by the manufacturer; substances for which no claim of efficacy is made are not subject to regulation by the EPA. Typically, these are substances or mixtures of substances that are used to destroy or suppress the growth of harmful microorganisms, whether bacteria, viruses, or fungi on inanimate objects and surfaces. In the US market, the EPA currently has more than 5000 registered antimicrobial products which contain about 275 different active ingredients. These products are sold as sprays, liquids, concentrated powders, and gases. In the US, approximately one billion dollars each year are spent on a variety of different types of antimicrobial products. Nearly 60% of antimicrobial products are registered to control infectious micoorganisms in hospitals and other health care environments.

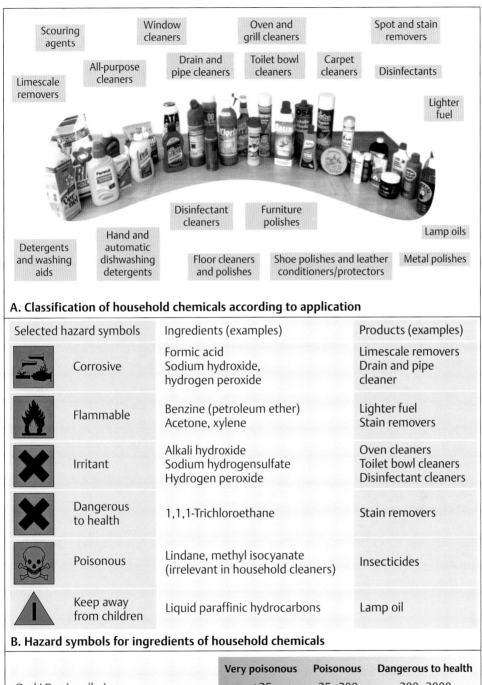

A. Classification of household chemicals according to application

Selected hazard symbols		Ingredients (examples)	Products (examples)
	Corrosive	Formic acid Sodium hydroxide, hydrogen peroxide	Limescale removers Drain and pipe cleaner
	Flammable	Benzine (petroleum ether) Acetone, xylene	Lighter fuel Stain removers
	Irritant	Alkali hydroxide Sodium hydrogensulfate Hydrogen peroxide	Oven cleaners Toilet bowl cleaners Disinfectant cleaners
	Dangerous to health	1,1,1-Trichloroethane	Stain removers
	Poisonous	Lindane, methyl isocyanate (irrelevant in household cleaners)	Insecticides
	Keep away from children	Liquid paraffinic hydrocarbons	Lamp oil

B. Hazard symbols for ingredients of household chemicals

	Very poisonous	Poisonous	Dangerous to health
Oral LD_{50} (mg/kg)	< 25	25–200	200–2000
Dermal LD_{50} (mg/kg)	< 50	50–400	400–4000
Inhalation LC_{50} (mg/L) (exposure time: 4h)	< 0.5	0.5–2.0	2–20

C. Toxicity of substances depending on the mode of uptake

◼ Health Hazards Posed by Household Chemicals

Over 13 million chemicals are known worldwide. About 600 000 new chemicals are still developed every year, and there are around 60 000 commonly used chemical substances with which the general public may come into contact. As ingredients of detergents, cleaners, and polishes, many chemicals are now being used in large quantities in every household, where they pose a potential hazard despite all preventive measures. Household products may cause adverse health effects and lethal poisoning in adults and, of particular concern, in small children.

The foundation for a realistic assessment of health risks posed by household chemicals is the knowledge gained from the system that analyzes and documents the data of poisoning cases reported to European poison control centers. Etiology and frequency of poisoning (in %) are similarly distributed in industrial countries. Using Germany (with many data) as an example, absolute numbers are given below.

Etiology of poisonings (A). Between 1990 and 2000, the German toxicology documentation center received a total of 10 507 reports on poisonings or suspected poisonings. However, this number suggests marked underreporting because, every year, the poison control centers receive 30 000 requests for information on poisonings by chemical substances. Despite obligatory notification, the number of poisonings or suspected poisonings in the private sector is estimated to be much higher than the number of reports actually received. Of the reports received during the period 1990–2000, 79% related to cases of accidental poisoning in the private sector; this was followed by poisonings after normal use (16%) and cases of suicide (11%).

Frequency of poisonings (B). Most reports in the period 1990–2000 related to adults (77%), and only 22% to children. Of the persons in question, 56% were male and 38% were female; the sex of the remaining individuals was not specified.

Range of noxious substances (C). Reports on poisonings with chemical products predominated (28%). They were followed by reports on basic materials (24%), pesticides (16%), and pharmaceuticals (14%).

Severity of poisonings (D). The health effects due to accidental poisoning are classified by their degree of severity (mild, moderate, severe, lethal). The majority of reports concerned only mild symptoms (67%), followed by moderate symptoms (24%). Cases with severe symptoms constituted only 8%, and those with lethal outcome about 1%.

Frequency of moderate and severe poisonings due to chemicals (E). Esters of phosphoric acid (insecticides) represent the group of substances posing the largest health hazard. They are followed by combustion gases, paints and paint thinners, liquid fuels, all-purpose cleaners, drain cleaners, disinfectants, herbicides, and technical solvents. Next in the frequency of severe cases are cleaning agents, because aspiration of surfactant-containing products creates special problems. Chemical burns caused by household cleaners have become very rare, especially in small children. More common are burns caused by industrial cleaners and liquid fuels, such as lamp oils.

In adults, poisonings with cleaning agents involve mainly drain cleaners and all-purpose cleaners. In children, drain cleaners, oven and grill cleaners, and automatic dishwasher detergents predominate.

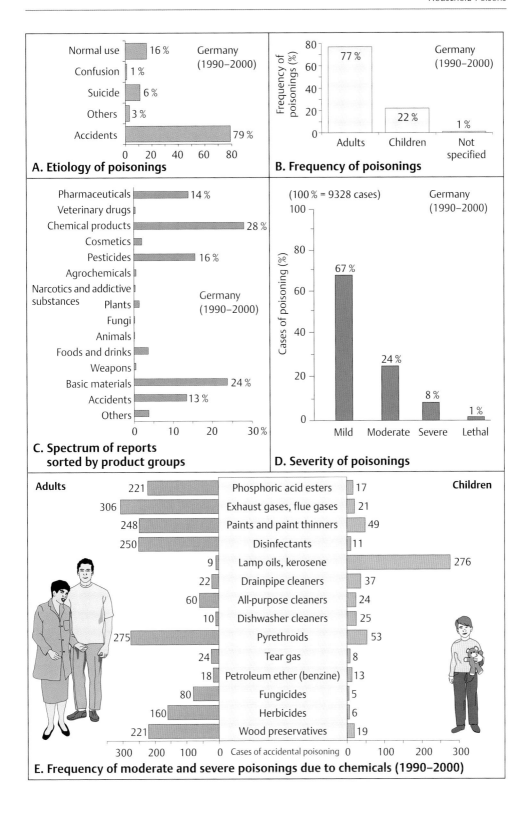

A. Etiology of poisonings

Normal use — 16 %
Confusion — 1 %
Suicide — 6 %
Others — 3 %
Accidents — 79 %

Germany (1990–2000)

B. Frequency of poisonings

Adults — 77 %
Children — 22 %
Not specified — 1 %

Germany (1990–2000)

Frequency of poisonings (%)

C. Spectrum of reports sorted by product groups

Pharmaceuticals — 14 %
Veterinary drugs
Chemical products — 28 %
Cosmetics
Pesticides — 16 %
Agrochemicals
Narcotics and addictive substances
Plants
Fungi
Animals
Foods and drinks
Weapons
Basic materials — 24 %
Accidents — 13 %
Others

Germany (1990–2000)

D. Severity of poisonings

(100 % = 9328 cases) Germany (1990–2000)

Cases of poisoning (%)

Mild — 67 %
Moderate — 24 %
Severe — 8 %
Lethal — 1 %

E. Frequency of moderate and severe poisonings due to chemicals (1990–2000)

Adults		Children
221	Phosphoric acid esters	17
306	Exhaust gases, flue gases	21
248	Paints and paint thinners	49
250	Disinfectants	11
9	Lamp oils, kerosene	276
22	Drainpipe cleaners	37
60	All-purpose cleaners	24
10	Dishwasher cleaners	25
275	Pyrethroids	53
24	Tear gas	8
18	Petroleum ether (benzine)	13
80	Fungicides	5
160	Herbicides	6
221	Wood preservatives	19

Cases of accidental poisoning

231

■ Toxicologically Important Ingredients of Household Chemicals

These ingredients are shown in (**A**). All other ingredients (e.g., enzymes, colors, fragrances, preservatives) play no important role in toxicology because of their low concentrations in household chemicals.

Surfactants

Surfactants are contained in almost all washing and cleaning agents and are the actual surface-active agents. They reduce the surface tension of water and increase its dirt-dissolving power. They are classified as follows:
- anionic surfactants (e.g., linear alkyl sulfonates)
- cationic surfactants (e.g., tetraalkyl ammonium chloride)
- amphoteric surfactants (e.g., betaines)
- nonionic surfactants (e.g., amine oxides).

Toxicity of surfactants. Common household cleaners, such as laundry and dishwashing detergents, and all-purpose cleaners, are generally of low systemic toxicity. Absorption of anionic and cationic surfactants through the skin is low. However, when in frequent contact with the skin, these surface-active substances may attack the lipid surface film of the skin. The resulting increase in permeability and loss of water may lead to roughness and scaling of the skin.

Severe skin lesions are likely only after intense and prolonged contact with concentrated solutions (**B**). Tolerance to surfactants declines from nonionic to anionic to cationic surfactants. When concentrated solutions of surfactants get into the eyes and are not immediately flushed out with water, eye damage is to be expected. Cationic surfactants, which are found mainly in fabric softeners, are absorbed to a lesser extent by the gastrointestinal tract when ingested, whereas anionic and nonionic surfactants are absorbed to a considerable extent. The symptoms after ingestion of surfactant-containing products reach from mild irritation of oral mucosa, esophagus, and stomach to chemical burns of the mucosae. These effects usually occur only after ingestion of powdered products (e.g.,

scouring agents). Mucosal irritation by liquid products (pH 7–9) is less severe than that caused by granulated products. Detergent builders (e.g., sodium silicates) present in powdered cleaning products make them more alkaline (pH 9.5–10.5); however, swallowing cleaners in powder form is difficult because of their consistency. In the case of liquid cleaners, it is rare for more than two sips to be ingested. (One sip is equivalent to 0.3–1.0 mL/kg BW.)

Major symptoms (B). Nausea, vomiting, diarrhea, and occasional abdominal pain occur after ingestion of highly alkaline, surfactant-containing cleaners. For adults, oral uptake of anionic surfactants is not dangerous as long as the amount is not greater than 1.0 g/kg BW. For children, the limit is 0.1–1.0 g/kg BW. Severe health effects may occur after inhalation of surfactant-containing dusts or aerosols, or after aspiration of surfactant-containing solutions. There is a risk of suffocation and development of pulmonary edema due to foam formation in the airways. Vomiting must not be induced after ingestion of foaming products, because there is a risk of aspiration and subsequent complications. Emptying of the stomach is only recommended if large quantities have been ingested, e.g., after attempted suicide with surfactant-containing cleaning products.

Therapy (B). After ingestion of surfactants, the immediate administration of fluid (e.g., water or tea) and a dose of antifoaming agent (dimeticon) within 1 h is sufficient in most cases.

Ingredients of household chemicals	Chemical substances (examples)	Products (examples)	Concentration of ingredients (%)
Surfactants	Sodium salts of fatty acids	Almost all washing and cleaning agents	0.5–40
Acids and acid salts	Citric acid Formic acid Hydrochloric acid Sodium hydrogen sulfate	Rinsing agents Limescale removers Urine stain removers Toilet bowl cleaners	10–30 10–90 5–40 5–40
Alkalis and alkali salts	Potassium hydroxide Sodium carbonate Sodium silicate Sodium hydroxide	Oven and grill cleaners Automatic dishwasher cleaners Blockage removers	2–10 5–30 20–60 25–90
Bleaching agents	Sodium perborate Sodium hypochlorite	Detergents Automatic dishwasher cleaners Drain cleaners	10–25 3–20 0–40
Solvents (water soluble)	Ethanol Isopropanol Butoxy ethanol	Floor cleaners Carpet cleaners Glass cleaners	0–10 5–25 0–30
Solvents (water insoluble)	Petroleum ether (benzine) Toluene Xylene	Furniture polishes Leather polishes Stain removers	0–50 5–80 95–100
Lamp oil (kerosene)	A mixture of paraffins (hydro-carbons C_{12}–C_{18})	Colored and scented lamp oils	99

A. Toxicologically important ingredients of household chemicals

Eye damage
Immediate flushing with water

Irritation of the mucosae in mouth, nose, throat, and esophagus

Risk of suffocation due to foaming and development of pulmonary edema following aspiration
Administration of dimeticon

Skin lesions on the hands
Prevention by avoiding concentrated solutions and wearing protective gloves

Drinking tea or water (dilution effect)

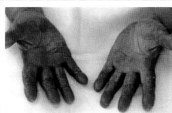

Skin lesions due to frequent contact with surfactants (rough hands)

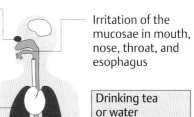

Gastrointestinal complaints (e.g., vomiting, diarrhea)
Restoring electrolyte balance

B. Toxicity of surfactants and treatment options in case of poisoning

Solvents (A)

Water-soluble organic solvents. These include *ethanol, isopropanol, acetone, and butoxyethanol* (also known as *butyl glycol* or *ethylene glycol monobutyl ether*). They are predominantly used as a 30% solution in cleaning and polishing agents for floors, carpets, and glass.

Depending on the amount taken up and the concentration of the alcohol component, the following symptoms may occur after ingestion of these solvents (ingestion of glass cleaners is common with adults): psychomotor stimulation, ataxia, disturbed balance, nausea and vomiting, acidosis, and localized irritation of the mucosae (see also addictive substances, p. 84). In children, small amounts of alcohols may lead to distinct signs of poisoning. Contamination of the eyes with neutral organic solvents may cause pain and, in case of substantial exposure, even corneal opacity. The damage is usually reversible because these substances are highly volatile.

Water-insoluble organic solvents. These include *hydrocarbons*, such as certain *aromatic compounds* (e.g., *benzene, toluene, xylene*). They are largely contained in special cleaning agents (stain removers, furniture polishes, and leather conditioners), which are toxic even in small amounts.

The clinical picture of acute poisoning is characterized by irritation of the mucosae and by narcotic and neurotoxic effects. Absorption of these solvents in the gastrointestinal tract is markedly increased by emulsifiers, which are often also present in cleaning products. Milk should not be administered, as it promotes absorption and increases the risk of vomiting. It is important to realize that there is a risk of aspiration, particularly in case of vomiting, which may lead to the development of chemical pneumonitis (e.g., after ingestion of benzene).

Alkalis (B)

The main active ingredients of alkaline cleaning products (e.g., all-purpose cleaners, alkaline disinfectant cleaners, automatic dishwasher detergents) include *sodium carbonate, sodium* and *calcium hypochlorite*, and *sodium silicate*. *Sodium* or *potassium hydroxide* is added to special products, such as drain and pipe cleaners, or oven and grill cleaners.

Toxicity. Irritation and burns to eyes, skin, and mucosa may occur, depending on the duration of exposure and the concentration of the alkaline cleaner. After ingestion of highly alkaline products (pH 10–13), considerable burns may occur to the upper intestinal tract resulting in necrosis (e.g., in case of automatic dishwasher cleaners containing a high portion of metasilicates). Furthermore, edema of the epiglottis may develop after vomiting.

First aid. The decisive first aid measure in case of alkali poisoning is the immediate administration of fluid (e.g., water). Induction of vomiting is contraindicated because of the risk of aspiration due to interference with the swallowing reflex. Gastric lavage would be too painful and is therefore not advised.

Acids (C)

The active ingredients of acid cleaning products (toilet bowl cleaners, acid disinfectant cleaners, limescale removers) are largely organic or inorganic acids, or acid salts such as *citrate, acetate, formate, hydrochloride, amidosulfate*, or *sodium hydrogen sulfate*.

Toxicity. Contact with acids may lead to irritation of skin, mucosa, and eyes. Ingestion of weak acids, such as hand dishwashing detergents or fabric softeners, may cause localized mucosal irritation and even vomiting and other gastrointestinal symptoms. Ingestion of highly acidic solutions may lead to burns of the upper intestinal tract followed by coagulative necrosis, and also to absorptive acidosis and, in case of organic acids, hemolysis.

First aid. As with other highly caustic substances, immediate administration of noncarbonated fluid is indicated.

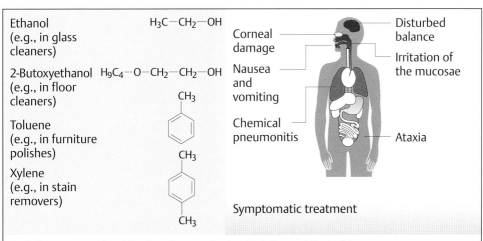

Ethanol (e.g., in glass cleaners) H_3C-CH_2-OH

2-Butoxyethanol (e.g., in floor cleaners) $H_9C_4-O-CH_2-CH_2-OH$

Toluene (e.g., in furniture polishes)

Xylene (e.g., in stain removers)

Corneal damage

Nausea and vomiting

Chemical pneumonitis

Disturbed balance

Irritation of the mucosae

Ataxia

Symptomatic treatment

A. Solvents contained in cleaning products: toxicity and first aid

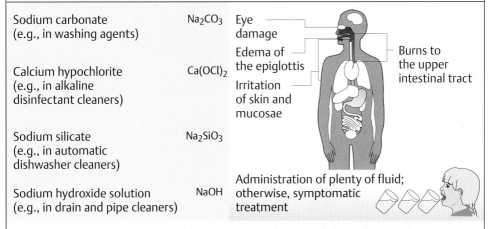

Sodium carbonate (e.g., in washing agents) Na_2CO_3

Calcium hypochlorite (e.g., in alkaline disinfectant cleaners) $Ca(OCl)_2$

Sodium silicate (e.g., in automatic dishwasher cleaners) Na_2SiO_3

Sodium hydroxide solution (e.g., in drain and pipe cleaners) $NaOH$

Eye damage

Edema of the epiglottis

Irritation of skin and mucosae

Burns to the upper intestinal tract

Administration of plenty of fluid; otherwise, symptomatic treatment

B. Alkaline substances contained in cleaning products: toxicity and first aid

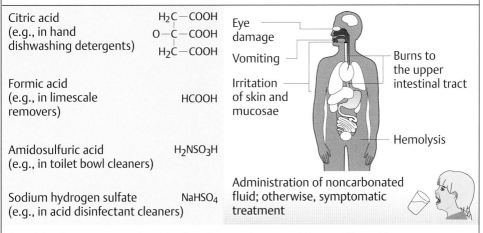

Citric acid (e.g., in hand dishwashing detergents)

Formic acid (e.g., in limescale removers) $HCOOH$

Amidosulfuric acid (e.g., in toilet bowl cleaners) H_2NSO_3H

Sodium hydrogen sulfate (e.g., in acid disinfectant cleaners) $NaHSO_4$

Eye damage

Vomiting

Irritation of skin and mucosae

Burns to the upper intestinal tract

Hemolysis

Administration of noncarbonated fluid; otherwise, symptomatic treatment

C. Acid substances contained in cleaning products: toxicity and first aid

Bleaching Agents (A)

Oxidizing agents. The bleaching activity of cleaners is due to *hypochlorite* or *peroxide* bleaching agents that also act as disinfectants (e.g., disinfectant cleaners). The following substances are used as peroxide bleaching agents: *hydrogen peroxide, sodium perborate,* and *salts of peroxysulfuric acid.* Substances used for bleaching generally irritate the skin and mucosa. Absorption takes place through the mucosa of the gastrointestinal tract, but not through intact skin. Theoretically, ingestion of products containing sodium perborate may lead to symptoms of boric acid poisoning as perborate is rapidly hydrolyzed in the body. This is to be expected only after uptake of unusually large quantities but not in case of accidental ingestion by children because they often ingest only small amounts. *Hydrogen peroxide* at the usual concentrations may cause oxygen emphysema of the mucosa. High concentrations of *sodium hypochlorite, isocyanuric acid and its salts,* and *sodium percarbonate* (e.g., in automatic dishwasher detergents, drain cleaners, spot-removal salts, or individual components of the building-block system for laundry detergents) may severely burn the mucosa. Toxic effects of hypochlorite-containing solutions are due to their high alkalinity and also to the strong oxidative effect of hypochloric acid: severe damage to the mucosa is possible at concentrations of more than 5%. Under no circumstances must hypochlorite-based cleaning products (e.g., alkaline disinfectant cleaners, dishwasher cleaners, or drain blockage removers) be used together with acid cleaners (e.g., toilet bowl cleaners, acetic acid, limescale removers, or rinsing agents based on citric acid). If they come into contact with each other, toxic *chlorine gas* is released, which is corrosive and irritates the mucosa. Heating of hypochlorite-containing cleaning solutions (e.g., by adding hot water) also results in chlorine gas formation. Should the occasion arise, administration of inhaled corticoid may become necessary. In case of dyspnea and persistent cough, treatment should be continued in hospital.

Reducing agents. The reducing agent in textiles decolorant is usually *sodium dithionite,* which is an irritant and dangerous to health. Dissolution of the dye of a fabric leads to the formation of *sulfur dioxide,* which irritates the eyes and airways.

Propellant Gases (B)

Certain products (e.g., oven and grill cleaners, floor foam cleaners, furniture polishes and leather conditioners/protectors) are marketed in metal or plastic spray containers together with a propellant gas. The propellant content is between 30% and 60% by weight (largely hydrocarbons, like *propane, butane, isobutane,* or *dimethyl ether*). These products are flammable and must not come into contact with open fire or heat. In gas ovens, some sprays (containing propane or butane) can form explosive mixtures with air. Inhalation of these gases may cause tickling of the throat and an urge to sneeze, vertigo, nausea, vomiting, and spasms of the intestinal and urinary tracts; the gases also irritate the airways. Accidental spraying into the eyes usually causes irritation. Providing fresh air alleviates the symptoms.

Lamp Oils (C)

Lamp oils are highly purified petroleum fractions (kerosene) or paraffin mixtures to which scents and colors have been added. Small children in particular may easily confuse the colored and perfumed liquids with fruit juice and drink them. Ingestions of lamp oils mainly leads to aspiration and the development of chemical pneumonitis, thus causing long-term damage. Perfumed paraffin-based lamp oils have been prohibited in the consumer sector throughout Europe and the United States since January 1, 2000.

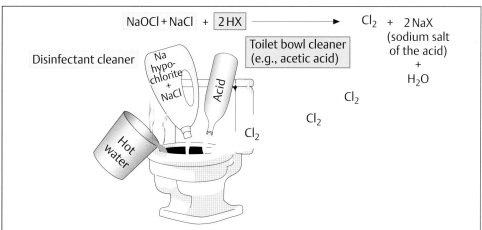

A. Formation of chlorine gas due to combined use of cleaning products

$$NaOCl + NaCl + 2HX \longrightarrow Cl_2 + 2NaX$$
(sodium salt of the acid) + H_2O

Disinfectant cleaner

Na hypo-chlorite + NaCl

Acid

Hot water

Toilet bowl cleaner (e.g., acetic acid)

Cl_2

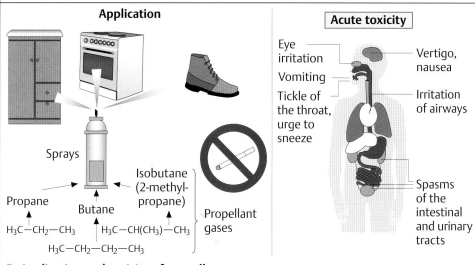

Application

Acute toxicity

Eye irritation
Vomiting
Tickle of the throat, urge to sneeze

Vertigo, nausea
Irritation of airways
Spasms of the intestinal and urinary tracts

Sprays

Propane
$H_3C-CH_2-CH_3$

Butane
$H_3C-CH_2-CH_2-CH_3$

Isobutane (2-methyl-propane)
$H_3C-CH(CH_3)-CH_3$

Propellant gases

B. Application and toxicity of propellants

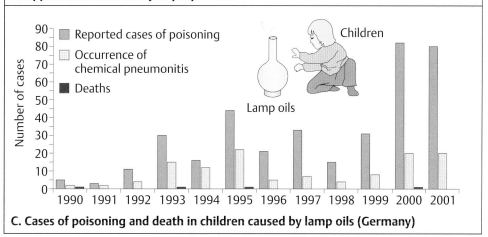

Number of cases

90 80 70 60 50 40 30 20 10 0

Reported cases of poisoning
Occurrence of chemical pneumonitis
Deaths

Children

Lamp oils

1990 1991 1992 1993 1994 1995 1996 1997 1998 1999 2000 2001

C. Cases of poisoning and death in children caused by lamp oils (Germany)

Chemical Warfare Agents I

History. Poisons were used in warfare even in antiquity. However, the misuse of poisons as weapons of mass destruction became only possible through the rapid development of chemistry in the 19th and 20th centuries, which widened the knowledge of their damaging effects and offered the possibility of large-scale production.

Modern chemical warfare was ushered in by the German chlorine gas attack in Flanders on April 22, 1915, although synthetic poisons had been used earlier in World War I by various parties.

Efforts to ban the use of poisons as warfare agents can be traced back to the ancient world. In modern times, the Hague Conferences of 1899 and 1907, the Geneva Protocol of 1925, and the Chemical Weapons Convention signatory conference held in Paris in 1993 led to a commitment to destroy stockpiles under international control. Despite the existing agreements on banning chemical warfare agents, chemical weapons were used during the Iran–Iraq war (1980–1988) and the Iraq–Kuwait conflict (1990–1991). The willingness to disobey the agreements, the slow disposal of hazardous materials, and the use of chemical warfare agents by terrorists (e.g., sarin and cyanide in Tokyo in 1995) show how important it is to keep up with the current state of knowledge about the dangers of these substances and means of protection, particularly as this knowledge is indispensable for achieving compliance with the international agreements on chemical weapons.

Classification (A). Chemical compounds that can be misused for warfare purposes are called chemical warfare agents. From the medical–toxicological point of view, their classification according to type and site of action is widely accepted, even though it is scientifically inaccurate (e.g., hydrogen cyanide is considered a blood agent, but blood constituents are not affected). We distinguish *incapacitating agents (hallucinogens), nerve agents, blister agents (vesicants), choking agents (lung irritants), blood agents,* and *tear gas (eye irritants, lacrimators).*

Uptake into the body. The uptake of chemical warfare agents occurs largely by inhalation and through the skin, and to a lesser extent by uptake in contaminated food and water.

Nowadays, the most important chemical warfare agents are liquids; they evaporate or disintegrate in the field at different rates (**B**). Substances that persist for days to weeks are called stationary agents, while those persisting only for minutes or hours are called nonstationary agents. Warfare agents buried or submerged in ammunition or containers retain their toxicity over many years or decades.

Protection against chemical warfare agents (C). Physical measures (e.g., wearing a protective suit) can prevent contact with the poison and its uptake into the body. For low-molecular-weight compounds (e.g., hydrogen cyanide, carbon monoxide), which are hardly adsorbed at all by activated charcoal, the filter of the gas mask must be specially impregnated in addition to containing the usual activated charcoal and aerosol filter portions.

A change of clothes and the use of decontamination agents prevent further uptake of poison into the body. Chemicals such as calcium chloride hypochlorite (chlorinated lime, CaCl [OCl]) are suitable for large-scale decontamination.

When the warfare agent has already entered the body, its effects can be alleviated or eliminated by administering specific antidotes (for individual substances, see the following pages).

Chemical warfare agents

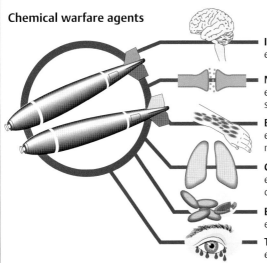

Incapacitating agents (hallucinogens)
e.g., 3-quinuclidinyl benzilate (BZ)

Nerve agents
e.g., tabun (GA), sarin (GB),
soman (GD), cyclosarin (GF), VX

Blister agents (vesicants)
e.g., mustard gas (HD) (synonym: yperite, S-Lost),
nitrogen mustard (HN-3) (synonym: N-Lost)

Choking agents (lung irritants)
e.g., phosgene (CG), diphosgene (DP),
chloropicrin (PS)

Blood agents
e.g., hydrogen cyanide (AC), chlorine cyanide (CK)

Tear gas (eye irritants)
e.g., chloroacetophenone (CN),
o-chlorobenzylidene malononitrile (CS)

A. Classification of chemical warfare agents

Chemical warfare agent	Weather conditions		
	15 °C	10 °C	–10 °C
	Dry, moderate wind	Rain, moderate wind	No wind, snow on the ground
Mustard gas	2–7 d	12–48 h	2–8 wk
Tabun	1–4 d	30 min–6 h	1–14 d
Sarin	15 min–4 h	15–60 min	1–2 d
Soman	2.5–5 d	3–36 h	1–6 wk
VX	3–21 d	1–12 h	1–16 wk

B. Retention time of liquid chemical warfare agents in the field

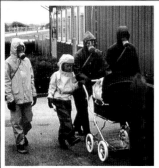
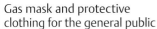
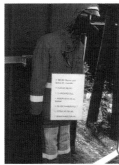
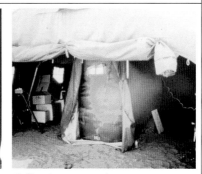

Gas mask and protective clothing for the general public

Special protective suit

Collective protection tent

C. Protective measures against chemical warfare agents

■ Chemical Warfare Agents II

Organophosphates

Nerve agents are organophosphorus compounds (see p. 200) that inhibit acetylcholine esterase (AChE).

Structure and properties. The basic structure was described by G. Schrader. *Tabun, sarin, cyclosarin, soman*, and *VX* are liquids of different volatilities and have hardly any noticeable odor (**A**).

Uptake and elimination. These highly lipophilic compounds are rapidly taken up by ingestion, inhalation, and through the skin and then distributed in the body. Their concentration in the blood rapidly declines due to spontaneous, ion-catalyzed enzymatic hydrolysis (A esterases: phosphoryl phosphatases) and binding to esterases (B esterases: choline esterases, carboxyl esterases).

Mechanism of action. Inhibition of AChE leads to accumulation of acetylcholine (ACh) in the area of cholinergic synapses, thus causing an uncontrolled increase in the activity of inner-vated organs and tissues, up to loss of function. The cholinergic stimulation affects also other neuronal systems (GABA, dopamine, gluta-mate), mainly in the central nervous system.

Symptoms. The clinical picture is characterized by peripheral muscarinic stimulation of exo-crine glands and smooth muscles, and also by nicotinic dysfunction of striated muscles and ganglia. The predominant effects on the central nervous system are inhibition of the respiratory drive and epileptiform stimulation with seiz-ures of the grand mal type (**B**).

Central and peripheral respiratory paralysis as well as bronchorrhea and bronchospasm may lead to death. Circulatory collapse may occur as a late complication.

Diagnosis and therapy. A distinct reduction in the activities of butyrylcholine esterase (plasma) and AChE (erythrocytes) indicates poisoning, with the latter reflecting more the activity in the synaptic cleft. Both enzyme activities should be assessed only in connection with the clinical symptoms. Adaptation processes at the receptors or treatment with atropine do not affect the activity.

Atropine (an antimuscarinic agent), *diazepam* (an anticonvulsive agent), and *oximes* (reactivators of AChE) are the first-line drugs for treatment (**C**).

Ventilation under increased oxygen pressure and cleaning of the bronchial tract can save lives.

Prognosis. If treatment is delayed and/or high levels of poison cause hypoxia, complicated reactions and adverse health effects may occur some time after exposure has occurred.

The "intermediary syndrome," characterized by weakness in neck muscles and auxiliary respiratory muscles, has been described for soman poisoning in dogs.

Occurrence of peripheral neuropathy 1–2 weeks after the poisoning is unlikely in humans. So far, it has only been described in chickens exposed to extremely high doses of tabun and soman.

There is no evidence that sarin and VX are teratogenic or mutagenic.

Nerve agents 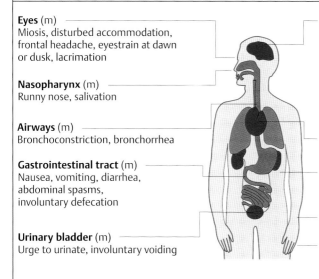	Oral LD$_{50}$ (mg/kg; humans)	Dermal LD$_{50}$ (mg/kg; humans)	Oral LD$_{50}$ (mg/kg; rat)	Volatility (mg/L; 20°C)	Inhalation LCt$_{50}$ (mg × min/m^3; humans, resting)
Tabun $(H_3C)_2N-\overset{\overset{O}{\|}}{P}-OC_2H_5$ with CN	5	12.6	300	3.7	0.6
Sarin $(H_3C)_2CH-O-\overset{\overset{O}{\|}}{P}-CH_3$ with F	0.14	24	100	1.1	11.3
Soman $(H_3C)_3C-\overset{\overset{CH_3}{\|}}{CH}-O-\overset{\overset{O}{\|}}{P}-F$ with CH$_3$	0.14	15	70	0.4	10
VX $H_3C-\overset{\overset{OC_2H_5}{\|}}{\underset{O}{P}}-S-CH_2-CH_2-N\overset{CH(CH_3)_2}{\underset{CH(CH_3)_2}{}}$	0.07	0.04	36	0.1	0.01

A. Toxicological and physical data of several nerve gases

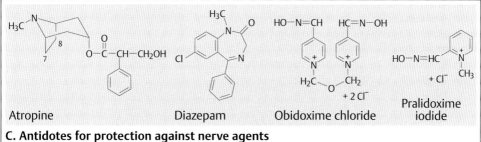

B. Acute toxicity of nerve agents

Eyes (m)
Miosis, disturbed accommodation, frontal headache, eyestrain at dawn or dusk, lacrimation

Nasopharynx (m)
Runny nose, salivation

Airways (m)
Bronchoconstriction, bronchorrhea

Gastrointestinal tract (m)
Nausea, vomiting, diarrhea, abdominal spasms, involuntary defecation

Urinary bladder (m)
Urge to urinate, involuntary voiding

CNS
– Respiration (m):
  reduced respiratory rate, central respiratory paralysis
– Activity (m + n):
  restlessness, weakness, tremor, ataxia, epileptiform seizures
– Behavior (m + n):
  nightmares, insomnia, instability

Heart (m)
Bradycardia

Skeletal muscles (n)
Weakness, fasciculation, peripheral respiratory paralysis

Sympathetic ganglia (n)
Temporary increase in blood pressure

Skin (m)
Sudden sweating

(m)–muscarinic
(n)–nicotinic

Atropine   Diazepam   Obidoxime chloride   Pralidoxime iodide

C. Antidotes for protection against nerve agents

241

■ Chemical Warfare Agents III

Alkylating Agents

Some sulfur and nitrogen compounds contain chloroethyl groups; they are known as sulfur and nitrogen mustards and are classified as blister agents. These compounds and their derivatives are also used as cytostatic agents.

Structure and properties (A). These alkaline agents are slowly evaporating liquids with a strong odor; e.g., dichlorodiethyl sulfide (sulfur mustard; S-Lost) smells of garlic or mustard, while nitrogen mustards (N-Lost) smell of fish.

Uptake and elimination. Mustards are highly reactive, lipophilic compounds that are readily taken up by all three pathways (ingestion, inhalation, and through the skin). They are quickly distributed in the body, bound to various compounds, and then rapidly eliminated. In the urine, mainly glutathione conjugates and the metabolite thiodiglycol are found.

Mechanism of action. In aqueous media, the chloroethyl groups react to form thiiranium-1,1-dioxide ions or aziridinium ions, which have a high affinity for nucleophilic centers. The amino, sulfhydryl, hydroxyl, carboxyl, phosphate, and imidazole groups of various molecules can be alkylated in this way. Every chloroethyl group may react, thus generating di- and trifunctional alkylations and crosslinks. Systemic toxicity is most likely due to alkylation of DNA, with particularly high affinity for guanine. With higher doses or concentrations, the binding to other molecules increases, resulting in binding of proteins and inhibition of the energy metabolism. These mechanisms may predominate at the sites of localized lesions.

Symptoms (B). Exposure to mustard agents typically goes unnoticed, although the odor may be observed. There is a symptom-free interval of several hours (or minutes, if the eyes have been exposed) inversely proportional to the dose or concentration. The maximum manifestation of acute damage is usually only found after 3–4 days. All tissues that have been exposed to the poison are affected.

Diagnosis and treatment. Diagnosis is based on the patient's history and also on the characteristic course and clinical picture of the poisoning. Detection of metabolites in the urine can be helpful.

Cooling preparations (powder, calamine lotion) help the itching of the skin. Skin lesions should be kept sterile and moist. The eyes should be flushed regularly. Atropine helps to prevent adhesions in the eyes, and antibiotics control infections. Regular bronchial lavage is indicated if there is pseudomembrane formation. It is essential to replenish electrolytes and water if there is diarrhea.

Prophylactic administration of antibiotics is controversial because it promotes microbial resistance, but targeted antibiotic treatment is often inevitable (**C**).

Prognosis. Both delayed development of lesions and delayed healing are characteristic. Necrotic areas reaching into the subcutis require weeks or months to heal.

Blister agent	Oral LD$_{50}$ (mg/kg; humans)	Dermal LD$_{50}$ (mg/kg)	Inhalation LCt$_{50}$ (mg × min/m^3)	Volatility (mg/L; 20°C)
$S(CH_2-CH_2-Cl)_2$ 2,2'-Dichlorodiethylsulfide (HD)	–	40–60	1500	0.625
$H_3C-CH_2-N(CH_2-CH_2-Cl)_2$ Ethyl(2,2'-dichlorodiethyl)amine (HN-1)	–	–	–	1.59
$H_3C-N(CH_2-CH_2-Cl)_2$ Methyl(2,2'-dichlorodiethyl)amine (HN-2)	–	15	1500	2.58
$Cl-CH_2-CH_2-N(CH_2-CH_2-Cl)_2$ 2,2',2''-Trichlorotriethylamine (HN-3)	2	15	20 mg/m^3 (20 min)	0.07

A. Toxicological, physical, and chemical data of blistering agents

Acute toxicity

Chronic toxicity

Eyes
Conjunctivitis, corneal clouding, photophobia, corneal erosion

Neurosis, depression, personality disorder

Airways
Cough, bronchitis, pseudomembrane, bronchial necrosis, pneumonia

Conjunctivitis

Bronchial spasms, bronchial cancer

Gastrointestinal tract
Nausea, vomiting, diarrhea

Chronic gastritis

Skin
Itching, redness, swelling, blistering, necrosis, pain

Pigment disorder of the skin, skin cancer, Bowen disease

Leukemia

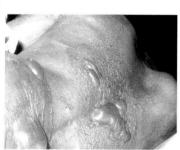

Lesions on the back caused by sulfur mustard

Systemic symptoms
Nausea, vomiting, fever, fatigue, leukopenia, thrombocytopenia

B. Toxicity of alkylating agents, such as blistering agents

Eyes:

Skin:

Lungs:

Gastrointestinal tract:

Sterile paraffin jelly, eye ointment, atropine eye drops

Cooling lotion/ powder, sterile moist compression

Codeine, cleaning of the bronchial tract, antibiotics

Replenishing of electrolytes and fluid

C. Treatment of poisoning with alkylating agents

■ Chemical Warfare Agents IV

Arsenic-Containing Compounds

Some trivalent dihalogenated organoarsenic compounds were used as blistering agents in World War I. Lewisite (2-chlorovinyldichloroarsine) (**A**) has not so far been used in warfare, although several countries have large stockpiles.

Monohalogenated arsenic compounds are also of military importance. Their primary effect is an intense, but reversible, stimulation of the mucosa associated with nausea and vomiting. These compounds are therefore classified as nasopharyngeal irritants. For arsenic toxicity, see p. 162.

Structure and properties. In the following sections, lewisite is described as an example.

Uptake and elimination. Lewisite is lipophilic and is rapidly taken up by ingestion, inhalation and through the skin. In aqueous media, it is quickly hydrolyzed to form the more lipophilic and similarly toxic oxide. Maximum accumulations of arsenic (5–7 times the concentration in the blood) have been found in the lungs, liver, kidneys, and the skin of rabbits about 4 h after administration of lewisite, and in the central nervous system and testes after 2–14 h (at about the same concentration as in the blood).

Mechanism of action. Lewisite and its oxide rapidly react in the tissues with molecules with sulfhydryl groups, preferentially at adjacent or nearby sites. Reaction with reduced lipoic acid in the pyruvate or ketoglutarate dehydrogenase complex leads to inhibition of the citrate cycle and energy metabolism. This may result in the inhibition of gluconeogenesis, thus leading to terminal hypoglycemia and increased pyruvate concentration in the blood. Inhibition of the β-oxidation of fatty acids has also been described.

Symptoms. With sufficient concentrations, lesions develop in all affected areas of skin and mucosa and other tissues are also damaged (**B**). The development and healing of skin lesions occurs much faster than with mustard agents (**C**).

The uptake of only 2 mL of lewisite through the skin may cause lethal poisoning in humans.

Therapy. Dithiols with adjacent sulfhydryl groups bind trivalent arsenic compounds (see arsenic, p. 162; for British antilewisite (BAL), see p. 176). Symptomatic topical and systemic treatments are the same as described for lesions caused by mustard agents, see p. 242). Timely administration of high doses of glucocorticoids is indicated because of the risk of toxic pulmonary edema.

Prognosis. With timely treatment, the prognosis is usually good, but deep skin lesions heal very slowly. The mutagenic and teratogenic effects of arsenic are undisputed. Studies have not revealed any evidence of carcinogenic effects (see also arsenic, p. 162).

Hydrogen Cyanide

Its high toxicity, high vapor pressure at room temperature (boiling point 26 °C), and immediate effect on the body resulted in the use of hydrogen cyanide (HCN) as a chemical weapon in World War I.

HCN and cyanide salts are widely used in industry (metal working) and in laboratories. (For toxicology of HCN, see p. 140.)

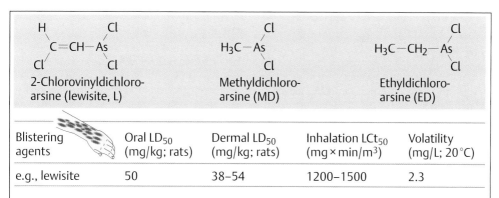

Blistering agents	Oral LD$_{50}$ (mg/kg; rats)	Dermal LD$_{50}$ (mg/kg; rats)	Inhalation LCt$_{50}$ (mg × min/m^3)	Volatility (mg/L; 20 °C)
e.g., lewisite	50	38–54	1200–1500	2.3

A. Properties and toxicity of lewisite and its derivatives

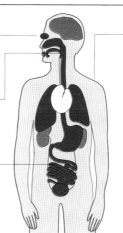

Eyes
Irritation, blepharospasm, corneal clouding, photophobia, corneal erosion

Airways
Irritation, cough, burning, pseudomembrane, bronchial necrosis, toxic pulmonary edema

Gastrointestinal tract
Nausea, vomiting, colics, diarrhea

 Carcinogenic and teratogenic

Skin
Irritation, burning, redness, swelling, blistering, necrosis

Systemic symptoms
Nausea, vomiting, weakness, petechiae, edema, toxic shock, damage to liver, kidneys, and brain, paresthesia, disturbed coordination

B. Acute toxicity of lewisite

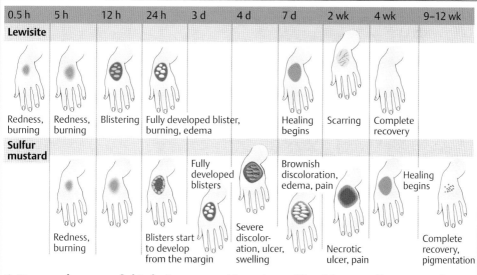

0.5 h	5 h	12 h	24 h	3 d	4 d	7 d	2 wk	4 wk	9–12 wk

Lewisite
Redness, burning — Redness, burning — Blistering — Fully developed blister, burning, edema — Healing begins — Scarring — Complete recovery

Sulfur mustard
Redness, burning — Blisters start to develop from the margin — Fully developed blisters — Severe discoloration, ulcer, swelling — Brownish discoloration, edema, pain — Necrotic ulcer, pain — Healing begins — Complete recovery, pigmentation

C. Temporal course of skin lesions caused by a drop of lewisite or sulfur mustard

■ Chemical Warfare Agents V

Lung Irritants

Poisons that damage the lungs, such as phosgene ($COCl_2$) and chlorine gas (Cl_2), played a major role as choking agents in World War I. They were responsible for around 80% of all casualties caused by chemical weapons. Their importance as warfare agents subsequently declined as a result of the development of more toxic, percutaneously acting agents. However, they still pose a risk in industry and trade (see household poisons, p. 236).

Hallucinogens

Currently, the most important incapacitating agents are central antimuscarinic agents (e.g., quinuclidinyl benzilate, BZ).

Under field conditions, they cause difficulty in concentration, misperception of sensory stimuli, bradykinesia, and—at higher concentrations ($> 10\,\mu g/kg$)—hallucination and delirium with peripheral antimuscarinic symptoms (e.g., tachycardia, heat accumulation, dry mouth, impaired vision) (**A**).

The effects may last 24 h or longer. Physostigmine is used as an antidote.

Eye Irritants

The most important representatives are ω-chloroacetophenone (CN) and o-chlorobenzylidene malononitrile (CS). In many countries, these lacrimatory agents (tear gas) are also used for self-defense and riot control (**B**). They are primarily taken up by inhalation. Little is known about the metabolism of CN; CS is largely metabolized in the liver.

Their mechanisms of action have not been established. CS and CN alkylate nucleophilic compounds (S_N2 type), preferentially those with thiol and amino groups. The main symptom of exposure is intense stimulation of the mucosae (eyes, nasopharyngeal space).

High concentrations cause headache (mucosal swelling of the sinuses), nausea and—in closed spaces—toxic pulmonary edema. Blisters develop preferentially on moist skin. Spray from gas cartridges at short range may lead to severe eye damage, even blindness (**C**).

Allergies and contact dermatitis have been described for CN and CS.

There is no evidence that these substances are carcinogenic, mutagenic, or teratogenic in humans. At cytotoxic doses, positive findings have been described sporadically; however, it should be noted that there has been little research into the effects of CN.

Herbicides

Various herbicides designed for civilian use have also been used in warfare, e.g., 2,4-dichlorophenoxy acetic acid (2,4-D), 2,4,5-trichlorophenoxy acetic acid (2,4,5-T), picloram, and cacodylic acid. The contamination of 2,4,5-T with highly toxic dioxins, which was detected only later, led to much personal injury when it was used as a defoliant during the Vietnam War (Agent Orange; see also biocides, p. 206, and PCBs, p. 114).

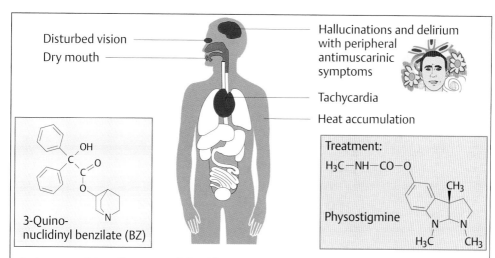

Disturbed vision

Dry mouth

Hallucinations and delirium with peripheral antimuscarinic symptoms

Tachycardia

Heat accumulation

3-Quino-nuclidinyl benzilate (BZ)

Treatment:

$H_3C-NH-CO-O$

Physostigmine

A. Acute toxicity of quinonuclidinyl benzilate (BZ)

	Eye irritants	Inhalation LCt_{50} $(mg \times min/m^3)$	Threshold (mg/m^3)	Volatility $(mg/L; 20\,°C)$
ω-Chloroacetophenone (CN)		4000–11000	0.15–0.4	105
o-Chlorobenzylidene malononitrile (CS)		25000	0.004	0.31–0.7

B. Properties and toxicity of the eye irritants CN and CS

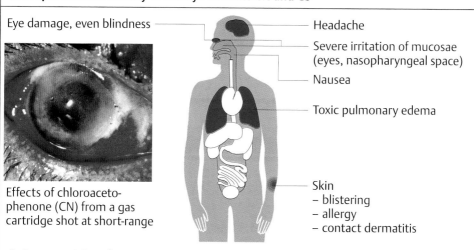

Eye damage, even blindness

Headache

Severe irritation of mucosae (eyes, nasopharyngeal space)

Nausea

Toxic pulmonary edema

Skin
– blistering
– allergy
– contact dermatitis

Effects of chloroaceto-phenone (CN) from a gas cartridge shot at short-range

C. Acute toxicity of irritants

■ Biological Warfare Agents I

Biological weapons are specific application devices (e.g., bomb, spraying device, letter bomb) (**A**) that release biological warfare agents (**B**). Biological warfare, as defined by the United Nations in 1969, is the use of any living organism or infective material derived from them (toxins) to cause disease or death in humans, animals, or plants and used specifically for this reason. Biological warfare agents are produced for *nonpeaceful* purposes. The "dirty dozen" (see **A** on p. 251) includes particularly dangerous pathogens and toxins. Apart from these, several other pathogenic human and animal viruses (**C, D**), bacteria, fungi, and toxins may be used for biological warfare. The release of highly virulent biological warfare agents puts the population at great risk and may reach the dimension of an international or national catastrophe. Biological weapons are therefore weapons of mass destruction. For example, the United Kingdom tested the anthrax bacillus on the Hebridean island of Gruinard in 1942; as a result, the island has been a restricted area for almost 50 years. The Soviet Union experimented with anthrax as well: 79 workers at a microbiological military facility near Yekaterinburg were infected with anthrax during a workplace accident in April 1979, and 68 of them died. To ban the threat of biological warfare, more than 170 states are currently signatories to the *Biological and Toxin Weapons Convention (BTWC)* of 1972. The convention prohibits the development, production, and stockpiling of biological weapons and toxin weapons. However, the situation has changed recently, and it is feared that biological weapons may be used in terrorist attacks (bioterrorism).

Recognizing the Release of Biological Weapons

So that a biological threat may be recognized immediately, national and international surveillance systems have been established which register outbreaks of rare diseases and sound the alarm when the release of a biological warfare agent is suspected. Nevertheless, the following peculiar features should lead one to suspect a bioterrorism attack:

- Sudden occurrence of diseases with similar symptoms.
- High incidence of rapidly progressing, refractory, and deadly diseases.
- Absence of typical host reservoirs and vectors.
- No endemic or enzootic occurrence of the disease; outbreak outside the usual season.
- No accidental release of pathogens or toxins.
- Spread of the disease in the direction of prevailing winds; special demographic distribution.

The release of biological warfare agents is usually quiet, odorless, and invisible, i.e., it is not perceived by the human senses. Usually the agents are released as aerosols (small droplets or particles suspended in air) which can easily enter the lungs. Currently, there are no early warning systems announcing the release of biological warfare agents. Despite considerable technical advances, the unequivocal detection of biological warfare agents is very difficult and is left to specialized laboratories. To prevent or contain an epidemic, the following measures are essential in the event of a bioterrorist attack:

- Report suspicious cases of disease immediately to public health authorities.
- Supply appropriate personal protection equipment immediately to medical staff and patients (protection against secondary contamination).
- Decontaminate exposed individuals immediately (remove clothes). Disinfect surfaces and materials regularly.
- Closely monitor and, if necessary, quarantine all individuals who have been exposed without protection, as they are at risk of contracting the disease.
- Administer protective vaccination (e.g., against smallpox) or postexposure chemoprophylaxis (e.g., against plague), if necessary.
- Isolate and treat diseased individuals in special hospital facilities.

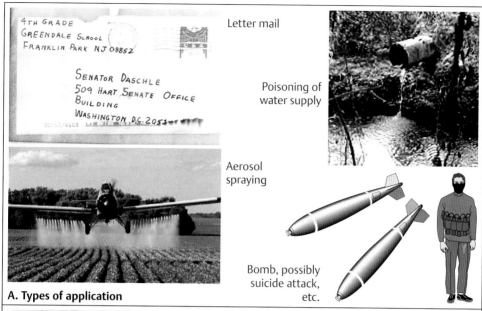

Letter mail

Poisoning of
water supply

Aerosol
spraying

Bomb, possibly
suicide attack,
etc.

A. Types of application

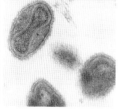

Viruses (< 0.5 µm)

Bacteria (> 1 µm)

Fungi (> 10 µm)

Biohazard logo

B. Types of pathogens

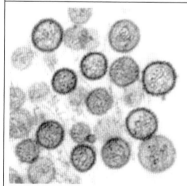

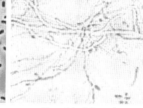

Structure of paramyxoviruses

Polymerase

Fusion protein

HN* protein

Matrix protein

Nucleocapsid and
(−)ssRNA** genome

* Hemagglutinin-neuraminidase protein
** Negative-sensed, single-stranded RNA

Electron micrograph of SNV particles.
Hantaviruses are enveloped single-
stranded RNA viruses. These rodent-borne
pathogens cause hantavirus pulmonary
syndrome (HPS) and hemorrhagic fever
with renal syndrome (HFRS).

**C. Sin nombre virus (SNV) of the genus
Hantavirus (family: Bunyaviridae)**

After incubation of less than 2 weeks, Nipah virus
disease begins in humans with acute encephalitis
accompanied by fever, headache, and vertigo. Early
on, the CSF shows abnormal signs of viral infection in
75 % of patients. Coma rapidly sets in within 24 to 48 h.

**D. Structure of Nipah virus
(family: Paramyxoviridae)**

■ Biological Warfare Agents II

Although bacteria, rickettsia, viruses, fungi, and toxins have very different characteristics, they share certain properties that facilitate their potential use as biological warfare agents. They can be dispersed as aerosols with a particle size of 1–5 µm, which facilitates deep penetration into the alveoli of the lungs. Uptake by ingestion of contaminated food is also possible, and penetration through the skin is possible in rare cases (e.g., the trichothecene mycotoxin T-2). So far, biological warfare agents have been naturally occurring organisms or toxins. However, genetic engineering, microencapsulation, or nanotechnology may lead to new, yet unknown types of pathogens. It is feared that the genetic manipulation of known pathogens could give rise to pathogens with increased virulence, resistance to therapeutic agents, increased stability in the environment, and changed antigenicity. The deployment of biological weapons is generally difficult to recognize, since delays in the onset of their effects frequently make it difficult to connect a particular disease outcome to a specific exposure. Furthermore, insufficient stability and storage properties, and sensitivity to certain weather conditions are major elements of uncertainty.

In addition to the "dirty dozen" (**A**), the US Centers for Disease Control and Prevention (CDC) have compiled a new list in which potential biological warfare agents are divided into three categories (A, B, and C) according to availability, mortality rate, risk of transmission, and treatment options (**B**).

Category A. The biological warfare agents of this group are rare in the United States. They represent a high national risk, since they are easily distributed or transmitted from person to person and have high mortality rates. They may cause widespread social panic and require special security preparations. These diseases (or pathogens, toxins) include anthrax (*Bacillus anthracis*), botulism (*Clostridium botulinum*), plague (*Yersinia pestis*), smallpox (*Variola major*), and viral hemorrhagic fevers (e.g., Ebola, Lassa, Marburg).

Category B. The biological warfare agents of this group are comparatively easy to distribute and result in moderate morbidity rates and low mortality rates. They require an increase in the diagnostic capacity of the CDC, or corresponding international institutions, and the installation of a surveillance system. These diseases (or pathogens, toxins) include brucellosis (*Brucella* sp.), ε-toxin poisoning (*Clostridium perfringens*), enteropathogens (e.g., *Salmonella* sp., *E. coli* O157:H7, *Shigella*), ornithosis (*Chlamydia psittaci*), Q fever (*Coxiella burnetii*), ricin toxin poisoning (*Ricinus communis*), intestinal diseases (*Staphylococcus* enterotoxin B), typhus (*Rickettsia prowazekii*), viral encephalitis (Venezuelan equine encephalitis viruses), and water safety threats (e.g., *Vibrio cholerae* and *Cryptosporidium parvum*).

Category C. The biological warfare agents of this group could possibly be used for mass distribution. They are characterized by high availability, easy production, and easy distribution. They have low morbidity and mortality rates but nevertheless have a huge impact on public health. Pathogens of this group include Nipah viruses or hantaviruses (see p. 249 **C, D**).

Diagnosis, detection, and treatment. It is essential for clinical diagnosis that physicians acquire specialized knowledge of the symptoms of diseases caused by biological warfare agents, as this is often not part of their professional training. Toxins and pathogens are detected by standard immunological methods (e.g., ELISA, immunofluorescence) or molecular biological methods (e.g., PCR). The required validated methods and suitably qualified personnel for detection, including the ability to carry out fine typing of pathogen isolates, are usually available only at highly specialized centers. Treatment of disease varies and depends on the biological warfare agents involved: it ranges from simple decontamination or disinfection to the administration of specific medications.

Pathogen	Transmission	Incubation period	Mortality rate (without treatment)	Therapy and prophylaxis
Smallpox *Orthopoxvirus variola* (variola virus)	Person to person	1–2 weeks	Up to 90%	Vaccination
Anthrax *Bacillus anthracis*	No direct transmission	1–6 days	Up to 80%	Antibiotic treatment
Plague *Yersinia pestis*	Person to person	1–3 days	90–100%	Antibiotic treatment
Tularemia (rabbit fever) *Francisella tularensis*	No direct transmission	2–10 days	Up to 60%	Antibiotic treatment
Brucellosis *Brucella* species	No direct transmission	2–3 weeks	Less than 5%	Antibiotic treatment
Q fever *Coxiella burnetii*	Person to person	9–40 days	Less than 2%	Antibiotic treatment
Glanders *Burkholderia mallei*	Person to person	10–14 days	Up to 50%	Antibiotic treatment
Encephalitis Encephalitis viruses	Person to person	1 week	Up to 50%	Antiviral treatment
Hemorrhage Hemorrhagic viruses	Person to person	4–21 days	Up to 100%	None
Ricin toxin *Ricinus communis*	No direct transmission	1 day	Up to 100%	None
Botulinum toxin *Clostridium botulinum*	No direct transmission	Up to 5 days	Up to 90%	Vaccination, antidote
Staphylococcus aureus toxin *Staphylococcus aureus*	No direct transmission	3–12 h	Up to 25%	None

A. The "dirty dozen" of biological warfare agents

Classification of biological warfare agents
as defined by the Centers for Disease Control and Prevention

A   B   C

- Easy to transmit
- High mortality
- Security problem

- Relatively easy to transmit
- Moderate mortality
- Easy to contain

- Easy to obtain
- Low mortality
- Difficult to transmit
- Easy to treat

B. Categories of biological warfare agents

■ Dental Restorative Materials I

Basics. Dental materials are classified according to their use (**A**):

1. *Direct restorative materials* are processed inside the patient's mouth (e.g., composites, amalgam, sealers).

2. *Indirect restorative materials* are fabricated outside the mouth (e.g., inlays, crowns, bridges, dentures).

3. *Auxiliary materials* are required for producing indirect restorative materials (e.g., impression materials, molding materials).

Composites (Plastics)

It was not until 1962 that the development of dental composites by R. Bowen opened the way for alternatives to amalgam fillings. Composites are synthetic polymers (**B**) consisting of an organic matrix into which inorganic filling materials are embedded. The monomers used for this purpose are usually (di)methacrylates (e.g., HEMA, TEGDMA, Bis-GMA). They can be divided into heavy *basic monomers* and light *comonomers*. The latter are included in the composites as diluting agents to facilitate processing of the viscous basic monomers. The composite matrix also contains photoinitiators or thermal initiators; in combination with suitable coinitiators or accelerators, they start the free radical polymerization of the methacrylates. Photostabilizers are added for color stability of the filling, and small amounts of inhibitors are added for adequate strength of the composites. In addition, composites may also contain other organic components, like softeners.

Inorganic filling materials consist of finely ground quartz or glass (macrofillers) and pyrogenic silicon dioxide particles (microfillers). The combination of macrofillers and microfillers results in hybrid composites. The admixture of pigments and heavy metal compounds makes it possible to produce different shades of color and to increase radio-opacity. Tight bonding of inorganic and organic phases is achieved through silanization of the filling materials by means of a polymerizable silane coupling agent. Provided in the form of a one-component system, the composite paste is directly filled into the cavity and hardened there by irradiation with white light.

Toxicity. The biological tolerance of composites creates some problems. This applies especially to the nerves of the dental pulp, since direct application of composites near the pulp may lead to pulpitis (**C**). Some studies on pulp damage by composite fillings have graded the effects from mildly damaging to severely damaging, depending on the composite. Possible causes include devitalization of the pulp (due to leaching of residual monomers and additives) and damage to the pulp (due to secondary caries caused by bacteria intruding into the cleft between filling and tooth and using the composite as a nutrient).

Saliva, as well as foods and beverages, may cause monomers and other composite ingredients to leach from the dental fillings, thus adding to normal abrasion and wear. Abraded particles less than 10 µm in size may even be inhaled and then enter the circulation via the lungs. Some composite ingredients have cytotoxic as well as allergenic effects. Allergies to synthetic polymers are more common than those to amalgam, and dentists are expecting a rise in allergies to certain composites. It is postulated that carcinogenic or mutagenic metabolites form when (co)monomers derived from dental fillings are degraded in the body.

Cast Gold

Gold alloys used for inlays also contain additives, such as copper, palladium, iridium, silver, and platinum. Allergic reactions to gold alloys have been known to occur (**D**).

Ceramics (Porcelain)

Porcelain-based inlays are secured with composites; at the interface with the tooth (dentin wound), synthetic polymers (see above) are required as an adhesive. The porcelain itself may contain small amounts of radioactive substances (**D**).

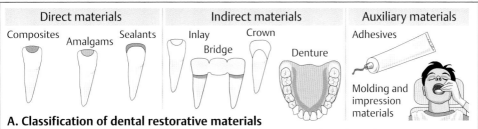

A. Classification of dental restorative materials

Direct materials	Indirect materials	Auxiliary materials
Composites, Amalgams, Sealants	Inlay, Crown, Bridge, Denture	Adhesives, Molding and impression materials

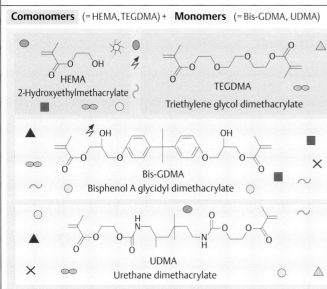

Comonomers (= HEMA, TEGDMA) + **Monomers** (= Bis-GDMA, UDMA)

HEMA
2-Hydroxyethylmethacrylate

TEGDMA
Triethylene glycol dimethacrylate

Bis-GDMA
Bisphenol A glycidyl dimethacrylate

UDMA
Urethane dimethacrylate

Other ingredients of composite fillings:

- photoinitiators (e.g., camphorquinone)
- thermal initiators (e.g., peroxides)
- accelerators (e.g., amines)
- photostabilizers (e.g., benzotriazoles)
- inhibitors (e.g., phenol derivatives)
- softeners (e.g., polyvinyl butyral)
- ground quartz
- silicon dioxide (silica)
- color pigments (e.g., iron oxide pigments, yttrium fluoride)
- silane coupling agents

B. Ingredients of dental composite fillings

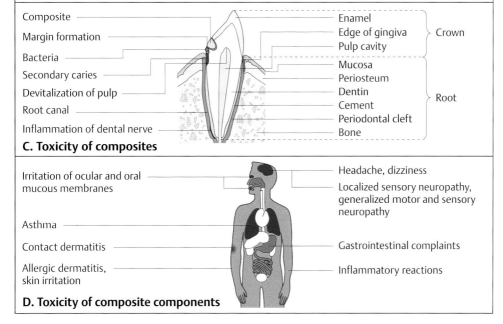

Composite
Margin formation
Bacteria
Secondary caries
Devitalization of pulp
Root canal
Inflammation of dental nerve

Enamel
Edge of gingiva — Crown
Pulp cavity

Mucosa
Periosteum
Dentin — Root
Cement
Periodontal cleft
Bone

C. Toxicity of composites

Irritation of ocular and oral mucous membranes

Asthma

Contact dermatitis

Allergic dermatitis, skin irritation

Headache, dizziness
Localized sensory neuropathy, generalized motor and sensory neuropathy

Gastrointestinal complaints

Inflammatory reactions

D. Toxicity of composite components

253

Dental Restorative Materials II

Amalgam

History and basics. In a Chinese manuscript dating from AD 659, Su Jing described a recipe for producing a silver–mercury paste. The word amalgam is derived from the Greek *amalos* for soft and *gamos* for combination. The oldest known amalgam filling was discovered in a molar of Princess Anna Ursula of Brunswick (1573–1601) excavated at Crailsheim in southern Germany (**B**).

There are frequent media reports about the health risks posed by amalgam fillings and the alleged threat to public health. Nevertheless, the toxicological assessment should be based on facts that are scientifically sound, namely:

1. the exposure to mercury derived from amalgam fillings

2. the contribution of this exposure to the total mercury load of the body

3. the comparison with current knowledge of toxicology and symptoms of mercury poisoning.

Dental amalgam contains mercury (Hg) and is prepared by mixing mercury with an alloy powder consisting of other metals, such as silver, copper, and zinc. The alloy–mercury ratio is 1 : 1.

Mercury exposure resulting from amalgam fillings. Amalgam fillings release mercury vapor (Hg^0) and mercury ions (Hg^{2+}) (**A**). The extent of exposure to Hg^0 from amalgam fillings can be determined by measuring the mercury concentration in the intraoral air ($0.2–5\,\mu g/m^3$). Chewing for just 10 min causes the mercury concentration to rise to $30\,\mu g/m^3$. Considering this increased release of Hg^0, the average absorption of mercury vapor by the pulmonary epithelium has been calculated to be $0.2–8\,\mu g/day$. Mercury ions are absorbed by the gastrointestinal tract at a rate of $0.5–6\,\mu g/day$ (**A**).

Total exposure of the body to mercury. In estimating the total mercury exposure of the body, the additional uptake of mercury with foods should be taken into account. In industrialized countries, an adult absorbs around $8\,\mu g/day$, depending on food intake (**C**). Mercury in foods is predominantly in the form of the highly toxic organic compound methylmercury (MeHg). Fatty fish have the highest methylmercury content (**D**). In countries with high fish consumption (e.g., Japan), people take up large quantities of mercury (**C**). This whole-body exposure, additional to that from amalgam, can be monitored by measuring the mercury levels in the blood (**A**).

Toxicology (A). According to documented cases of poisoning with mercury vapor in humans, the first signs of poisoning occur at about $2000\,\mu g/m^3$ air. The World Health Organization (WHO) has established a limit of $50\,\mu g/day$ for the total uptake of mercury, with no more than $33\,\mu g/day$ of this coming from organic mercury compounds. The critical amount of uptake of methylmercury with food, as specified by WHO, is $400\,\mu g/day$, and the WHO limit for mercury in the blood is $20\,\mu g/L$. Information from mass poisonings in humans has suggested that the first signs of methylmercury poisoning occur at mercury concentrations of more than $300\,\mu g/L$ blood.

Conclusions. 1. In principle, the use of mercury in the human body is not generally recognized as safe.

2. Amalgam fillings contribute to the total human exposure to mercury; the amount of mercury released is minute but measurable.

3. The amount of mercury released from amalgam fillings is not expected to be associated with mercury poisoning.

Dental fillings made of amalgam

		Number of amalgam fillings			Guidance values		First symptoms
		0–2	3–12	>12			
Hg^0 concentration in intra-oral air	$\mu g/m^3$	0.2	3–14	5–30		–	2000
Absorbed Hg^0	$\mu g/d$	0.2	5	8	–	–	–
Absorbed Hg^{2+}	$\mu g/d$	0.5	4	6	–	–	–
Absorbed Hg (food)	$\mu g/d$	8	8	8	–	–	–
Σ absorption $Hg^0 + Hg^{2+}$ + Hg (food)	$\mu g/d$	~9	~17	~22	WHO 50/33	Critical amount of MeHg 400	–
Hg concentration in the blood	$\mu g/L$	0.3	2	3	WHO 20	International value 50	300

A. Total mercury exposure of individuals with amalgam fillings

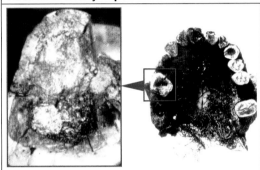

The oldest known amalgam filling in the maxilla of Princess Anna Ursula of Brunswick (1573–1601)

B. The oldest amalgam filling in the world

μg Hg/d

Mean mercury absorption from food in different countries

C. Mercury absorption from food

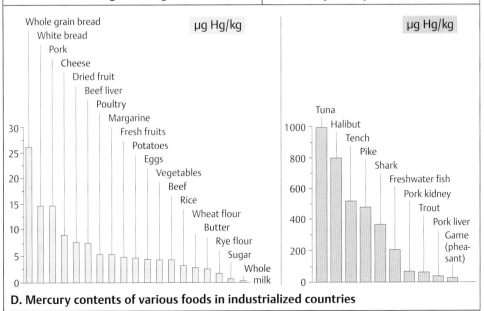

D. Mercury contents of various foods in industrialized countries

Animal Poisons (Zootoxins)

Basics. In Europe, the most common zootoxin poisonings are the result of bee or wasp stings. Poisonings due to exotic animals occur regularly because of the increasing numbers of poisonous animals kept in zoos or in an aquarium or terrarium in private households, and as a result of increasing international travel.

Venomous animals. These animals produce their poison in special tissues and use an active delivery system, such as a sting or fang. Venom apparatus is found in all classes of the animal kingdom. The venom is used for defense against predators and, predominantly, for catching prey.

Poisonous animals. These do not have a special venom apparatus but can store poison in their body. The poison is either produced by other organisms inhabiting the animal's body (e.g., dinoflagellates and bacteria) or is taken up through the food chain and from the environment, thus giving the animal a certain protection from predators. We humans experience the poisonous effects only at the end of the food chain after ingesting the toxin with our food (e.g., ciguatoxin and maitotoxin in fish, saxitoxin in shellfish; see also environmental toxicology, p. 62).

Toxinology is the science of toxic substances produced by plants, animals, and microbes. These include *poisons* (mixtures of various poisonous substances, such as the venoms of bees and snakes) and *toxins* (natural, chemically pure, and unambiguously defined substances that are poisonous, such as melittin and apamin in bee venom).

The chemical composition of zootoxins is usually complex. The ingredients include alkaloids, biogenic amines, glycosides, ketones, hydrocarbons, peptides, and proteins.

Venomous Marine Animals

Every year, these marine animals cause approximately 50 000 accidents to humans worldwide. To this may be added approximately 20 000 cases of poisoning per year that are due to the consumption of poisonous animals. Marine animals produce the most powerful zootoxins (e.g., saxitoxin, tetrodotoxin, palytoxin; see also p. 62).

Cnidarians (Cnidaria)

There are around 10 000 species of cnidarians, including jellyfish, corals, sea anemones, and hydras. Cnidarians have long tentacles equipped with nematocysts. Inside the nematocyst (**A**) is a long tube with a barbed structure at the end, containing a mixture of powerful toxins. The nematocysts explode in response to danger or when catching prey, and the toxin mixture is shot into the skin of the target. The poisons consist of proteins, including *cytolysins* (MW > 10 000), which damage the cell membrane and thereby interfere with the ionic currents, and *neurotoxins* (MW < 6000), which inactivate sodium channels, thus leading to continuous stimulation and, as a result, muscular paralysis.

Examples of species containing such toxins are the Portuguese man-of-war (*Physalia physalis,* **B**), the mauve stinger (*Pelagia noctiluca,* **C**), the box jellyfish (*Chironex fleckeri,* **D**), and the snakelocks sea anemone (*Anemonia viridis,* previously *Anemonia sulcata,* **E**).

Toxicity. In humans, contact with these poisons generally leads to local skin irritation. Allergic and anaphylactic reactions that are particularly dangerous for allergic individuals deserve special mention. In addition, the following symptoms may occur: severe pain, edema, contact dermatitis, urticaria, muscle spasms, circulatory insufficiencies, nausea, kidney failure, cardiovascular symptoms up to cardiac arrest or respiratory paralysis.

First aid. This includes immediate inactivation of any nematocysts still present in tentacles adhering to the skin. Here, the following measures have proved helpful: rubbing with household vinegar (5 % solution), baking powder (ammonium bicarbonate), magnesium sulfate solution, or, if nothing else is available, abrasion with sand.

Therapy. Application of analgesic lidocaine ointment is recommended; otherwise, the treatment is symptomatic.

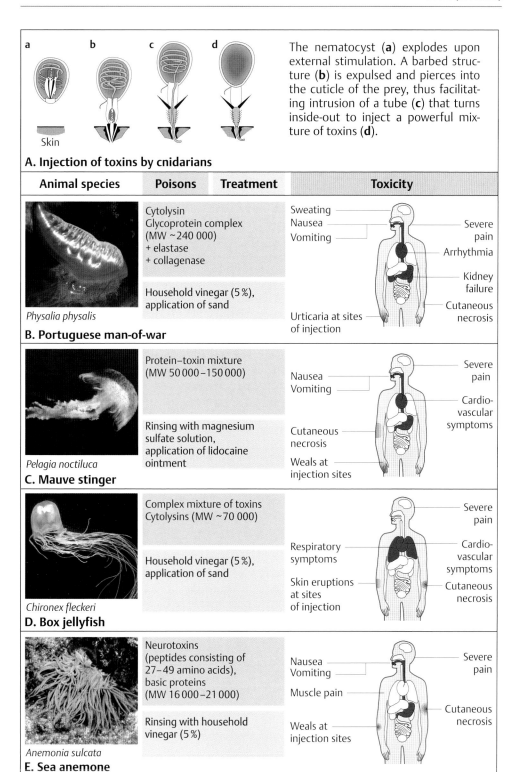

The nematocyst (**a**) explodes upon external stimulation. A barbed structure (**b**) is expulsed and pierces into the cuticle of the prey, thus facilitating intrusion of a tube (**c**) that turns inside-out to inject a powerful mixture of toxins (**d**).

A. Injection of toxins by cnidarians

Animal species	Poisons	Treatment	Toxicity
Physalia physalis **B. Portuguese man-of-war**	Cytolysin Glycoprotein complex (MW ~240 000) + elastase + collagenase / Household vinegar (5%), application of sand		Sweating, Nausea, Vomiting — Severe pain, Arrhythmia, Kidney failure, Cutaneous necrosis; Urticaria at sites of injection
Pelagia noctiluca **C. Mauve stinger**	Protein–toxin mixture (MW 50 000–150 000) / Rinsing with magnesium sulfate solution, application of lidocaine ointment		Nausea, Vomiting — Severe pain, Cardiovascular symptoms; Cutaneous necrosis; Weals at injection sites
Chironex fleckeri **D. Box jellyfish**	Complex mixture of toxins Cytolysins (MW ~70 000) / Household vinegar (5%), application of sand		Severe pain, Respiratory symptoms, Cardiovascular symptoms, Skin eruptions at sites of injection, Cutaneous necrosis
Anemonia sulcata **E. Sea anemone**	Neurotoxins (peptides consisting of 27–49 amino acids), basic proteins (MW 16 000–21 000) / Rinsing with household vinegar (5%)		Nausea, Vomiting — Severe pain, Muscle pain, Cutaneous necrosis, Weals at injection sites

Mollusks (Mollusca)

These include cone snails (Conidae) (**A**), which are much sought-after collector's items because of their rich coloring, but are also very dangerous. Although only a few of the 300 or so species are harmful to humans, the most beautiful ones are unfortunately also the most poisonous.

These snails have a poison gland and an arrow-like tooth through which they can inject poison into their target when sensing danger (e. g., someone touching the shell) or when catching prey. All snail poisons are proteins and may include up to 50 toxins, depending on the species. The main components are conotoxins (alkaline, stable peptides consisting of 13–29 amino acids). They are highly neurotoxic, block neuromuscular transmission, and inhibit the flow of sodium ions at the muscle cell membrane.

Toxicity. A sting by a snail frequently causes acute pain locally. The following symptoms may occur after around 20 min: numbness, difficulty in swallowing, impaired speech, muscular paralysis, and dyspnea. Because of paralysis of the respiratory muscles, humans may die within 5 h after injection of the poison.

First aid and therapy. No incision should be made at the site of the sting and no tourniquet should be applied. In case of respiratory failure, perform mouth-to-mouth resuscitation immediately. Further treatment is symptomatic.

Annelids (Annelida)

Annelid worms are found in all oceans. The bearded fireworm (*Hermodice carunculata*) (**B**) is a popular fishing bait, and careless handling frequently leads to poisoning in humans. Fireworms are a type of bristleworm (Polychaeta). They reach almost 40 cm in length and have groups of white bristles (chaetae) along each side, which are flared in defense. These bristles are hollow and filled with venom; they easily penetrate the skin. The poison is a mixture of proteins. The main component is glycerotoxin (MW ~ 300 000); it stimulates the release of neurotransmitters at the synapses.

Toxicity. Poisoning is characterized by burning pain at the site of contact, headaches, and vomiting.

Therapy. Treatment is usually not required.

Echinoderms (Echinodermata)

Echinoderms include sea cucumbers, sea urchins, and starfish. The crown-of-thorns starfish (*Acanthaster planci*) (**C**) has spines that, in humans, cause painful wounds upon contact and introduce venom at the same time. These spines are covered with tissue containing poison glands; this tissue remains in the wound and thus causes the poisoning. A glycoprotein toxin (MW ~ 25 000) and phospholipase A have been isolated from the mixture of poisons.

Toxicity. Nausea, vomiting, and cardiovascular symptoms are common.

Therapy. Treatment is usually not required.

Fish (Pisces)

Only around 200 out of more than 20 000 fish species can cause poisoning in humans. They either deliver their venom by bony fin rays connected to poison glands, or secrete poisonous substances upon contact. These poisons are exclusively for defense and largely represent mixtures of very labile proteins. Fish species with poisonous fin rays include stingrays (Dasyatidae), dogfish sharks (Squalidae), morays (Muraenidae), weaverfish (Trachinidae), surgeonfish (Acanthuridae), and scorpionfish (Scorpaenidae, e.g., the radial firefish, **D**).

Trunkfish (Ostraciidae) (**E**) secrete venom from glands in their skin (ichthyocrinotoxins, e.g., pahutoxin), and contact may lead to poisoning in humans. The poison is used for defense against predators; it also protects the skin from infections (antibiotic activity).

Toxicity. In humans, contact with fish poisons primarily causes allergic reactions.

Therapy. Treatment is usually not required.

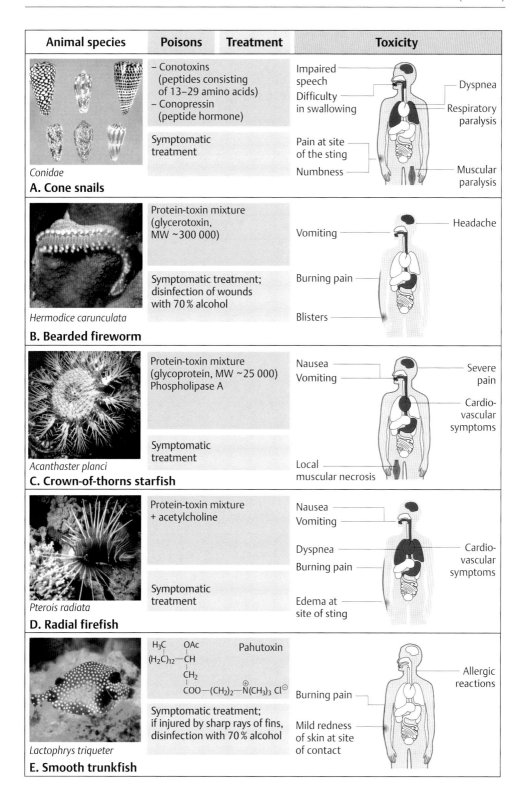

Animal species	Poisons	Treatment	Toxicity
Conidae **A. Cone snails**	– Conotoxins (peptides consisting of 13–29 amino acids) – Conopressin (peptide hormone)	Symptomatic treatment	Impaired speech · Difficulty in swallowing · Dyspnea · Respiratory paralysis · Pain at site of the sting · Numbness · Muscular paralysis
Hermodice carunculata **B. Bearded fireworm**	Protein-toxin mixture (glycerotoxin, MW ~300 000)	Symptomatic treatment; disinfection of wounds with 70 % alcohol	Vomiting · Headache · Burning pain · Blisters
Acanthaster planci **C. Crown-of-thorns starfish**	Protein-toxin mixture (glycoprotein, MW ~25 000) Phospholipase A	Symptomatic treatment	Nausea · Vomiting · Severe pain · Cardio-vascular symptoms · Local muscular necrosis
Pterois radiata **D. Radial firefish**	Protein-toxin mixture + acetylcholine	Symptomatic treatment	Nausea · Vomiting · Dyspnea · Burning pain · Cardio-vascular symptoms · Edema at site of sting
Lactophrys triqueter **E. Smooth trunkfish**	Pahutoxin $(H_2C)_{12}-\overset{\overset{\displaystyle H_3C}{\mid}}{C}H\overset{\overset{\displaystyle OAc}{\mid}}{}$ CH_2 $COO-(CH_2)_2-\overset{\oplus}{N}(CH_3)_3\ Cl^{\ominus}$	Symptomatic treatment; if injured by sharp rays of fins, disinfection with 70 % alcohol	Allergic reactions · Burning pain · Mild redness of skin at site of contact

Poisonous Marine Animals

These animals cause poisoning in humans after consumption (see environmental toxicology, p. 62). Raw slices cut from the pufferfish (Tetraodontidae) are called *fugu* and are considered a delicacy in Japan. Only licensed cooks may prepare this poisonous fish, but even so, there are around 80 deaths per year. Moderate consumption causes mild intoxication, which is a desired effect. The main component of the poison is tetrodotoxin produced by bacteria (e.g., *Bacillus* species) inhabiting the skin of the pufferfish (**A**). Its high toxicity is due to blockage of sodium transport, which ultimately leads to muscular paralysis.

Toxicity. The signs occurring 10–20 min after consumption of fugu include paresthesia of the lips and tongue, nausea, muscle spasms, breathing difficulties, and paralysis of the respiratory muscles.

Therapy. Treatment consists of immediate gastric lavage, followed by symptomatic treatment.

Venomous and Poisonous Land Animals

Most of these animals transmit their poison by sting or bite.

Scorpions (Scorpiones)

There are about 1500 species of scorpions (**B**), about 25 of which can kill a person by a sting. In Mexico alone, there are approximately 100 000 accidents per year, of which about 800 are fatal. Deadly accidents due to native species also occur in Europe. Scorpions have a spine with two ducts from paired poison glands. Scorpion venom consists of highly active polypeptide toxins, for example, neurotoxins affecting sodium transport and neurotransmitter function.

Toxicity. In humans, these neurotoxins cause vomiting, hyperglycemia, hypertension, tachycardia, and finally death by circulatory failure.

Therapy. Specific antisera are available.

Spiders (Araneae)

There are about 30 000 species of spiders, some 300 of which may be harmful to humans. Dangerous species include banana spiders, sac spiders, bird spiders, spitting spiders, funnel weavers, cobweb weavers, and wolf spiders. The venom is produced in glands located primarily in the cephalothorax; it is injected by fangs during a bite. The amount of venom injected is about 0.2 mg, consisting predominantly of peptides, proteins, and polyamines. They act as neurotoxins or necrotizing toxins (necrotoxins). The black widow (*Latrodectus mactans*, a cobweb weaver) (**C**), is the only dangerous spider native to Europe. The main component of its venom, a polypeptide (latrotoxin) consisting of 42 amino acids, causes a massive release of neurotransmitters from synapses and thus induces muscle spasms in humans.

Toxicity. After 10–15 min, the bitten person complains about extreme sensitivity to pain; the eyelids and conjunctiva are swollen, and the face is disfigured by grimaces (*latrodectism*).

Therapy. Specific antisera are available.

Insects (Insecta)

With more than 1.5 million species, insects represent the largest group of animals. Bees (Apidae) (**D**) and wasps (Vespidae) (**E**) are considered the most important poisonous animals in Europe. A bee injects about 100 µg of venom per sting. To receive a lethal dose, a person would need 1000 stings.

Toxicity. About 4% of the general public have allergic reactions to bee stings.

Bee venom is the best researched animal poison. It consists of enzymes (e.g., phospholipase A_2, the most important allergen), peptides (e.g., melittin, which amounts to 50% dry weight, consists of 26 amino acids, and is responsible for the painful effect), histamines, monosaccharides, and lipids.

Therapy. Application of ice packs is recommended. Allergic reactions are treated by administering epinephrine, antihistamines, and corticosteroids.

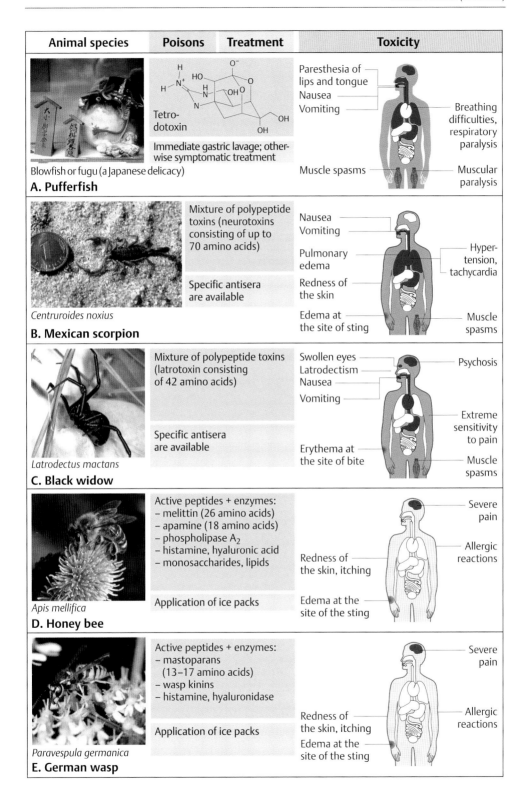

Animal species	Poisons	Treatment	Toxicity
A. Pufferfish Blowfish or fugu (a Japanese delicacy)	Tetrodotoxin	Immediate gastric lavage; otherwise symptomatic treatment	Paresthesia of lips and tongue; Nausea; Vomiting; Breathing difficulties, respiratory paralysis; Muscle spasms; Muscular paralysis
B. Mexican scorpion *Centruroides noxius*	Mixture of polypeptide toxins (neurotoxins consisting of up to 70 amino acids)	Specific antisera are available	Nausea; Vomiting; Pulmonary edema; Hypertension, tachycardia; Redness of the skin; Edema at the site of sting; Muscle spasms
C. Black widow *Latrodectus mactans*	Mixture of polypeptide toxins (latrotoxin consisting of 42 amino acids)	Specific antisera are available	Swollen eyes; Latrodectism; Nausea; Vomiting; Psychosis; Extreme sensitivity to pain; Erythema at the site of bite; Muscle spasms
D. Honey bee *Apis mellifica*	Active peptides + enzymes: – melittin (26 amino acids) – apamine (18 amino acids) – phospholipase A_2 – histamine, hyaluronic acid – monosaccharides, lipids	Application of ice packs	Severe pain; Allergic reactions; Redness of the skin, itching; Edema at the site of the sting
E. German wasp *Paravespula germanica*	Active peptides + enzymes: – mastoparans (13–17 amino acids) – wasp kinins – histamine, hyaluronidase	Application of ice packs	Severe pain; Allergic reactions; Redness of the skin, itching; Edema at the site of the sting

Amphibians (Amphibia)

Amphibians produce poisons in cutaneous glands for protection from predators and from skin infections. The skin secretion of the European spotted salamander (*Salamandra salamandra*) contains central-acting, spasmolytic steroid alkaloids (e.g., samandarin) (**A**). The poison of the tropical harlequin poison frog (*Dendrobates histrionicus*) (**A**) contains complex alkaloids, such as the highly poisonous batrachotoxin (used by the Indians of Colombia as a blow dart poison; the subcutaneous LD_{50} for mice is 2 µg/kg BW). The poison of a single frog is sufficient to kill 20 000 mice or 10 humans.

Toxicity. The toxins interfere with sodium transport and may lead to paralysis and cardiac arrest. Poisoning in humans is extremely rare. Contact with the skin secretion leads to irritation of the mucosae.

Therapy. Since there are no antisera, treatment is only symptomatic.

Reptiles (Reptilia)

Of 2000 species of lizards, only two are venomous. One of them is the Gila monster (*Heloderma suspectum*) (**B**). Its venom consists of serotonin and proteins (e.g., hyaluronidase, kallikreine) and is injected into its prey through grooves in the teeth of the lower jaw.

Toxicity. The poisoning is characterized by nausea, vomiting, and headache.

Therapy. Treatment is usually not required.

Snakes (Serpentes)

Snakes have venom glands and hollow teeth (fangs) in their upper jaw by which they inject venom into their prey. Only around 10% of almost 4000 species are venomous. About 2 million accidents per year are caused by snake bites worldwide, and about 2.5% of those are fatal. The mortality due to snake bites is around 1% for adders, 32% for cobras, and 100% for the black mamba. Venomous snakes include vipers/adders (Viperidae, e.g., rattlesnakes and the common viper, or adder, which is native to Eu-

rope), mole vipers (Atractaspididae, e.g., burrowing adder), calubrid snakes (Colubridae, e. g., oriental whipsnake), and elapid snakes (Elapidae, e.g., cobras, mambas, Indian kraits, coral snakes, and sea snakes).

Snake venoms contain various toxins, which are peptides consisting of up to 74 amino acids. They are predominantly neurotoxins and result in rapid paralysis of the prey or attacker. The toxins of elapid snakes block the acetylcholine receptors at neuromuscular endplates, thus causing rapid paralysis. Almost 30 different enzymes with various activities have been isolated from snake venoms. The following enzymes are contained in almost all snake venoms:

- *Proteolytic enzymes* degrade proteins and produce severe necrosis and suffusions, causing the skin to lift in blisters (e.g., after bites by rattlesnakes) (**C**).
- *Nucleotidases* degrade DNA and energy carriers (ATP) and are therefore cytotoxic.
- *Collagenases and hyaluronidases* damage the tissue and thereby facilitate rapid penetration of the venom into the body.
- *Phospholipase A_2* hydrolyses phospholipids with multiple consequences. The venom of vipers (e.g., that of the adder) (**D**) also contains *coagulation enzymes* that affect blood clotting.

Snakes will bite only when seriously threatened; frequently, they do not even inject their venom. About 50% of all defensive bites are nonpoisonous.

Toxicity. The various compositions of snake venoms lead to many symptoms of poisoning. The black mamba (*Dendroaspis polylepis*), native to South Africa (**E**), ejects about 1 g venom per bite; the lethal dose in humans is about 120 mg. The adder native to Europe (*Vipera berus*) ejects only about 10 mg poison, and the lethal dose is about 75 mg.

Therapy. Antisera are now available against almost all snake venoms. However, they should only be applied in life-threatening conditions, since allergic reactions associated with anaphylactic shock and death may occur after administration of the serum (foreign proteins). Such reactions occur in about 0.3% of cases.

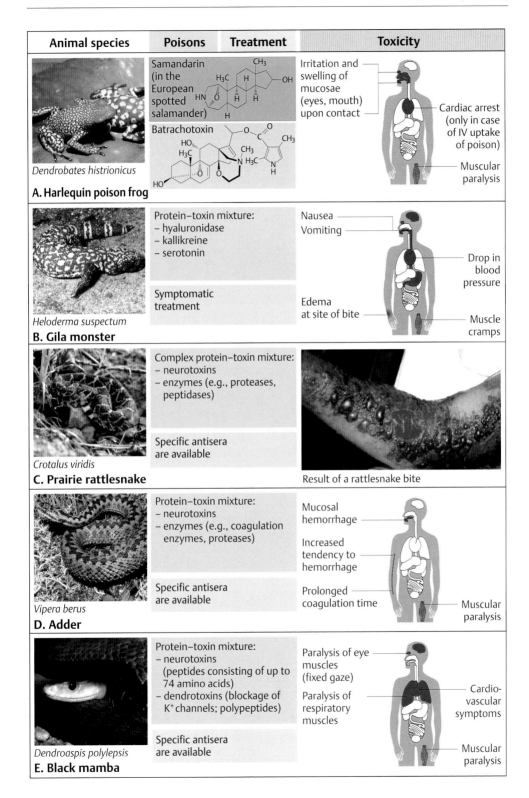

Animal species	Poisons	Treatment	Toxicity

A. Harlequin poison frog
Dendrobates histrionicus

Samandarin (in the European spotted salamander)

Batrachotoxin

Irritation and swelling of mucosae (eyes, mouth) upon contact

Cardiac arrest (only in case of IV uptake of poison)

Muscular paralysis

B. Gila monster
Heloderma suspectum

Protein–toxin mixture:
– hyaluronidase
– kallikreine
– serotonin

Symptomatic treatment

Nausea
Vomiting
Drop in blood pressure
Edema at site of bite
Muscle cramps

C. Prairie rattlesnake
Crotalus viridis

Complex protein–toxin mixture:
– neurotoxins
– enzymes (e.g., proteases, peptidases)

Specific antisera are available

Result of a rattlesnake bite

D. Adder
Vipera berus

Protein–toxin mixture:
– neurotoxins
– enzymes (e.g., coagulation enzymes, proteases)

Specific antisera are available

Mucosal hemorrhage
Increased tendency to hemorrhage
Prolonged coagulation time
Muscular paralysis

E. Black mamba
Dendroaspis polylepsis

Protein–toxin mixture:
– neurotoxins (peptides consisting of up to 74 amino acids)
– dendrotoxins (blockage of K^+ channels; polypeptides)

Specific antisera are available

Paralysis of eye muscles (fixed gaze)
Paralysis of respiratory muscles
Cardio-vascular symptoms
Muscular paralysis

■ Birds (Aves)

Hooded Pitohui (*Pitohui dichrous*) (A) and Blue-capped Ifrita (*Ifrita kowaldi*) (B)

Birds with poisonous substances in their feathers and on their skin live in the rain forest of Papua New Guinea. Five poisonous species belong to the genus *Pitohui*, and one to the genus *Ifrita*. These birds use the highly toxic homobatrachotoxin for their protection (the intravenous LD_{50} for mice is $2\,\mu g/kg$ BW). This toxin is probably produced by the birds from their diet; it belongs to the group of toxins that had previously only been found in poison dart frogs (see p. 262). The birds show the highest toxin concentration in their feathers and on the skin of abdomen, breast, and legs (a total of ~ $30\,\mu g$ toxin per bird). The substance can therefore easily be rubbed on to the eggs or the nest for protection from predators and parasites. The natives call the pitohui "garbage bird" because of its bitter taste; it can only be eaten when carefully skinned and specially prepared. Eating the meat causes burning in the mouth. In humans, contact with the feathers leads to inflammatory reactions at the site of contact. If inhaled, the poisons trigger allergic symptoms (e.g., sneezing, coughing).

Toxicity. The toxin interferes with sodium transport, thus leading to paralysis. The effect is similar to that of batrachotoxin from poison dart frogs (see p. 262).

Therapy. Treatment is only symptomatic.

■ Mammals (Mammalia)

Platypus (Ornithorhynchus anatinus) (C)

Only the male platypus has venom glands. They are located in the upper thighs and are connected by means of a duct to a horny spine on the inside of the ankles. This poison spur sits in a fold of the skin and can be erected. The venom (containing a neurotoxin, among others) is used for paralyzing larger prey (e.g., frogs) and also for defense. It is ejaculated by means of a vigorous push from the hind leg. The venom glands enlarge at the beginning of the mating season, indicating that they also play a role in mating behavior. During the mating season, males often use their poison spur during aggressive confrontations. It is possible that the venom delivery system has developed for protection against a predator that has long since died out. A single contact with the venom is not life-threatening to humans but may kill a small mammal, such as a small dog. In humans, the parts of the body injured by the poison spur show severe swelling. The pain lasts for about a day, but the wound remains sensitive to touch for a longer period. Healing of the injury may take several weeks.

Northern Short-Tailed Shrew (*Blarina brevicauda*) (D)

This shrew is the only venomous mammal naturally occurring in North America. The venom is produced in the salivary glands of the lower jaw, which open between the incisors, and is continuously secreted into the saliva during chewing. It contains a neurotoxin for paralyzing the prey and a hemotoxin for faster distribution of the venom. The anesthetized insects remain alive for 3–5 days and thus provide the shrew with fresh food in case of food shortages. The venom also protects the shrew from predators. In humans, it causes inflammation at the site of the bite, lasting for 7 days.

Haitian Solenodon (*Solenodon paradoxus*) (E)

The solenodon, an animal resembling a large shrew, also produces a venom that mixes with the saliva and contains a neurotoxin, among other components. The venom is produced in the ducts of the salivary glands of the lower jaw; these are located on both sides at the root of each incisor. The saliva is channeled through a deep groove in the incisor (the scientific name *Solenodon* means groove-toothed). The venom is used in the same way as in the northern short-tailed shrew.

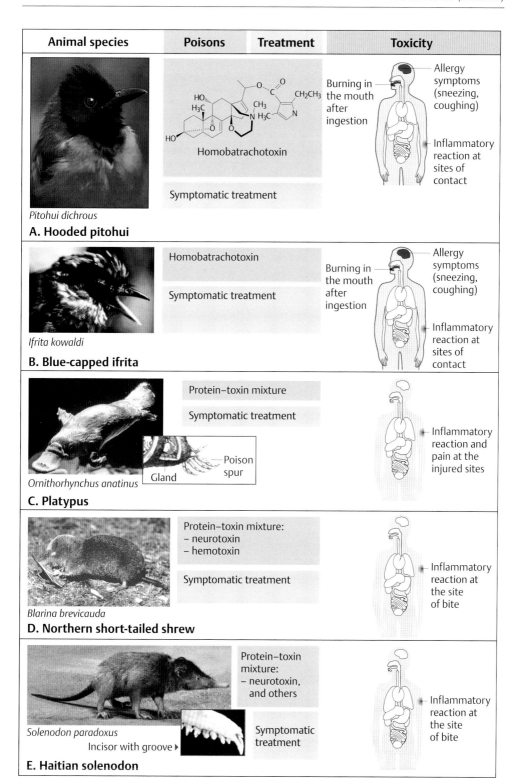

Animal species	Poisons	Treatment	Toxicity

A. Hooded pitohui
Pitohui dichrous

Homobatrachotoxin

Symptomatic treatment

Burning in the mouth after ingestion

Allergy symptoms (sneezing, coughing)

Inflammatory reaction at sites of contact

B. Blue-capped ifrita
Ifrita kowaldi

Homobatrachotoxin

Symptomatic treatment

Burning in the mouth after ingestion

Allergy symptoms (sneezing, coughing)

Inflammatory reaction at sites of contact

C. Platypus
Ornithorhynchus anatinus

Protein–toxin mixture

Symptomatic treatment

Gland — Poison spur

Inflammatory reaction and pain at the injured sites

D. Northern short-tailed shrew
Blarina brevicauda

Protein–toxin mixture:
– neurotoxin
– hemotoxin

Symptomatic treatment

Inflammatory reaction at the site of bite

E. Haitian solenodon
Solenodon paradoxus
Incisor with groove ▶

Protein–toxin mixture:
– neurotoxin, and others

Symptomatic treatment

Inflammatory reaction at the site of bite

Plant Poisons (Phytotoxins)

Basics. As early as 1500 BC, the poisonous saffron crocus (*Crocus sativus*) was mentioned in an Egyptian medical document, the Ebers papyrus. In ancient Athens, Socrates (470–399 bc) was sentenced to death by drinking a cup of poison hemlock (*Conium maculatum*).

More than half a million plant species are known today, and one plant in ten is poisonous. Only about 1000 species, however, have been studied in detail for their ingredients. In Europe, there are around 50 plant families with poisonous species. The toxicity of poisonous plants is graded as follows: extremely poisonous (+++, milligram quantities may have life-threatening effects), very poisonous (++, severe signs of poisoning), and poisonous (+). The poisonous substances of plants are divided into **alkaloids**, **triterpene glycosides**, **cyanogenic glycosides**, and **other poisonous substances**. Poisonous plants mostly contain several of these substances. At proper dosages, some are used for medical purposes (see pharmaceuticals, p. 68): *dosis sola facit venenum*—only the dose makes the poison (Paracelsus, 1493–1541).

Alkaloids

Aconitine

Aconitine is the primary active principle of monkshood (*Aconitum napellus*) (**A**) and larkspurs (*Delphinium* sp.), both of which belong to the family Ranunculaceae. Monkshood is one of the most poisonous plants in Europe. The poison is largely located in the tuberous roots, at concentrations of 0.2–3.0%.

Toxicity. Uptake of 6 mg of the toxin may be lethal to humans. The toxin is also absorbed through intact skin. After a few minutes, it causes burning in the mouth and tingling in fingers and toes, sweating, bradycardia, diarrhea, and colics. Lethal doses lead to respiratory paralysis and cardiac arrest. The oral LD_{50} for mice is 1 mg/kg BW.

First aid and therapy. Treatment consists of fluid supply and gastric lavage with potassium permanganate, followed by administration of 10 g activated charcoal. In case of severe bradycardia, atropine (see p. 68) is given.

Chelerythrine

Chelerythrine is the most active alkaloid of greater celandine (*Chelidonium majus*) (**B**); the plant contains up to 2%. When parts of the plant are broken, they exude an orange-yellow, milky juice.

Toxicity. Ingestion by humans causes vomiting, gastroenteritis, and diarrhea. At higher doses, the toxin causes paralysis of the vasomotor and respiratory centers. The subcutaneous LD_{50} for mice is 95 mg/kg BW.

First aid and therapy. Treatment involves induced vomiting, gastric lavage with potassium permanganate, and instillation of 10 g activated charcoal.

Coniine

Coniine is the primary active principle of poison hemlock (*Conium maculatum*) (**C**); the seeds contain up to 3.5%.

Toxicity. The toxin is rapidly absorbed by the mucosae and also through intact skin. Coniine is a neurotoxin that causes paralysis of the motor nerve endings and interferes with chemoreceptors of the carotid sinus. The first symptoms are burning in the mouth, paralysis of the tongue, and vomiting; these are followed by paralysis, coldness, and numbness, and finally death by respiratory paralysis (0.5–5 h after taking a lethal dose of ~0.5 g). The oral LD_{50} for mice is 100 mg/kg BW.

First aid and therapy. Treatment is the same as for chelerythrine poisoning.

Cytisine

Cytisine is present mainly in the pods of common laburnum (golden chain tree; *Laburnum anagyroides*) (**D**) and Spanish broom (*Spartium junceum*). The seedpods contain up to 3%.

Toxicity. Like nicotine (see p. 154), the toxin blocks ganglia and causes vomiting, tachycardia, hallucination, and—at lethal doses—central respiratory paralysis (in small children after ingestion of 3–4 laburnum seedpods, in adults after ingestion of 15–20 seedpods).

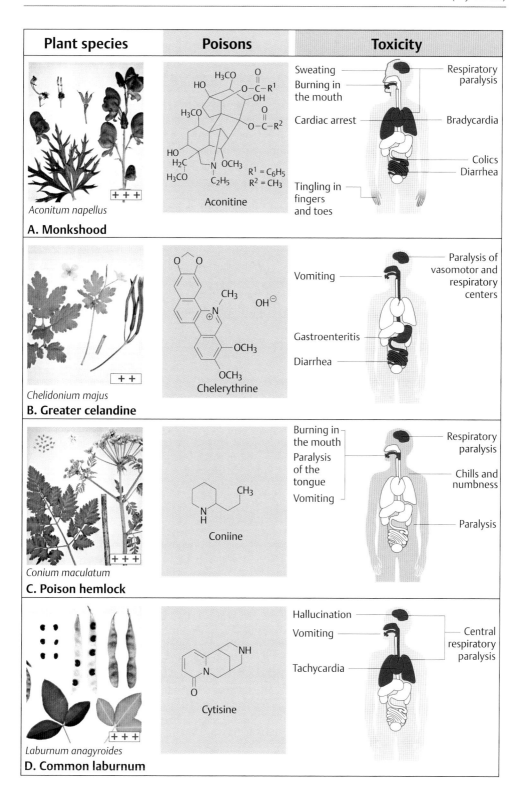

Plant species	Poisons	Toxicity

A. Monkshood
Aconitum napellus

Aconitine

$R^1 = C_6H_5$
$R^2 = CH_3$

Sweating — Burning in the mouth — Respiratory paralysis — Cardiac arrest — Bradycardia — Colics — Diarrhea — Tingling in fingers and toes

B. Greater celandine
Chelidonium majus

Chelerythrine

Vomiting — Paralysis of vasomotor and respiratory centers — Gastroenteritis — Diarrhea

C. Poison hemlock
Conium maculatum

Coniine

Burning in the mouth — Paralysis of the tongue — Vomiting — Respiratory paralysis — Chills and numbness — Paralysis

D. Common laburnum
Laburnum anagyroides

Cytisine

Hallucination — Vomiting — Tachycardia — Central respiratory paralysis

267

First aid and therapy. Treatment is the same as for chelerythrine poisoning. Administration of biperiden is needed in case of spasms, and intubation and oxygen therapy in case of respiratory paralysis.

Evonine and Evonoside

Evonine (a polyester alkaloid) and evonoside (a glycoside) are found in all parts, but particularly in the fruits, of the European spindletree (*Euonymus europaea*) (**A**). The fruits are divided into four parts, somewhat resembling a priest's hat (the German name is *Pfaffenhütchen*). In the past, a powder made from the plant has been used against lice and scabies mites.

Toxicity. Ingestion of two fruits causes severe signs of poisoning in small children, and about 36 fruits lead to death in adults. The first signs appear after a latency period of around 15 h. They include nausea, gastrointestinal symptoms with colics and hemorrhagic diarrhea; these are followed by arrhythmia, paralysis of the masticatory muscles, and tonic-clonic seizures.

First aid and therapy. Treatment involves induced vomiting followed by drinking of warm tea, or gastric lavage with potassium permanganate followed by electrolyte replacement. Diazepam is given in case of seizures.

Hyoscyamine

Hyoscyamine (see p. 68) is an active alkaloid of the following members of the family *Solanaceae*: henbane (*Hyoscyamus niger*) (**B**), deadly nightshade (*Atropa belladonna,* p. 69 **A**), mandrake (*Mandragora officinarum*, p. 3 **B**) and thornapples (*Datura* sp.). Since hyoscyamine racemizes to form atropine, the symptoms of poisoning are similar to those of atropine poisoning. Hence, henbane extract is used in the same way as belladonna extract; indications include eye injuries and spasms, particularly those of the smooth muscles. The action of hyoscyamine is parasympatholytic (anticholinergic), since it displaces acetylcholine. Daily doses of more than 3.6 mg over a prolonged period of time may lead to dependency.

Toxicity. The minimum toxic dose of hyoscyamine is about 5 mg. Higher doses lead to hallucination, mydriasis, impaired speech, tachy-

cardia, and finally coma and respiratory paralysis. The lethal oral dose for adults is approximately 10 mg; around 15 seeds of henbane are lethal to small children.

First aid and therapy. Treatment involves induced vomiting and, possibly, gastric lavage with a paraffin-lubricated tube, followed by IM or IV administration of 2 mg physostigmine.

Imperialine

Imperialine is found primarily in the bulbs of crown imperial (*Fritillaria imperialis*) (**C**) and snake's head, or toad lily (*Fritillaria meleagris*), with the bulbs containing 0.1–2.0%. These two members of the lily family (Liliaceae) are widespread in Europe and are also popular garden plants. Both species give off an unpleasant pungent odor that repels even voles. The flowers, leaves, and stems of crown imperial contain also the contact allergen tulipalin A, which may cause sensitization upon frequent contact.

Toxicity. Poisoning manifests itself by vomiting, spasms, a drop in blood pressure, and finally cardiac arrest.

First aid and therapy. Treatment consists of induced vomiting and administration of 10 g activated charcoal. A spasmolytic agent may also be indicated.

Lycorine

Lycorine is found in all parts and, in particular, in the bulbs of daffodil (*Narcissus pseudonarcissus*) (**D**), snowdrop (*Galanthus nivalis*), spring snowflake (*Leucojum vernum*), bush lily (*Clivia miniata*), and amaryllis (*Hippeastrum* sp.). The bulbs contain 0.1–1.0% of the toxin. Poisoning generally occurs after eating the bulbs, which are often mistaken for onions, or—in case of small children—after drinking water from the flower vase.

Toxicity. The following symptoms occur after ingestion: nausea, vomiting, a heavy sensation in the legs, and central nervous dysfunction. Eating just one daffodil bulb may be lethal to small children. Daffodil dermatitis (contact dermatitis due to alkaloids in the plant sap) is one of the most common occupational diseases of florists and gardeners.

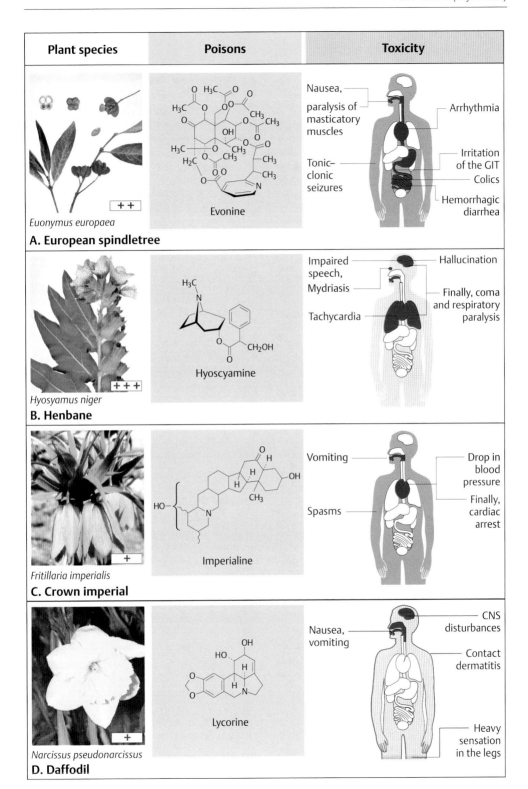

Plant species	Poisons	Toxicity
Euonymus europaea **A. European spindletree**	Evonine	Nausea, paralysis of masticatory muscles; Tonic–clonic seizures; Arrhythmia; Irritation of the GIT; Colics; Hemorrhagic diarrhea
Hyosyamus niger **B. Henbane**	Hyoscyamine	Impaired speech, Mydriasis; Tachycardia; Hallucination; Finally, coma and respiratory paralysis
Fritillaria imperialis **C. Crown imperial**	Imperialine	Vomiting; Spasms; Drop in blood pressure; Finally, cardiac arrest
Narcissus pseudonarcissus **D. Daffodil**	Lycorine	Nausea, vomiting; CNS disturbances; Contact dermatitis; Heavy sensation in the legs

First aid and therapy. Treatment consists of induced vomiting, fluid supply, and instillation of 10 g activated charcoal.

α-Solanine

α-Solanine is found in all parts, except the tubers, of the potato plant (*Solanum tuberosum*) (**A**) and in all parts, except the ripe fruits, of the tomato plant (*Lycopersicon lycopersicum*). Potato eyes and sprouts exposed to the light contain up to 5% solanine. The toxin is a powerful topical irritant and protoplasmic poison.

Toxicity. Since solanum alkaloids are heat-resistant, green potatoes may be poisonous even after frying. The following symptoms appear after ingestion: nausea, diarrhea, mydriasis, vertigo, spasms, fever, dyspnea, and finally respiratory paralysis. Even a 0.2 g dose of solanine causes considerable gastrointestinal irritation and hemolysis in adults. The intraperitoneal LD_{50} for mice is 42 mg/kg BW.

Therapy. Treatment involves induced vomiting and gastric lavage, followed by administration of 10 g activated charcoal. Physostigmine is given in case of anticholinergic symptoms.

Sparteine

Sparteine is primarily contained in the seeds (up to 0.2%) of lupines (*Lupinus polyphyllus*) (**B**) and in all parts of the common broom (*Cytisus scoparius*). Recently, there have been frequent poisonings in Asia where lupin seeds have been used as a soybean substitute for producing tofu and tempeh. Sparteine is almost completely absorbed by the gastrointestinal tract.

Toxicity. In humans, the ingestion of 0.01–0.1 g sparteine causes a drop in heart rate and blood pressure. An overdose leads to curare-like paralysis, spasms, and death by respiratory paralysis after 2–3 h. The oral LD_{50} for mice is 220 mg/kg BW.

Therapy. Treatment consists of induced vomiting, followed by gastric lavage with potassium permanganate, and finally administration of 10 g activated charcoal. Orciprenaline or lidocaine is given in case of arrhythmia.

Taxines

Taxines are present in all parts of yew trees (e. g., European yew, *Taxus baccata*), except in the edible, red, berry-like structure surrounding a single seed (**C**). The plants contain up to 2%, with the leaves and seeds being particularly poisonous. Native Americans use extracts from the Pacific yew (*Taxus brevifolia*) as a remedy for rheumatism.

Toxicity. Painful diarrhea, mydriasis, and vertigo occur in adults 1 h after ingestion, followed by bradycardia, arrhythmia, and possibly coma and death by circulatory collapse and respiratory paralysis after just 2 h. The cardiac effect of taxines is even more powerful than that of digitalis alkaloids. The lethal dose for adults is contained in 50–100 of the needle-like leaves. The intravenous LD_{50} of taxines for rats is 4.5 mg/kg BW.

Therapy. Treatment consists of induced vomiting or gastric lavage, followed by administration of 10 g activated charcoal. Diazepam is given in case of spasms.

Veratrum Alkaloids

Veratrum alkaloids are present in all parts of white hellebore (*Veratrum album*) (**D**), with the tubers containing up to 2%. The primary active compounds are alkaloids, such as protoveratrine A and B, and germerine. The plant is easily mistaken for yellow gentian (*Gentiana lutea*) when not in bloom; as a result, a poisonous liquor is sometimes distilled from hellebore roots. Veratrum alkaloids are rapidly absorbed by the mucosa and intact skin.

Toxicity. Veratrum alkaloids stimulate the peripheral sensory nerve endings, thus leading to itching, burning, and redness of the skin. When they get into the eyes, they cause severe lacrimation and pain. Complete anesthesia may develop later. Large quantities of these alkaloids lead to reduced diuresis, spasms, and possibly collapse. The lethal dose for adults is 1–2 g; death by circulatory collapse and respiratory paralysis occurs after 3–12 h.

Therapy. Treatment as for taxine poisoning. If respiratory paralysis is eminent, intubation and oxygen therapy are indicated.

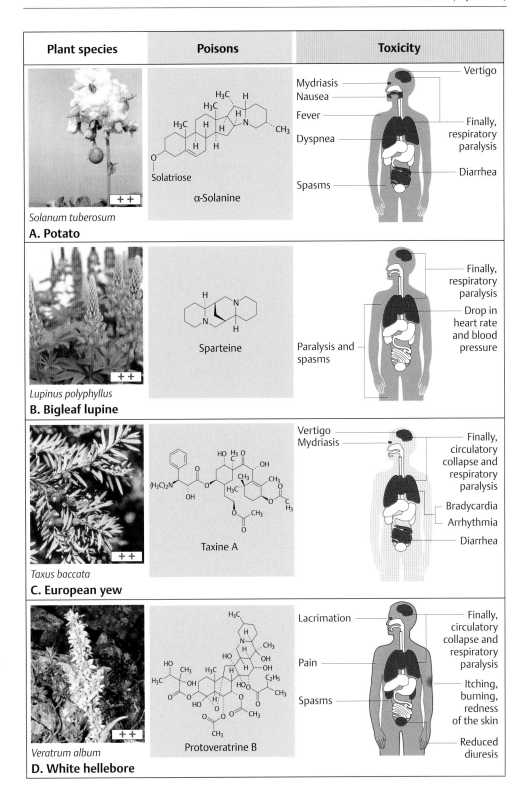

Plant species	Poisons	Toxicity
Solanum tuberosum **A. Potato**	Solatriose α-Solanine	Vertigo, Mydriasis, Nausea, Fever, Dyspnea, Finally, respiratory paralysis, Diarrhea, Spasms
Lupinus polyphyllus **B. Bigleaf lupine**	Sparteine	Finally, respiratory paralysis, Drop in heart rate and blood pressure, Paralysis and spasms
Taxus baccata **C. European yew**	Taxine A	Vertigo, Mydriasis, Finally, circulatory collapse and respiratory paralysis, Bradycardia, Arrhythmia, Diarrhea
Veratrum album **D. White hellebore**	Protoveratrine B	Lacrimation, Finally, circulatory collapse and respiratory paralysis, Pain, Itching, burning, redness of the skin, Spasms, Reduced diuresis

Triterpene Glycosides

Adonitoxin

Adonitoxin is present in all parts of spring pheasant's eye (*Adonis vernalis*) (**A**); the plant contains up to 1%. Adonitoxin is a cardiac glycoside of the cardenolide series, which also includes the active ingredients of foxglove (*Digitalis purpurea* and *D. lanata*, see p. 79 **A**). Since it has fewer side effects than digitalis toxins, the use of *Adonis vernalis* as a medicinal plant is on the rise. The advantage of drugs derived from *Adonis*, as compared with those from *Digitalis*, is that their action is faster and shorter; prolonged application does therefore not lead to accumulation.

Toxicity. Even 2 g of *Adonis* leaves are toxic to humans. Typical signs of poisoning include nausea, vomiting, colic, and dyspnea.

First aid and therapy. Treatment consists of induced vomiting, followed by administration of 10 g activated charcoal. Atropine is administered for treating vagotonic cardiac symptoms, and sedatives are given for central sedation. The heart recovers only slowly from nonlethal poisoning. The intravenous LD_{50} of adonitoxin for cats is 0.19 mg/kg BW.

Convallatoxin

Convallatoxin is a cardenolide glycoside. It is present in all parts of lily of the valley (*Convallaria majalis*) (**B**), particularly in the flowers (up to 0.7%) and fruits (up to 0.2%). So far, 38 different glycosides have been found in this plant, with convallatoxin being the main one. Only 10% of the toxin is absorbed by the human gastrointestinal tract; hence, rapid emptying of the gastrointestinal tract is an important measure. In the past, pulverized flowers of lily of the valley were frequently used as a sneezing powder. Today, the active glycoside is used for treating acute cardiac insufficiency, arrhythmia, neurocirculatory asthenia, and atherosclerosis at menopause.

Toxicity. Convallatoxin acts like a typical digitalis glycoside. After ingestion of larger quantities of the toxin (e.g., after eating leaves, flowers, or 3–5 berries, or after drinking water from the flower vase, usually in the case of small children), the following signs of poisoning occur: nausea, vomiting, diarrhea, impaired vision, and vertigo. Lethal doses (such as a handful of berries) lead to bradycardia, ventricular fibrillation, and finally cardiac arrest.

First aid and therapy. Treatment consists of gastric lavage with potassium permanganate, followed by administration of 10 g activated charcoal. Atropine or orciprenaline is given in case of bradycardia.

Oleandrin

Oleandrin is a cardenolide present in all parts of oleander (*Nerium oleander*) (**C**), with the leaves containing up to 1.5%. The glycoside content is highest at flowering time.

Toxicity. Signs of poisoning include nausea, headache, diarrhea, mydriasis, and arrhythmia. After ingestion of lethal doses, cardiac insufficiency and death by cardioplegia occur after 2–3 h. Lethal poisonings due to toxin contained in the wood regularly occur in California in individuals who cut branches from oleander shrubs and use them as sticks for barbecuing meat. In sheep, 1–5 g oleander leaves are lethal. The intravenous LD_{50} of oleandrin for cats is 0.3 mg/kg BW.

First aid and therapy. Treatment is the same as for convallatoxin poisoning.

Cyanogenic Glycosides

Prunasin

Prunasin is mainly found in the seeds and leaves (up to 1.5%) of many members of the rose family (Rosaceae), e.g., cherry laurel (*Prunus laurocerasus*) (**D**), and amygdalin is present in the seeds of many stone fruits, with the seeds containing up to 0.2% hydrogen cyanide.

Toxicity. Nausea, vomiting, tachycardia, and spasms occur after ingestion of leaves or up to 10 seeds; ingestion of more than 10 seeds may lead to respiratory and cardiac arrest.

Therapy. Treatment is the same as for hydrogen cyanide poisoning (see p. 140).

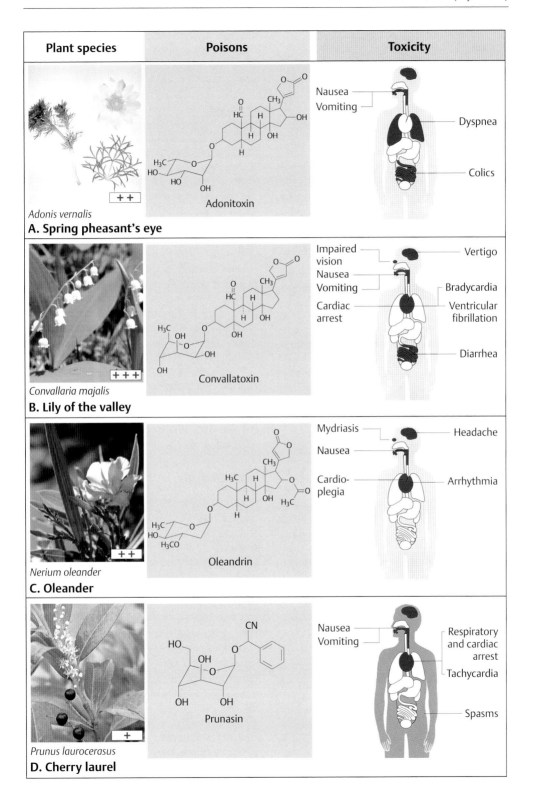

Plant species	Poisons	Toxicity

A. Spring pheasant's eye

Adonis vernalis

++

Adonitoxin

Nausea
Vomiting
Dyspnea
Colics

B. Lily of the valley

Convallaria majalis

+++

Convallatoxin

Impaired vision
Nausea
Vomiting
Cardiac arrest
Vertigo
Bradycardia
Ventricular fibrillation
Diarrhea

C. Oleander

Nerium oleander

++

Oleandrin

Mydriasis
Nausea
Cardio-plegia
Headache
Arrhythmia

D. Cherry laurel

Prunus laurocerasus

+

Prunasin

Nausea
Vomiting
Respiratory and cardiac arrest
Tachycardia
Spasms

Other Poisonous Substances

Basics. Other poisonous substances in plants include toxic essential oils, toxic proteins (toxalbumins), hemolytic saponins, and acrid, pungent, or bitter substances.

Aethusin

Aethusin is a polyacetylene derivative (polyyne) present in all parts of fool's parsley (*Aethusa cynapium*) (**A**). The scientific name *Aethusa* is derived from the Greek word for "burn," referring to the pungent taste. Fool's parsley is frequently mistaken for wild carrot and then causes severe poisoning. Unlike wild carrot, fool's parsley has characteristic long, pendulant leaflets drawn to one side under each umbellule.

Toxicity. The first symptoms of poisoning include burning in the mouth, vomiting, abdominal pain, headache, cold sweat, and mydriasis. This is followed by impaired vision and clouded consciousness, spasms, and finally respiratory paralysis. The lethal dose for cattle is 15 kg fool's parsley per animal.

First aid and therapy. Treatment after ingestion of fool's parsley by humans consists of induced vomiting or gastric lavage with potassium permanganate, followed by administration of 10 g activated charcoal. Acidosis is neutralized with sodium bicarbonate (the pH of the urine should be 7.5).

Andromedotoxin

Andromedotoxin is a diterpene derivative present in all parts of rhododendron plants (*Rhododendron* sp.) (**B**) and of Japanese andromeda and mountain fetterbush (*Pieris* sp.), and also in the leaves of mountain and sheep laurels (*Kalmia* sp.). Poisonings occur on ingestion of honey containing andromedotoxin.

Toxicity. The signs of poisoning include vomiting, gastroenteritis, spasms, sweating, bradycardia, and finally respiratory paralysis. The intraperitoneal LD_{50} for mice is 1.28 mg/kg BW.

Therapy. Treatment consists of induced vomiting, followed by increased fluid supply and administration of 10 g activated charcoal. Diazepam is given in case of spasms.

Cicutoxin

Cicutoxin is a polyacetylene derivative present in all parts of water hemlocks (*Cicuta virosa* and *C. maculata*) (**C**). Water hemlocks were used in ancient times as medicinal plants, e.g., for treating pain associated with fractures.

Toxicity. Burning in the mouth, mydriasis, and vertigo appear as early as 20 min after ingestion of the toxin. Cicutoxin is a powerful convulsive poison (seizures associated with bruxism and foam formation every 15 min). It causes hyperactivity of the vasomotor and respiratory centers as well as the vagal nuclei. The stimulation is followed by paralysis of the vital centers—the higher the dose, the faster the effect—finally leading to death by central respiratory paralysis.

First aid and therapy. Treatment consists of induced vomiting, followed by gastric lavage and enema with chloral hydrate. The seizures are treated with thiobarbiturates. Forced diuresis is recommended.

Cucurbitacins

Cucurbitacins are bitter substances with a tetracyclic triterpene structure. They are found in all parts of squirting cucumber (*Ecballium elaterium*) (**D**), bryonies (*Bryonia* sp.), hedge hyssop (*Gratiola officinalis*), and in small quantities also in the fruits of colocynth (*Citrullus colocynthis*).

Toxicity. Vomiting, salivation, diarrhea, colics, and spasms occur after ingestion. The dried latex of the squirting cucumber fruit causes irritation with blistering and necrosis of the skin upon contact. Oral doses of more than 0.6 g of the fresh latex may cause death in humans. The oral LD_{50} of cucurbitacin E for mice is 340 mg/kg BW.

First aid and therapy. Treatment consists of induced vomiting, followed by drinking plenty of tea and administration of 10 g activated charcoal. Diazepam is indicated in case of spasms. Cutaneous and mucosal blisters require sterile coverings.

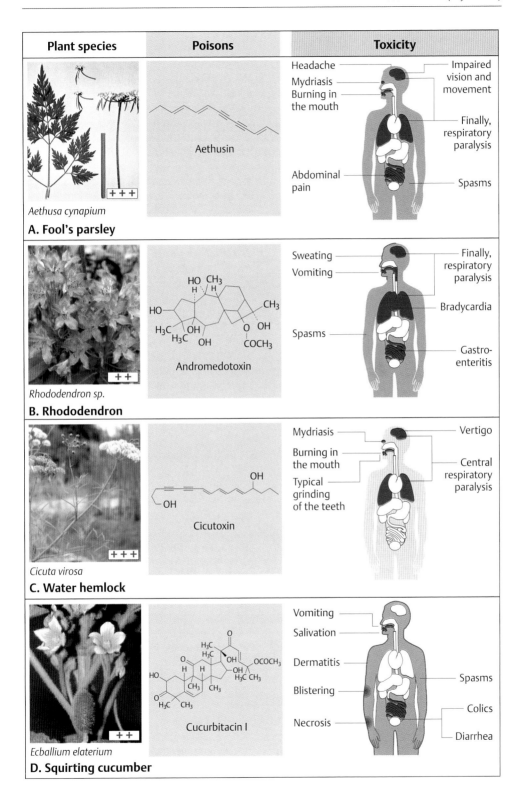

Plant species	Poisons	Toxicity

A. Fool's parsley
Aethusa cynapium
+++
Aethusin

Headache — Impaired vision and movement
Mydriasis
Burning in the mouth
Finally, respiratory paralysis
Abdominal pain
Spasms

B. Rhododendron
Rhododendron sp.
++
Andromedotoxin

Sweating — Finally, respiratory paralysis
Vomiting
Bradycardia
Spasms
Gastro-enteritis

C. Water hemlock
Cicuta virosa
+++
Cicutoxin

Mydriasis — Vertigo
Burning in the mouth
Central respiratory paralysis
Typical grinding of the teeth

D. Squirting cucumber
Ecballium elaterium
++
Cucurbitacin I

Vomiting
Salivation
Dermatitis
Spasms
Blistering
Colics
Necrosis
Diarrhea

Daphnetoxin, Mezerein, Daphnin

Daphnetoxin (a cyclopentenone derivative), mezerein (a terpene), and daphnin (a cumarin derivative) are present largely in the red berries and the bark of the paradise plant (*Daphne mezereum*) (**A**) and rose daphne (*Daphne cneorum*). The common feature of these plants is their silk-like, tough bast layer. Berries and bark contain up to 20% toxins. Hippocrates recommended the use of paradise plant as a laxative.

Toxicity. The signs of daphne poisoning in humans include sneezing, nausea, fever, gastroenteritis, colics, spasms, kidney damage, tachycardia, and finally circulatory collapse. Contact with these plants causes erysipelas-like erythema with blistering of skin and mucosa. The lethal dose for adults is 10–12 berries, and for children just 6 berries. The mortality due to daphne poisoning is very high (30%). Furthermore, mezerein is a carcinogen.

First aid and therapy. Treatment consists of induced vomiting, followed by fluid supply. The gastrointestinal irritation is treated with mucilage, and spasms with diazepam.

Euphorbol

Euphorbol is a triterpene found in members of the spurge family (Euphorbiaceae), such as cypress spurge (*Euphorbia cyparissias*, **B**) and poinsettia (*Euphorbia pulcherrima*). Spurges also contain phorbols (tiglianes). The milk sap (latex) of these plants has a pungent taste; it has been used in the past as an emetic and laxative.

Toxicity. Spurge latex is a cutaneous irritant. Contact with the skin leads to blistering and necrosis. Contact with the mucosae causes tissue damage; in the eyes, this may lead to blindness. The following symptoms are observed after ingestion: mydriasis, stomach ache, diarrhea, arrhythmia, delirium, paralysis, and finally death by circulatory arrest after 1–3 days.

First aid and therapy. Treatment consists of induced vomiting, followed by fluid supply and administration of 10 g activated charcoal. The gastrointestinal irritation is treated with mucilage, and spasms with diazepam.

Protoanemonin

Protoanemonin is a lactone found in all parts of plants belonging to the buttercup family (Ranunculaceae), such as *Ranunculus acris* (**C**), anemones (*Anemone* sp.), pasque flowers (*Pulsatilla* sp.), hepaticas (*Hepatica* sp.), clematis (*Clematis* sp.). It is also contained in the tuberous roots of hellebores (*Helleborus* sp.).

Toxicity. Protoanemonin is a powerful irritant of the skin and mucosae. Members of the buttercup family are thought to contribute to the induction of "meadow dermatitis," a reaction often occurring after sunbathing. Ingestion of the poison leads to kidney dysfunction (oliguria, anuria) and affects the central nervous system, initially causing central stimulation and then paralysis up to respiratory arrest.

First aid and therapy. Treatment consists of induced vomiting or gastric lavage, followed by administration of 10 g activated charcoal. Gastrointestinal irritation is treated with antacids. Monitoring the kidney function is essential.

Ricin

Ricin is a toxic protein (toxalbumin) in the seeds of the castor oil plant (*Ricinus communis*) (**D**) and croton plants (*Croton* sp.). The German names *Wunderbaum* and *Wunderstrauch*, respectively, indicate the multiple uses of the oil recovered from their seeds. In medicine, it has been used for a long time as a mild laxative. Ricin is one of the most potent poisons because it inhibits protein synthesis. It was patented as a warfare agent (respiratory poison) in 1962. Like all toxalbumins, it is well absorbed by the gastrointestinal tract.

Toxicity. The first sign of poisoning is nausea; this is followed by vertigo, diarrhea, nephritis, blood clotting (thrombosis), and death by circulatory collapse after 48 h. The lethal dose for adults is 5 µg/kg. A single swallowed seed may be lethal. The intravenous LD_{50} for mice is 12 µg/kg BW.

First aid and therapy. Treatment consists of induced vomiting, followed by fluid supply and administration of 10 g active charcoal.

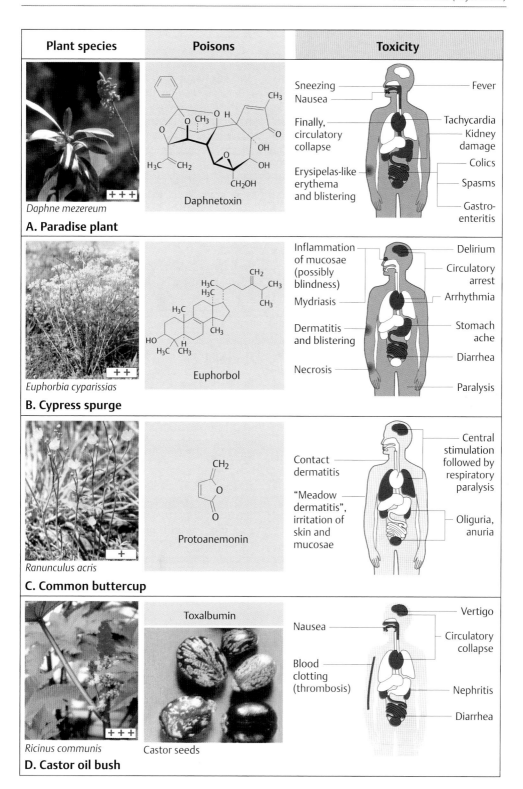

Plant species	Poisons	Toxicity

A. Paradise plant

Daphne mezereum +++

Daphnetoxin

Sneezing — Fever
Nausea
Finally, circulatory collapse — Tachycardia — Kidney damage
Erysipelas-like erythema and blistering — Colics — Spasms — Gastro-enteritis

B. Cypress spurge

Euphorbia cyparissias ++

Euphorbol

Inflammation of mucosae (possibly blindness) — Delirium — Circulatory arrest
Mydriasis — Arrhythmia
Dermatitis and blistering — Stomach ache — Diarrhea
Necrosis — Paralysis

C. Common buttercup

Ranunculus acris +

Protoanemonin

Contact dermatitis — Central stimulation followed by respiratory paralysis
"Meadow dermatitis", irritation of skin and mucosae — Oliguria, anuria

D. Castor oil bush

Ricinus communis +++

Toxalbumin

Castor seeds

Nausea — Vertigo — Circulatory collapse
Blood clotting (thrombosis) — Nephritis — Diarrhea

Sabinene, Thujone

Sabinene and thujone are poisonous monoterpenes. They are contained in the essential oils present in all parts of plants belonging to the cypress family (Cupressaceae) and especially in the needles of savin juniper (*Juniperus sabina*) (**A**) and white cedar (*Thuja occidentalis*) (**B**). The shrubs and trees of the cypress family contain up to 5% essential oil, and up to 20% of this is toxin. Thujone is also contained in the flowers of common tansy (*Tanacetum vulgare*) and in the essential oils of sages (*Salvia* sp.) and wormwoods (*Artemisia* sp.). Members of the cypress family also contain the fungicide thujaplicine; this guarantees excellent durability of the wood, which is therefore often chosen for construction. The poisonous berry-like cones of *Juniperus sabina* have an oval, flattened shape and are blue with a whitish waxy bloom. This distinguishes them from the nonpoisonous round, dark-blue cones of *Juniperus communis* (**A**), which are a popular flavouring (juniper berries). Sabinene and thujone are rapidly absorbed by the gastrointestinal tract—but also by the intact skin and mucosae—and distributed in the body. They are largely excreted by the kidneys.

Toxicity. In adults, the first symptoms of poisoning after ingestion of the lethal dose (6 drops of pure essential oil, or about 7 g of the tips of *Juniperus sabina* branches) include nausea, arrhythmia, and gastroenteritis. They are followed by cramps, kidney damage, and finally death by central paralysis after one day. Contact with the skin leads to dermatitis, blistering, and necrosis at the sites of contact. The subcutaneous LD_{50} of α-thujone for mice is 88 mg/kg BW.

First aid and therapy. Treatment consists of induced vomiting or gastric lavage, followed by administration of 10 g activated charcoal. Cramps are treated with diazepam. Electrolytes should be replenished. Monitoring kidney function is essential.

Ursolic Acid

Ursolic acid is a triterpene found in many plants, e.g., English holly (*Ilex aquifolium*) (**C**), alpenrose (*Rhododendron ferrugineum*), rhododendrons (*Rhododendron* sp.), southern catalpa (*Catalpa bignioides*), and black crowberry (*Empetrum nigrum*). Holly branches with characteristic mucronate-dentate leaves and red berries are a popular Christmas decoration. Time and again, the temptingly red berries cause poisoning in small children. The leaves of *Ilex paraguayensis* are used in South America for preparing the stimulating yerba maté tea.

Toxicity. Signs of poisonings include vomiting, pain, bradycardia, kidney damage, gastroenteritis, and diarrhea. For adults, 20–30 holly berries are lethal; just 2 berries cause vomiting in children.

First aid and therapy. Treatment consists of induced vomiting or gastric lavage, followed by fluid supply and administration of 10 g activated charcoal. Monitoring of kidney function is essential.

Urushiol

Urushiol III is a pyrocatechol derivative found in all parts of the eastern poison oak (*Toxicodendron quercifolium*) (**D**); the plant contains up to 4%. The toxin-containing yellow-white milk sap, which turns black when exposed to air, is characteristic.

Toxicity. The following signs occur after ingestion of the poison: irritation in the mouth, throat, and gastrointestinal tract, followed by vomiting, severe colic, kidney damage, and hemorrhagic diarrhea. Urushiol is a strong skin irritant in just microgram quantities. Picking the leaves causes inflammation of the skin (dermatitis) with itching, redness, and blistering. If the milk sap gets in the eyes (e.g., by wiping the eyes), corneal clouding and even blindness may result. A single contact with the leaves of poison oak may lead to sensitization within a few days, thus triggering a severe allergic reaction at the next contact.

First aid and therapy. It is important to rinse the poison off the skin with soap and water, or even better, with alcohol or ether. Zinc oxide powder is used to treat the itching. Otherwise, treatment is the same as in the case of ursolic acid.

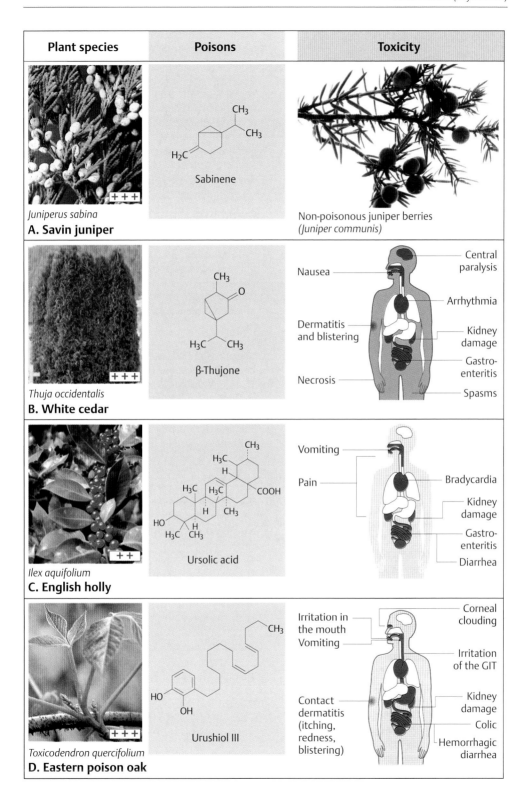

Plant species	Poisons	Toxicity

A. Savin juniper
Juniperus sabina

Sabinene

Non-poisonous juniper berries
(*Juniper communis*)

B. White cedar
Thuja occidentalis

β-Thujone

- Nausea
- Dermatitis and blistering
- Necrosis
- Central paralysis
- Arrhythmia
- Kidney damage
- Gastro-enteritis
- Spasms

C. English holly
Ilex aquifolium

Ursolic acid

- Vomiting
- Pain
- Bradycardia
- Kidney damage
- Gastro-enteritis
- Diarrhea

D. Eastern poison oak
Toxicodendron quercifolium

Urushiol III

- Irritation in the mouth
- Vomiting
- Contact dermatitis (itching, redness, blistering)
- Corneal clouding
- Irritation of the GIT
- Kidney damage
- Colic
- Hemorrhagic diarrhea

279

■ Fungal Poisons (Mycotoxins)

Basics. In Europe, intoxications from poisonous mushrooms accounts for approximately 1–3% of all poisonings. There are about 100 mushroom species in Europe that are poisonous, about 50 species that are toxic only when eaten raw, and another 30 or so species that are suspected to be poisonous. Many cases of mushroom poisoning are not caused by toxic mushrooms but are the result of eating spoiled mushroom meals, i.e., they are actually caused by ingesting bacterial toxins or mycotoxins produced by lower fungi (mold fungi, or ascomycetes) (see toxins in food, p. 210). The content of toxic substances in poisonous mushrooms varies considerably. Depending on their effects on the body, the toxins from higher fungi (basidiomycetes) are divided into **parenchymal poisons, neurotoxins, gastrointestinal irritants, and toxins with other effects.**

■ Parenchymal Poisons

Parenchymal poisons damage or destroy vital organs.

Amatoxins, Phallotoxins

Amatoxins are thermostable cyclic octapeptides, and phallotoxins are cyclic heptapeptides. Both cyclopeptides are contained in amanita mushrooms, such as death cap (*Amanita phalloides*) (**A**) and the European destroying angel (*Amanita virosa*) (**B**).

Toxicity. Amatoxins (e.g., α- and β-amanitins) inhibit DNA-dependent RNA polymerase II. The resulting collapse of protein synthesis damages liver and kidney cells. Phallotoxins (e.g., phalloidin) destroy intestinal cells by binding to actin, thus preventing its depolymerization. The first signs of poisoning appear after a latency period of about 12 h; they include diarrhea and vomiting, dehydration, impaired blood clotting, necrosis of liver and kidneys, and finally death due to anuria, uremia, or hepatic coma after 3–10 days. The lethal dose for adults is 0.1 mg amatoxins/kg BW and 5 mg phallotoxins/kg BW. Since 100 g of fresh amanita mushrooms contains up to 17 mg amanitin, eating a single mushroom can be fatal. The mortality from exposure to amanitin is about 10–15% in adults and 50% in small children.

Therapy. Treatment consists of induced vomiting or gastric lavage, followed by administration of activated charcoal. Administration of penicillin G and silibinin is indicated after ingestion of lethal doses. These drugs inhibit the uptake of amanitin into liver cells. In cases of hepatic failure, liver transplantation is required.

Gyromitrin

Gyromitrin (acetaldehyde-*N*-methyl-*N*-formyl-hydrazone) is found primarily in the false morel (*Gyromitra esculenta*) (**C**). It is partly metabolized in the body to monomethylhydrazine. Since the toxin is thermolabile and volatile, false morels can be largely detoxified by boiling them twice in water.

Toxicity. The first signs of poisoning appear 2–20 h after ingestion. They are similar to those of amanita poisoning. In addition, they include restlessness, delirium, spasms, and coma.

Therapy. Treatment is the same as for amanita poisoning.

Orellanines

Orellanines are thermostable toxins found largely in the fool's webcap (*Cortinarius orellanus*) (**D**), the dry substance of which contains up to 1% toxin.

Toxicity. The course of poisoning with this toxin is particularly dangerous because the first signs only appear 3–14 days after exposure. They include headache, severe thirst, and polyuria, followed by irreversible damage to the kidneys and finally death by uremia.

Therapy. Treatment is symptomatic.

Fungus species	Poisons	Toxicity

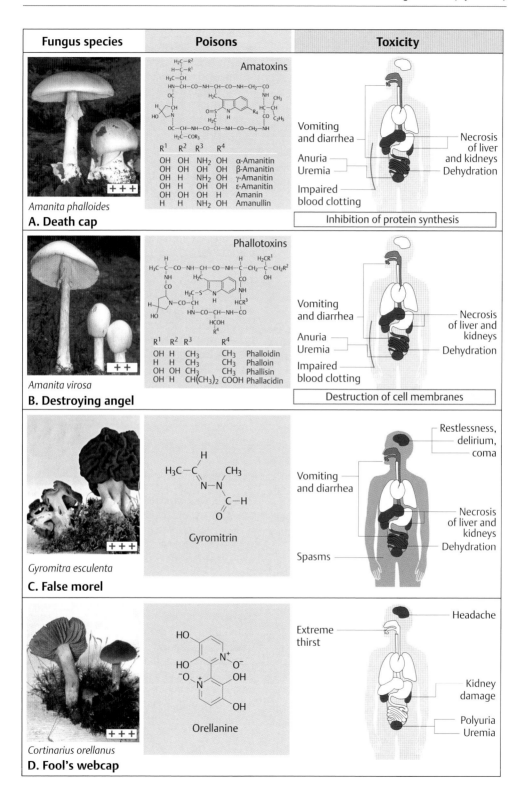

Amanita phalloides **A. Death cap**	Amatoxins — Vomiting and diarrhea, Anuria, Uremia, Impaired blood clotting, Necrosis of liver and kidneys, Dehydration — Inhibition of protein synthesis
Amanita virosa **B. Destroying angel**	Phallotoxins — Vomiting and diarrhea, Anuria, Uremia, Impaired blood clotting, Necrosis of liver and kidneys, Dehydration — Destruction of cell membranes
Gyromitra esculenta **C. False morel**	Gyromitrin — Restlessness, delirium, coma, Vomiting and diarrhea, Spasms, Necrosis of liver and kidneys, Dehydration
Cortinarius orellanus **D. Fool's webcap**	Orellanine — Extreme thirst, Headache, Kidney damage, Polyuria, Uremia

▓ Neurotoxins

Bufotenin

Bufotenin is found in the citron amanita (*Amanita citrina*) (**A**). The mushroom has a yellowish cap and a characteristic odor of raw potatoes.

Toxicity. Bufotenin causes tachycardia. It acts primarily on the smooth muscles of blood vessels (constriction). Persons with hypertension are particularly at risk.

Therapy. Treatment consists of induced vomiting or gastric lavage, followed by administration of activated charcoal.

Ibotenic Acid, Muscimol

Ibotenic acid and muscimol are isoxazoles present in the panther cap (*Amanita pantherina*) (**B**) and fly agaric (*Amanita muscaria*) (**B**). The fly agaric is well-known and hardly ever eaten as a result of mistaken identity; poisonings are therefore extremely rare. However, it is used increasingly as a narcotic. The poisonous *A. pantherina* differs from the edible European blusher (*Amanita rubescens*) (**B**) by the well-defined margins of cap and bulb, and also by its color. Fresh fly agaric contains muscimol and its precursor ibotenic acid (α-amino-3-hydroxy-5-isoxazoleacetic acid) at a concentration of about 500 mg/kg. The panther cap contains slightly more. Both mushrooms also contain small amounts of muscarine (2–3 mg/kg), but this adds little to their toxicity.

Toxicity. Eating 10 fly agaric mushrooms is fatal for adults. After eating just one or two, the first signs of poisoning appear 0.5–2 h after ingestion; they include increased glandular secretion, impaired coordination of movements (ataxia), and characteristic toxic psychosis. Initially, the psychosis resembles alcohol intoxication and is associated with euphoria, vertigo, and insecure gait; this is followed by agitation with muscle spasms, impaired vision, and hallucination up to sleepiness and coma. Vomiting has not been observed. Poisoning with the panther cap usually runs a more severe course than that with fly agaric.

Therapy. Treatment consists of induced vomiting or gastric lavage, followed by administration of activated charcoal. Sedatives are used for symptomatic treatment of the agitation. Diazepam is given in case of spasms. Atropine is contraindicated.

Muscarine

Muscarine is found in around 50 species of fibercaps (e.g., *Inocybe erubescens*) (**C**) and in several clitocybe species (*Clitocybe* sp.). It was the first mycotoxin to be identified, in 1869. Eating about 50 g of these mushrooms is fatal. Fibercaps contain up to 200 times more muscarine than the fly agaric.

Toxicity. Muscarine causes excessive glandular secretion (sweat, saliva, and tears) 0.5–2 h after ingestion. This is followed by gastroenteritis, impaired vision, bradycardia, bronchospasm, dyspnea, and circulatory insufficiency, possibly leading to death by circulatory paralysis after 8–9 h.

Therapy. Immediate administration of atropine has priority over other treatment. As a competitive antagonist, atropine displaces muscarine from the acetylcholine receptors.

Psilocybin

Psilocybin is contained (up to 1%) in the liberty cap (*Psilocybe semilanceata*) (**D**) and (up to 0.1%) in the girdled panaeolus or banded mottlegill (*Panaeolus cinctulus*). It is used increasingly as a narcotic (see also p. 92).

Toxicity. In adults, 6 mg psilocybin leads to mild mood alteration, and 10 mg causes acute toxic psychosis. The psychotropic effect corresponds to that of mescaline and LSD; for example, colored images appear after 1 h, with distorted perception of time and space, euphoria and dysphoria, visual and auditory hallucinations. The following symptoms may also be observed: vomiting and diarrhea, and a tingling sensation in the limbs.

Therapy. Treatment is typically not necessary, since the narcotic condition does not persist for long.

Toxins acting extracellularly	Toxins acting intracellularly
Pore-forming toxins (lysins)	**ADP-ribosyl transferases**
α-Toxins from *Staphylococcus aureus*	Diphtheria toxin
Streptolysin O	Botulinum toxin type C_2
Pneumolysin	Cholera toxin
Tetanolysin	Pertussis toxin
	Glycosidases
Indirect toxins	Shiga toxin, shiga-like toxins
Enterotoxins from	**Neurotoxic proteases**
Staphylococcus aureus	Tetanus toxin
Lipopolysaccharides (endotoxins)	Botulinum neurotoxins of types A, B, C_1, D, E, F, and G

A. Classification of bacterial toxins

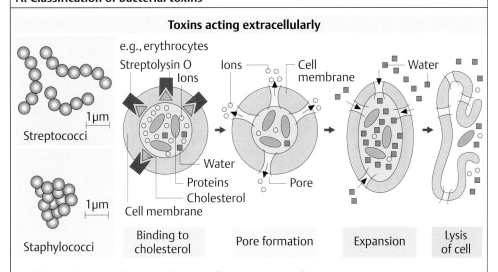

B. Effects of streptolysin O, the pore-forming toxin of streptococci

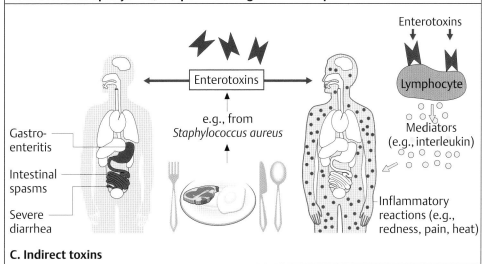

C. Indirect toxins

■ Toxins Acting Intracellularly

Toxins with intracellular effects bind to specific receptors located either on or in the outer cell layer (e.g., cell membrane) of the target cells (e.g., human blood cells, mucosal cells), and then enter the cells in ingenious ways and cause various harmful effects.

All these toxins are proteins. Almost all of them consist of two protein components: one is responsible for receptor binding and facilitation of transport into the cell (kinetic portion), and the other causes damage inside the cell (active portion). Before any damage can be done, the protein must be enzymatically cleaved into its two components. Some intracellularly active toxins can also get into the cell by creating pores in the cell membrane.

ADP-Ribosyl Transferases

ADP-ribosyl transferases belong to those bacterial toxins that transfer adenosine diphosphate ribosyl groups to amino acids (e.g., arginine, cysteine) of regulatory guanosine triphosphate (GTP)-binding proteins, or to structural proteins in the cytoskeleton (e.g., actin), and thus influence cellular function.

Diphtheria toxin is synthesized by *Corynebacterium diphtheriae*, a Gram-positive, irregular rod-shaped bacterium (**A**). The pathogen of diphtheria was discovered by Löffler in 1884. Diphtheria toxin is formed only by rods infected with a certain bacteriophage. It grows preferentially on the nasopharyngeal mucosae of humans and is transmitted by droplet infection from person to person. The incubation time is 3–5 days. The toxin causes inflammatory changes in the tissue of the pharyngeal cavity, thus leading to local fibrinous exudates and leukocyte invasion. The gray pseudomembranes thus formed on the tonsils and pharyngeal mucosa and in the larynx may cause respiratory obstruction and even death by suffocation. Arrhythmia and paralysis of the limbs also occur (**A**). The toxin is made up of 535 amino acids and is capable of forming pores, but it also enters the cells by adsorptive endocytosis. In the cytosol, the toxin transfers ADP-ribosyl groups from NAD^+ to elongation factor 2, which is responsible for the translocation (movement of ribosomes along the mRNA) of the nascent polypeptide chain, thus inhibiting protein biosynthesis in the target cell (**A**). A single toxin molecule can destroy a cell, and 7 µg of toxin is enough to kill a person.

Therapy. Treatment consists of administering diphtheria antitoxin. Active immunization against diphtheria is possible with attenuated toxin (toxoid).

Botulinum toxin C_2 is synthesized by *Clostridium botulinum*. The toxic protein binds to receptors on the cell membrane and enters the cell via endocytosis. Inside the cell, it prevents the formation of actin filaments (F-actin) by transferring ADP-ribosyl groups to actin monomers (G-actin). Normally, the monomers aggregate to form microfilaments, the basic scaffold of the cytoskeleton (**B**). Collapse of the microfilament network finally leads to cell death. Symptoms of intoxication in humans include hypotension, hemorrhage, and pulmonary edema (**B**). Since *Clostridium botulinum* occurs in the soil, fruits and vegetables may be contaminated at any time. The bacterium also forms spores that are particularly resistant to heat. The toxin, however, is heat labile and is destroyed in freshly cooked foods. The bacterium produces several other botulinum toxins, but these are largely neurotoxins (see neurotoxic proteases, p. 292).

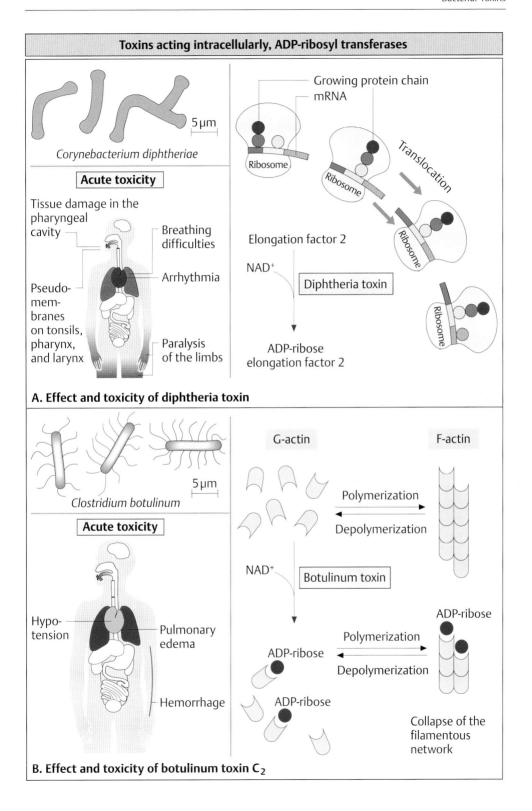

Toxins acting intracellularly, ADP-ribosyl transferases

Corynebacterium diphtheriae

5 µm

Acute toxicity

Tissue damage in the pharyngeal cavity

Breathing difficulties

Arrhythmia

Pseudo-membranes on tonsils, pharynx, and larynx

Paralysis of the limbs

Growing protein chain

mRNA

Ribosome

Translocation

Elongation factor 2

NAD⁺

Diphtheria toxin

ADP-ribose elongation factor 2

A. Effect and toxicity of diphtheria toxin

Clostridium botulinum

5 µm

Acute toxicity

Hypo-tension

Pulmonary edema

Hemorrhage

G-actin

F-actin

Polymerization

Depolymerization

NAD⁺

Botulinum toxin

ADP-ribose

Polymerization

Depolymerization

ADP-ribose

ADP-ribose

Collapse of the filamentous network

B. Effect and toxicity of botulinum toxin C₂

Cholera toxin is synthesized by *Vibrio cholerae*, the pathogen of cholera. This Gram-negative, curved, rod-shaped bacterium with a polar flagellum (**A**) was discovered by Robert Koch in 1883. The bacteria are ingested with contaminated water or food and multiply rapidly in the intestinal mucosa of humans. They cause severe vomiting and diarrhea within a few hours, with a daily water loss of up to 10 L (**A**). Patients may collapse and die within a few hours because of huge losses of minerals and water.

The toxin consists of two protein components. The active portion transfers an ADP-ribosyl group to the membrane-bound stimulatory G-protein (G_s). Normally, G_s activates the enzyme adenylate cyclase, which cleaves adenosine triphosphate (ATP) into diphosphate (PP, pyrophosphate) and cyclic adenosine monophosphate (cAMP). As an intracellular messenger, cAMP controls several functions (**A**). The G_s protein contains a guanosine diphosphate (GDP) group, which is replaced by guanosine triphosphate (GTP) after stimulation of a membrane receptor (formation of GTP–G_s). GTP–G_s then stimulates adenylate cyclase to form cAMP. The GTP–G_s protein furthermore contains GTPase activity, which is used to hydrolyze its own GTP to GDP, thus reducing activity and thereby also neutralizing the stimulation of adenylate cyclase. The formation of cAMP is thus either stimulated or inhibited, depending on the need for it. Cholera toxin transfers an ADP-ribosyl group to the GTP–G_s protein to form the GTP–G_s/ADP-ribosyl protein. This binding causes the protein to lose only its GTPase activity, with the active component remaining in the active state. As a result, adenylate cyclase is permanently activated and cAMP continuously formed (**A**). The uninterrupted formation of cAMP leads to activation of transport mechanisms in the intestine, which transfer ions and water from the blood into the intestinal lumen.

Therapy. Treatment consists of immediate replenishment of water and minerals by infusion, correction of acidosis, and administration of antibiotics (e.g., tetracycline). If infected individuals are left untreated, the mortality is up to 50%. Travelers to cholera-endemic countries (e.g., India, Pakistan, Burma) are recommended to obtain active immunization before traveling.

Pertussis toxin is synthesized by *Bordetella pertussis*, a Gram-negative rod-shaped bacterium with a capsule but without a flagellum (**B**). This bacterium, which is the pathogen of whooping cough, was discovered by Bordet in 1906 and named after him. It preferentially grows in the nasopharyngeal cavity of humans and is transmitted in the expiratory aerosol from person to person. The toxin causes mucosal irritation and severe coughing fits (**B**). In infants, it leads to bronchitis; 60% of all pertussis-related deaths occur in early infancy. The mortality in the first year of life is 1–2%; later, it is less than 1 in 1000. Whooping cough usually lasts for about 3 months and leaves behind strong immunity.

The toxin (molecular weight 105 kDa) enters the cell after binding to certain receptors. The toxin transfers an ADP-ribosyl group to inhibitory G-proteins (G_i), which are then no longer activated and therefore have no inhibitory effect. The GDP–G_i/ADP-ribosyl protein formed cannot bind GTP, thus causing permanent activation of adenylate cyclase (**B**).

A new, noncellular vaccine has been available since 1996. It consists of cell constituents of inactivated pathogens and has very few side effects.

Therapy. Treatment consists of administering antibiotics (e.g., tetracycline).

Toxins acting intracellularly, ADP-ribosyl transferases

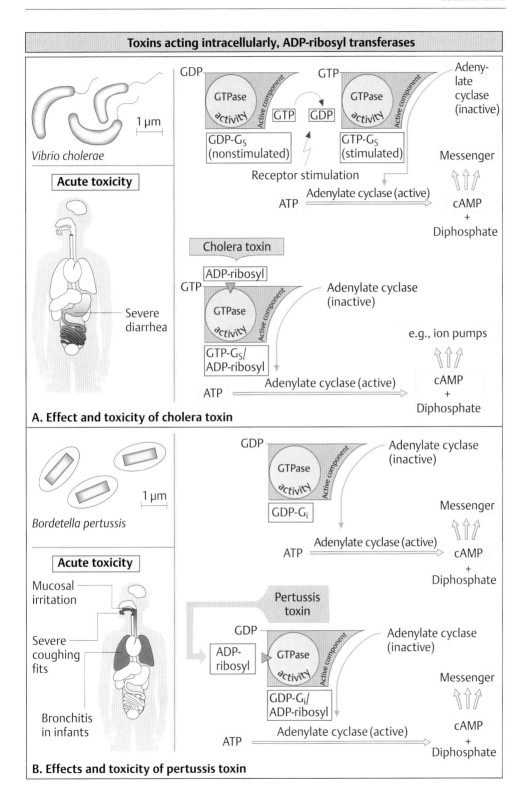

A. Effect and toxicity of cholera toxin

B. Effects and toxicity of pertussis toxin

Glycosidases

Some bacterial toxins are glucosidases that cleave glycosidic bonds between sugars (e.g., ribose) and nucleic acid bases (e.g., adenine) in target cells.

Shiga toxin is synthesized by *Shigella dysenteriae*, and **shiga-like toxins** are produced by various strains of *Escherichia coli*. The two groups of toxins have almost identical profiles of action. Shigellae are Gram-negative, aflagellate, rod-shaped bacteria (**A**). They are the pathogens of bacterial dysentery. Shigella infections are always transmitted by mouth. The disease process manifests predominantly in the colon and leads to acute colitis rather than enteritis. Unlike amoebic dysentery, the disease begins with acute nausea and severe colic, followed by excruciating tenesmus. *E. coli* is a Gram-negative, flagellate rod-shaped bacterium (**A**) and is predominantly taken up with contaminated drinking water.

The active portion of these bacterial toxins enters the target cell by adsorptive endocytosis. Once inside the cell, the toxin inhibits protein synthesis by glycosidic cleavage of adenine–ribose bonds in the 28S rRNA component of eukaryotic ribosomes (**A**).

Therapy. Treatment consists of administration of antibiotics (e.g., tetracycline); otherwise, it is mainly symptomatic.

Neurotoxic Proteases

Neurotoxic proteases cleave specific peptide bonds in the proteins of nerve tissues. All of these neurotoxins possess a homologous, zinc-binding amino acid sequence.

Tetanus toxin, or tetanospasmin, is synthesized by *Clostridium tetani*. The bacterium is the pathogen of tetanus, a disease caused mainly by injuries to the skin and contamination of the wound. The toxin enters the spinal cord through peripheral nerve endings and retrograde axonal transport. It then crosses the synaptic cleft and the presynaptic membrane of interneurons and stops these neurons from releasing inhibitory neurotransmitters (e.g., glycine, GABA). As a result, motor neurons are no longer inhibited, and continuous stimulation of the muscle causes sustained contraction (muscle stiffness) (**B**). In humans, the toxin causes tonic (tetanic) contractions of voluntary muscles, which usually start in the face and lead to generalized spasms and, finally, death by suffocation (**B**). Tetanus still occurs occasionally in Europe. In developing countries, up to 10% of live-born children still die of tetanus due to infection of the umbilical cord (neonatal tetanus).

Therapy. Treatment consists of administration of immune serum (antitoxin). Active immunization against tetanus is possible with attenuated toxin (toxoid).

Botulinum toxins A–G are synthesized by *Clostridium botulinum* (for botulinum toxin C_2, see p. 288). Intoxication takes place when the toxins are ingested along with food (see p. 210). The genes for these toxins are transferred to the bacterium by a bacteriophage. The molecular weight of the toxins is approximately 150 kDa; the toxins enter the target cells through a pore in the membrane or by receptor-mediated endocytosis. Botulinum toxins inhibit the release of acetylcholine at neuromuscular endplates (**C**), thus leading to paralysis of the striated muscles. In humans, the first symptoms include double vision due to dysfunction of the eye muscles, difficulty in swallowing, and impaired speech (**C**). Botulinum toxins are the most effective biological poisons. The fatal dose for humans is 0.1 µg toxin when ingested, and only 1/1000 of this dose when inhaled. Just 1 g toxin is therefore sufficient to kill at least 10 million people.

Therapy. Treatment consists of the administration of antitoxin; otherwise, it is mostly symptomatic.

Toxins acting intracellularly, glycosidases

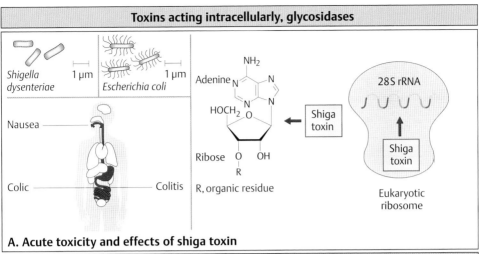

A. Acute toxicity and effects of shiga toxin

Toxins acting intracellularly, neurotoxic proteases

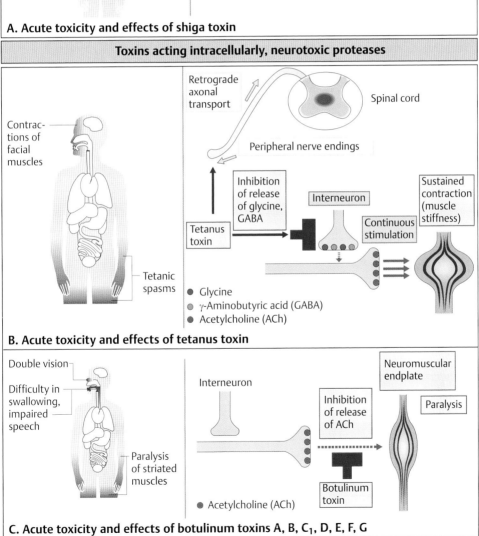

B. Acute toxicity and effects of tetanus toxin

C. Acute toxicity and effects of botulinum toxins A, B, C$_1$, D, E, F, G

▦ Radiation

Basics

The current state of knowledge about various types of radiation is far better than our scientific understanding of the effects of other toxic agents.

Depending on the type of radiation, excessive exposure may lead to complex clinical pictures in humans.

Ionizing radiation. This includes high-energy electromagnetic radiation (X-rays, γ-rays) and particulate radiation (α-rays, β-rays, protons, neutrons, and heavy ions). When high-energy radiation passes through matter, it causes ionization of atoms or molecules.

Nonionizing radiation. This includes short-wave radiation (ultraviolet, laser, and radar) as well as radio waves, microwaves, and electric and magnetic fields.

Units of measurement. Radioactivity is expressed as the number of atomic nuclei disintegrating per unit of time: 1 becquerel (*Bq*) equals 1 disintegration per second, and 1 curie (*Ci*) is the activity of 1 g of radium-226 (^{226}Ra), equaling 3.7×10^{10} Bq.

Radiation carries energy that can be absorbed by matter. The absorbed radiation energy per unit of mass is measured in *gray (Gy)*; when 1 kg of irradiated matter absorbs 1 J of energy, the *energy dose* is 1 J/kg = 1 Gy. (Formerly, this was measured as *radiation absorbed dose*, or *rad*; 1 Gy = 100 rad.) The intensity of the biological effects of ionizing radiation depends not only on the absorbed energy but also on the type of radiation. Different types of radiation have quantitatively different biological effects, depending on the ionization density in matter (number of ionization results per unit length within the matter). This fact is taken into account when using the quality factor Q (Q factor) (**A**). The energy dose multiplied by the Q factor is called the *equivalent dose*, and is measured in *sievert (Sv)*. (Formerly, this was measured as *roentgen equivalent for man*, or *rem*; 1 Sv = 100 rem). In medicine, the unit Gy is often used, since the radiation applied here is usually one with a Q factor of 1.

The biological effects of ionizing and nonionizing radiations on living tissues also depend on the length of time for which a certain dose is applied. The intensity of the effects differs, depending on whether the dose is applied for a short period of time or over a prolonged period (**B**). The dose per unit of time is called *dose rate*. It is measured in *Gy* or *Sv per year*. When only a part of the body is irradiated (partial body exposure), the effects are considerably less severe than with whole body irradiation (whole body exposure).

Tissues differ in their sensitivities to radiation in the following order: gonads > mammary gland > lungs, red bone marrow > thyroid gland, bones > other tissues. The *effective equivalent dose* (in Sv) is the sum of all partial body exposures, based on the sensitivities of the organs, plus the whole body exposure. It is a measure of the radiological risk to an individual person.

A feature of radioactive disintegration is the *physical half-life*, i. e., the time in which half of a given amount of radioactive element will disintegrate (**C**). The *biological half-life* is the time in which half of the administered radionuclide will be eliminated from the body (e.g., in urine, feces) (**D**). The abilities of α-, β-, and γ-radiations to penetrate matter differ considerably. The *half-value thickness* is the thickness of shielding that reduces the activity of a radionuclide by one-half (**E**).

Type of radiation	Quality factor	Type of radiation	Quality factor
X-Rays	1	Thermal neutrons	2.3
γ-Rays	1	Fast neutrons	10
β-Rays	1	α-Rays	20

A. Quality factors for various types of radiation

1/4 h + 1/4 h + 1/4 h + 1/4 h

1/2 h + 1/2 h

1 h

4 days (low-dose rate)   2 days (medium-dose rate)   1 day (high-dose rate)

Low effect
(e.g., no sunburn)   Medium effect   Strong effect
(e.g., sunburn)

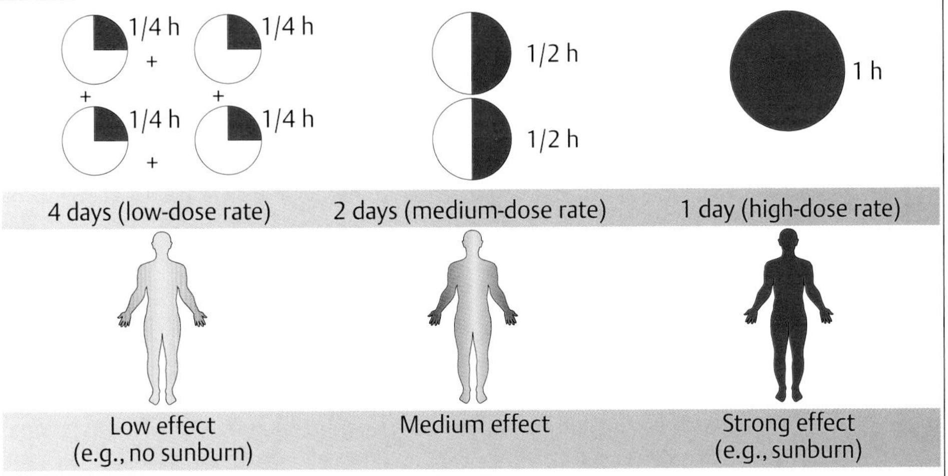

The same dose at lower dose rates is less effective.

B. Dose rates

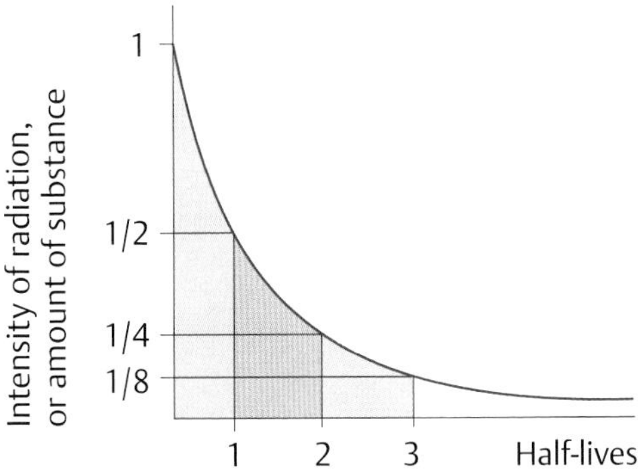

Intensity of radiation, or amount of substance

1
1/2
1/4
1/8

1   2   3   Half-lives

C. Physical half-life

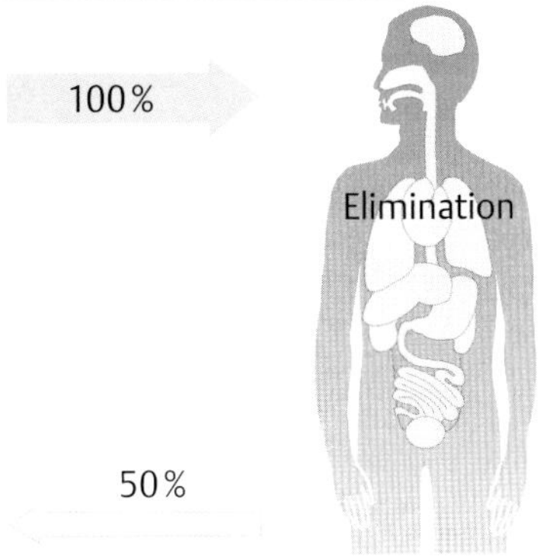

100%

Elimination

50%

D. Biological half-life

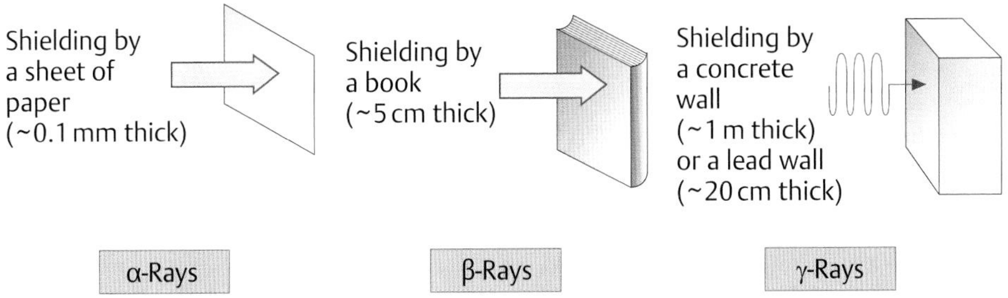

Shielding by
a sheet of
paper
(~0.1 mm thick)

Shielding by
a book
(~5 cm thick)

Shielding by
a concrete
wall
(~1 m thick)
or a lead wall
(~20 cm thick)

α-Rays   β-Rays   γ-Rays

E. Thickness of shields for various types of radiation

■ Ionizing Radiation

Life on Earth has evolved under the constant influence of radiation coming in part from outer space, and in part from various types of terrestrial rocks. In addition to this external radiation, humans are exposed to internal radiation because the body takes up radioactive substances.

Exposure to external radiation. This includes cosmic radiation emanating from outer space or from the Sun (primary cosmic radiation: protons, 86%; α-particles, 12%; heavy nuclei, 1%; electrons, 1%). For example, free protons with high energy can impact atomic nuclei in the Earth's upper atmosphere, thus forming secondary particles that induce further transformations and then release various types of radiation. The hard component of this secondary radiation consists largely of high-energy mesons, which can penetrate meter-thick walls of concrete. The soft, low-energy component consists of electrons, positrons, and γ-rays. These are partly absorbed in the atmosphere, with the dose rate of this cosmic radiation depending on the altitude. At sea level, the annual dose for humans is around 0.3 mSv, whereas on a mountain at 3000 m altitude it is 1.4 mSv (**A**). Frequent flyers have an increased exposure to cosmic radiation (~0.005 mSv/h of flight).

Terrestrial radiation originates from radioactive substances that are present in the soil, water, or air, or are continuously formed there, e.g., potassium (^{40}K), rubidium (^{87}Rb), thorium (^{232}Th), uranium (^{238}U, ^{235}U), carbon (^{14}C), and tritium (^{3}H). Human exposure to radiation takes place outdoors (~0.52 mSv/year) as well as indoors due to radiation released from building materials (~0.18 mSv/year) (**B**).

Exposure to internal radiation. This is due to ingestion and/or inhalation of radioactive substances, e.g., ^{40}K, ^{14}C, ^{226}Ra, radon (^{222}Rn), and ^{3}H. Upon uptake, ^{40}K and ^{14}C are evenly distributed in the body, whereas ^{226}Ra is deposited preferentially in the bones, and the gaseous ^{222}Rn in the airways. In Germany, the incorporation of naturally radioactive substances in humans leads to an average exposure of about 0.2 mSv/year. Depending on building materials

and geographical location, the partial body exposure (e.g., of airways to α-radiation from ^{222}Rn) maybe as high as 10 mSv/year. In some countries (e.g., Sweden) the exposure to ^{222}Rn may be even higher because buildings are so well insulated. As a rule of thumb, a reduction in the ventilation rate by one-half increases the radiation exposure of the lungs by a factor of two.

In addition to this exposure to natural radiation, humans are exposed to radiation from artificial sources, such as ionizing radiation in medicine and technology, or from nuclear weapon tests and nuclear plants. The most important source of radiation exposure (~0.5 mSv/year) is diagnostic X-rays (**C**). Compared with this, other civil radiation exposures are minor (<0.02 mSv/year). The radiation exposure of humans due to nuclear power plants is 0.005 mSv/year, constituting an extremely small proportion (**C**). These exposures to very low levels of radiation result almost exclusively from iodine in the thyroid gland, strontium in the bones, and cesium in the muscles, i.e., in the target organs of these radionuclides.

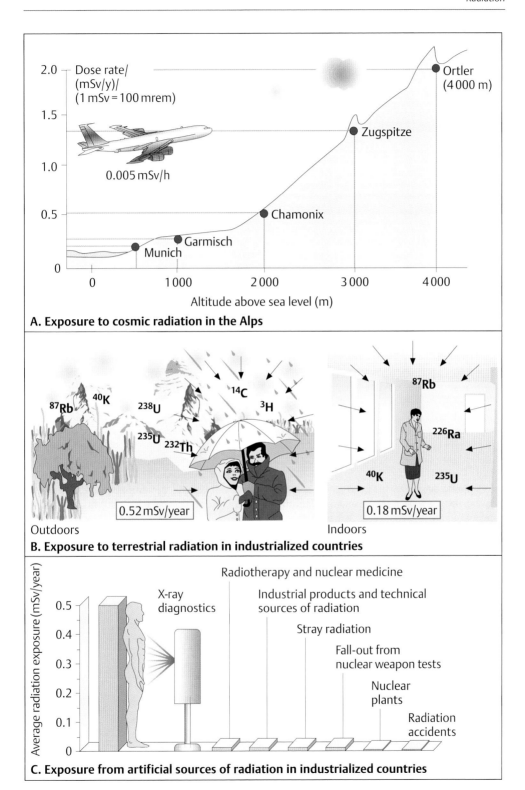

A. Exposure to cosmic radiation in the Alps

B. Exposure to terrestrial radiation in industrialized countries

C. Exposure from artificial sources of radiation in industrialized countries

Effects of Ionizing Radiation

External and internal ionizing radiation lead to the formation of free radicals and peroxides in the body, where they trigger various harmful reactions (**A**) (see formation of radicals and their effects, p. 147 **B**). There is somatic and genetic damage, which may appear early or late. Early somatic damage manifests itself several weeks after exposure to radiation at the latest, whereas late damage appears years or decades later. After the dropping of atom bombs in August, 1945, the leukemia rates in Hiroshima and Nagasaki did not increase until 1950, with a peak being registered 5 years after that. Other cancerous diseases had an even longer latency period, with the peak not appearing until 1970.

Early somatic damage. The relationship between dose and effect has been well documented for early somatic radiation-induced damages. After exposure to about 0.25 Sv (threshold dose) (**B**), a delay in the rate of cell division is observed in radiation-sensitive organs, such as bone marrow, spleen, lymph nodes, mucosae, gonads, and hair follicles. Exposure to higher doses (1–6 Sv) leads to the development of radiation sickness (see p. 182). For acute whole body irradiation, the fatal dose for humans is around 6–10 Sv (**B**).

Late somatic damage. This is largely characterized by the development of anemia, sterility, leukemia, and tumors (e.g., of the thyroid gland). The threshold dose for late damage is more difficult to determine than that for early damage, since these diseases also occur spontaneously. This situation results in a stochastic (random) distribution of cancer cases; i.e., there is no dose–effect relationship. The severity of the disease does not increase with increasing doses as in the case of (nonstochastic) early damage, but the probability of developing leukemia or other cancers is increased.

Genetic radiation damage. This affects DNA (e.g., germ line mutations). A change in the nucleotide sequence of a single gene does not necessarily mean that the change has a detectable phenotypic effect, such as a different gene product or loss of function. The number of mutations usually increases linearly with the radiation dose. Radiation exposure of 50 mSv leads to 15–25 DNA single-strand breaks and 1–2 double-strand breaks within a single cell; however, most of this damage is rapidly repaired (e.g., 90% of single-strand breaks within the first hour). The capacity of the repair systems is crucial in assessing the radiation risk. This capacity is reduced in rare genetic diseases, such as ataxia teleangiectasia, Fanconi's anemia, and progeria. Individuals with these diseases are therefore especially sensitive to ionizing radiation. Calculations of the radiation-induced genetic risk for the average population have shown that, after 1 Sv of radiation exposure, genetic damage occurs with a frequency of 20–50 per 10 000 individuals.

Low-dose, fractionated whole body irradiation can, however, also contribute to the stimulation of the immune system and thus lead to rapid wound healing.

Therapy. Treatment of radiation accidents is primarily geared to the excretion of radionuclides. Uptake and absorption of radionuclides can be inhibited by administering laxatives and the corresponding nonradioactive nuclides (e.g., iodine for radioactive iodine) or chelators (e.g., the zinc salt of diethylenetriaminepentaacetic acid for plutonium). Acute radiation syndrome can only be treated by bone marrow transplantation. In addition, antibiotics and immunosuppressants should be administered to suppress rejection reactions against the transplant (**C**).

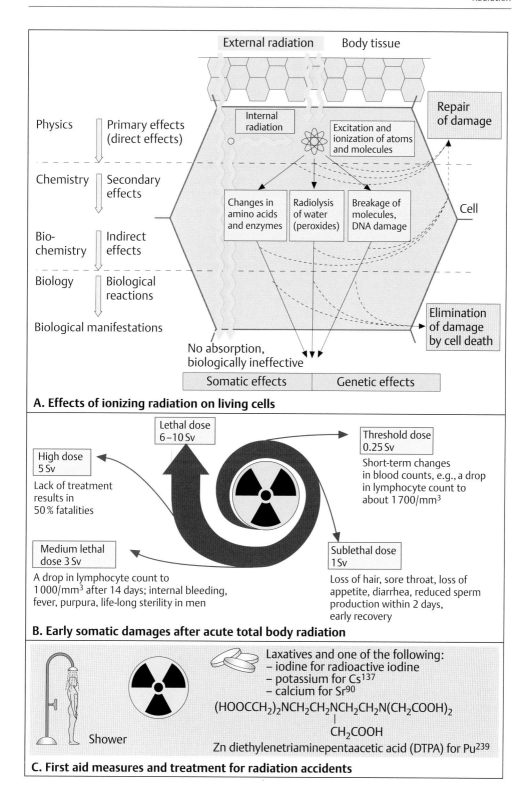

A. Effects of ionizing radiation on living cells

Physics — Primary effects (direct effects)

Chemistry — Secondary effects

Bio-chemistry — Indirect effects

Biology — Biological reactions

Biological manifestations

External radiation / Body tissue

Internal radiation

Excitation and ionization of atoms and molecules

Changes in amino acids and enzymes

Radiolysis of water (peroxides)

Breakage of molecules, DNA damage

Repair of damage

Cell

Elimination of damage by cell death

No absorption, biologically ineffective

Somatic effects / Genetic effects

B. Early somatic damages after acute total body radiation

Lethal dose 6–10 Sv

Threshold dose 0.25 Sv
Short-term changes in blood counts, e.g., a drop in lymphocyte count to about 1 700/mm^3

High dose 5 Sv
Lack of treatment results in 50 % fatalities

Medium lethal dose 3 Sv
A drop in lymphocyte count to 1 000/mm^3 after 14 days; internal bleeding, fever, purpura, life-long sterility in men

Sublethal dose 1 Sv
Loss of hair, sore throat, loss of appetite, diarrhea, reduced sperm production within 2 days, early recovery

C. First aid measures and treatment for radiation accidents

Shower

Laxatives and one of the following:
– iodine for radioactive iodine
– potassium for Cs^{137}
– calcium for Sr^{90}

$(HOOCCH_2)_2NCH_2CH_2NCH_2CH_2N(CH_2COOH)_2$
$|$
CH_2COOH

Zn diethylenetriaminepentaacetic acid (DTPA) for Pu^{239}

■ Nonionizing Radiation

Ultraviolet radiation. This includes wavelengths of 200–280 nm (UVC), 280–320 nm (UVB), and 320–400 nm (UVA). UVB and UVC are largely absorbed by the Earth's atmosphere and contribute to the formation of ozone (see p. 152). UVB light promotes the synthesis of vitamin D_3, while UVA promotes its degradation. Excessive UVA exposure (e.g., in tanning parlors) and simultaneous use of UVB sunscreen lotion can result in dramatically reduced vitamin D_3 levels in the blood, thus affecting calcium and phosphate metabolism (e.g., development of osteoporosis). Low-dose UVA irradiation is successfully used for the treatment of psoriasis. UVC light inactivates cells and induces mutations (e.g., formation of thymine dimers in DNA). A well-known skin reaction following UVB exposure is sunburn (solar dermatitis), which manifests itself as redness, edematous swelling, and a burning sensation. UV light stimulates melanin production in the skin (tanning). People with low melanin production in their skin (blond, fair-skinned individuals) are especially sensitive to UV light. High exposure to UV light may lead to the development of keratosis and teleangiectasia. Both are considered precursors to tumors (e.g., melanoma). Excessive exposure to UV light (e.g., in tanning parlors) increases the risk of skin cancer.

Laser (**l**ight **a**mplification by **s**timulated **e**mission of **r**adiation, 180–1000 nm). A laser beam consists of parallel, monochromatic, bundled light that, depending on its energy, causes damage in tissues (e.g., necrosis). Laser light is used in surgery for the coagulation of blood vessels and for treating retinal detachment.

Radar, radio waves, and microwaves. These are high-frequency electromagnetic waves. The radiant power of various equipment is measured in watts (W): traffic radar, 25 mW; radiotelephones, 2 W; microwave ovens, 1 kW; radio broadcast transmitters and military systems, about 2 MW (**A**). In the human body, waves with a radiant power of 70–280 W/h result in heating, differences in membrane potentials, and cataracts in eye lenses. The actual radiation exposure of the general public, however, is far below 7 W.

Electric and magnetic fields. These are generated when current flows through power lines (electrosmog) and are measured in tesla (T). In street cars and subways, magnetic flux densities (magnetic inductions) measure up to 80 µT, in magnetic suspension railways (monorails) up to 1 T, and in MRI equipment even up to 4 T. High-voltage transmission lines produce the highest electrical field strength (expressed in V/m) at the site of highest transit. The field strength decreases linearly with distance. The electrical field strength along electrified railway lines is ~ 0.8 kV/m at head level. Depending on the distance from household devices (50 Hz and 220 V), an electrical field strength of up to 0.5 kV/m (heating blanket) and a magnetic flux density of up to 2000 µT (hair dryer) can be measured (**B**). With the usual alternating current (50 Hz), 3% of the general population show a vibration of body hair at 1 kV/m, and 50% show it at 10 kV/m.

Magnetic fields induce currents in conductive media (including the human body). Depending on the electric current density (expressed in mA/m^2), these currents have biological effects, such as changes in enzyme activities and ion flux (**C**). The recommended limits for electrical field strength (2–5 kV/m) produce a current density of about 1 mA/m^2 in the body. This corresponds to the natural current density in the body (**C**). A connection between daily exposure to magnetic fields and the occurrence of health defects has not been documented.

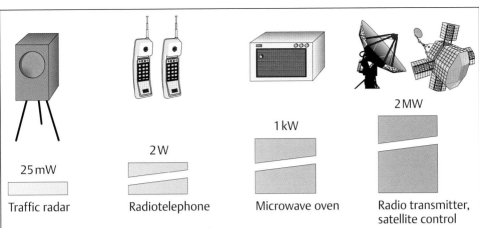

A. Power emitted by various types of equipment

Household appliances

Appliance	Electric field strength kV/m, distance 30 cm	Magnetic current density	
		µT at 3 cm	µT at 30 cm
Electric blanket	0.50	1 – 20	–
Boiler	0.26	–	–
Stereo receiver	0.18	2.5 – 50	0.04 – 2
Iron	0.12	8 – 30	0.12 – 0.3
Refrigerator	0.12	0.5 – 1.7	0.01 – 0.25
Hand mixer	0.10	60 – 700	0.6 – 10
Hair dryer	0.08	6 – 2000	0.01 – 7
Toaster	0.08	7 – 18	0.06 – 0.7
Coffee machine	0.06	0.3 – 1.5	0.1 – 0.2
Vacuum cleaner	0.05	200 – 800	2 – 20
Microwave oven	–	73 – 200	4 – 8

B. Electrical field strength and magnetic flux density

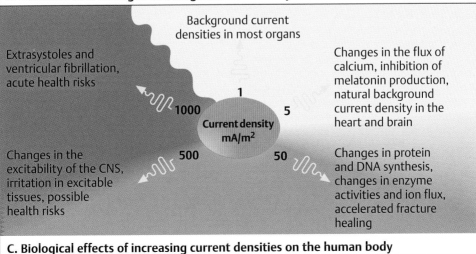

C. Biological effects of increasing current densities on the human body

▪ Noise

Basics

Noise is a mixture of sound waves in the audible frequency range, from 16 Hz to 20 kHz. These sound waves travel with a velocity of 332 m/s in air at 0°C. The sound pressure level is expressed in decibel (dB). The hearing sensitivity does not correspond to the physically measurable level of sound pressure. Using an assessment scale, the physical measuring result is adjusted to the hearing sensitivity of humans and expressed in $dB_{(A)}$.

The unit of the level of loudness is the *phon*. Only at a frequency of 1 kHz does the phon scale correspond to the decibel scale.

The limit value at which the sound pressure level is still just tolerable for the human ear is 85 $dB_{(A)}$, while the threshold of pain is reached at 130 $dB_{(A)}$ (**A**). Most relevant to environmental medicine is the noise of traffic (e.g., cars, airplanes, trains), followed by leisure noise (e.g., sports activities, restaurants, discotheques) and industrial noise (e.g., production plants).

The length of exposure to noise is important for the human sensation of stress. The guidance values for noise emission are 74 $dB_{(A)}$ for cars and 80 $dB_{(A)}$ for trucks.

▪ Effects of Noise

Prolonged exposure to noise adversely affects human health by leading to irritability and impairing sleep and recovery from illness. This results in underperformance and mental disorders. Symptoms of anxiety (e.g., nervousness) and impaired articulation of speech are frequently observed in children. In addition, humans find it very difficult to get used to constant acoustic impulses during sleep (~ 40 $dB_{(A)}$). The shortening of REM sleep—the stage that is most important for recovery—results in frequent periods of wakefulness, thus leading to severe health disturbances, such as frequent headaches, increased heart rate and respiratory rate, and decreased blood flow (stress reactions).

Constant noise pollution also increases the risk for humans of developing hypertension and coronary heart disease. In a person constantly subjected to noise of 66 $dB_{(A)}$ and more, the risk of cardiac infarction is increased to almost twice the normal risk.

Noise leads to measurable changes in physiological parameters in the human body. Studies have shown that constant noise pollution of 65–70 $dB_{(A)}$ causes increased plasma viscosity and increased levels of cholesterol and total triglycerides in the blood (**B**).

▪ Noise Reduction Measures

A reduction in noise emission can be achieved by developing quieter engines (e.g., for cars, trucks, trains and airplanes), improved car tires, and optimized road surfacing (reduced tire noise). The emission of noise can be reduced by installing sound barriers (walls and windows) as well as using noise protection headphones. In zones around recreation areas, hospitals, and care facilities, the emission limit is 45 $dB_{(A)}$ during the day and 35 $dB_{(A)}$ at night.

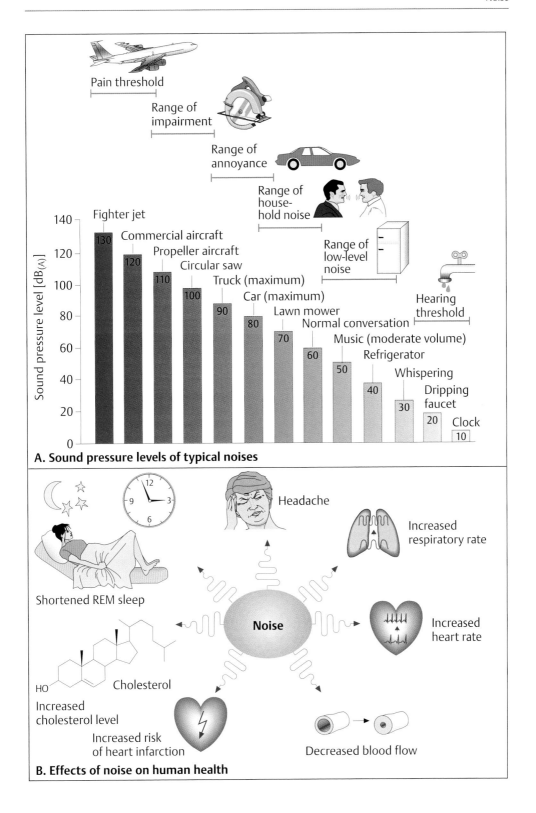

A. Sound pressure levels of typical noises

B. Effects of noise on human health

■ Glossary and Abbreviations

absorption: the passage of a substance across the absorption barriers (skin, mucosae) into the circulation (e.g., blood and/or lymphatic system).

absorption facilitators: various substances that mediate the penetration of active ingredients into the deeper skin layers. They include agents that reduce surface tension and thus facilitate wetting (emulsifiers) as well as lipid-soluble substances (e.g., lecithin, cholesterol, lanolin, or isopropyl fatty acid ester) which facilitate the absorption of fat-soluble active ingredients.

abundance: the number of organisms per unit area or unit space. Also, the number of individuals in a stock or population (population density).

abuse: the improper use of pharmaceuticals or recreational drugs (e.g., alcohol, tobacco). It is defined by WHO as the use of drugs without medical indication or in excessive doses.

accumulation: the quantitative increase of a substance in the body.

acme: the highest point of a fever curve; the crisis or critical stage of a disease.

acne: various diseases of the sebaceous follicle (pilosebaceous unit), characterized by disturbed secretion (parasecretion) and disturbed keratinization (parakeratosis) with subsequent inflammation and scarring.

acupuncture: an old Asian healing method based on the assumption that energy travels along specific channels (or meridians) on the body. There are 14 channels, each of which is assigned to a specific organ (e.g., heart channel, lung channel). Approximately 700 well-defined acupuncture points are located on these channels. The purpose of treatment is to stimulate or calm down the disturbed flow of energy through a specific organ by inserting needles into the corresponding acupuncture points.

acute toxicity testing: a toxicity test involving the one-off administration of a test substance

and subsequent observation for a period of up to 14 days ($\rightarrow$ LD$_{50}$).

adaptation: the adjustment of organs or organisms to specific environmental conditions by practice or habituation.

additive effects: synergistic effects; $\rightarrow$ synergism.

adenoma: a benign epithelial tumor originating from endocrine or exocrine glands or from the gastrointestinal mucosa. An adenoma may develop into a malignant tumor (adenocarcinoma).

ADI: acceptable daily intake. This is an estimate of the amount of a substance in food or drinking-water that can be ingested daily over a lifetime by humans without appreciable health risk. The ADI concept has been developed principally by WHO and FAO and is relevant to chemicals such as food additives, residues of pesticides, and veterinary drugs in foods. ADI values (usually expressed as mg/kg BW) are calculated on the basis of laboratory toxicity data ($\rightarrow$ NOAEL), and from data on human experience, if available, and incorporate a $\rightarrow$ safety factor. For contaminants in food and drinking water, the term tolerable daily intake ($\rightarrow$ TDI) is used. Related term: $\rightarrow$ RfD.

administration: the application of a substance to the body. Routes of administration include: PO, per os (by mouth, into the gastrointestinal tract); SC, subcutaneous (under the skin); IM, intramuscular (into a muscle); IV, intravenous (into the bloodstream); IP, intraperitoneal (into the peritoneal cavity).

adverse health effects: all temporary and permanent undesired changes resulting from chemicals, radiation, accidents, or lifestyle.

agonist: a substance that activates a receptor in the same way as a physiological mediator.

ALARA: as low as reasonably achievable. This term was first introduced in the US legislation on nuclear energy. It means that the environmental risks of radiation should be reduced as much as technically possible and economically feasible; certain health risks are knowingly accepted.

allergen: a particular → antigen that can trigger an allergic immune reaction (by stimulating the synthesis of IgE antibodies) and an immediate (type I) hypersensitivity reaction of the skin and mucosae. Allergens are usually polypeptides or proteins (molecular weight 5000–50 000), and their sensitization potency is determined by their chemical structure and the combination of antigenic determinants (→ epitope). We distinguish between major, intermediate, and minor allergens depending on their frequency, binding affinity to basophilic granulocytes and mast cells, and ability to stimulate IgE synthesis.

allergy: a state of hypersensitivity against a particular antigen (→ allergen) resulting in harmful immune reactions upon subsequent exposure. It leads to disturbances in skin, mucosae, and respiratory tract (e.g., urticaria, eczema, edema, conjunctivitis, hay fever, asthma).

allopathy: a term used in → homeopathy for the treatment of diseases by conventional means, i.e., with remedies having opposite effects to the symptoms.

ALT: alanine aminotransferase. Synonym: glutamic pyruvic transaminase (→ GPT).

Ames test: a procedure for detecting the mutagenic effects of various substances on microorganisms (e.g., salmonella) or on cultured cells or tissues. The test, named after its inventor Bruce Ames, is used for the direct detection of mutagenic and teratogenic effects of chemicals, e.g., in cigarette smoke. Since it is assumed that there is a connection between mutagenicity and carcinogenicity, this test is also used for identifying potentially carcinogenic substances.

annoyance: a negative emotional response originating from unwanted or irritating environmental stimuli, which are experienced as being forced upon oneself. A feeling of unease caused by substances or circumstances that have a negative effect on the individual or the group. The term *annoyance* always refers to a stimulus, while the term → *existential orientation* does not.

anosmia: the absence of the sense of smell. See also → cacosmia, → hyposmia, → hyperosmia, → parosmia.

antagonism: the opposing actions of two functional units (→ agonist, → antagonist). The inhibition or cancellation of the effect of a physiological transmitter by a drug. 1. *competitive a.:* blocking of the receptor leads to the inhibition or stimulation of cellular activity, depending on the type of receptor; an increase in agonist concentration causes displacement of the competitive antagonist from the receptor. 2. *noncompetitive a.:* a change in the molecular structure of the receptor prevents a cellular response; binding of the agonist to the receptor is not affected. 3. *functional a.:* activation of another system that has the opposite effect; inhibition of the cellular response is caused by blocking other receptors of the same cell, or it is mediated by other cells.

antagonist: a pharmaceutical agent that is structurally adapted to an inactive configuration of a receptor and thus prevents its activation.

anthroposophical medicine: an attempt, based on the anthroposophical philosophy of Rudolf Steiner (1861–1925), to widen the scientific image of human nature by adding a spiritual dimension. In terms of → nosology, a distinction is made between a nervous/sensory pole and a metabolic/motor pole, with mutual influence on and compensation by the rhythmic systems (respiratory and cardiovascular systems). Ethical considerations deal with the meaning of illness and life after death. Treatment mainly includes the use of herbal and mineral remedies as well as naturopathic methods and artistic exercises (e.g., eurythmy therapy, anthroposophical therapeutic speech).

antidote: a remedy for counteracting poison. A substance that reduces the effects of a poison.

antigen: a substance that is recognized by the body as being foreign and therefore triggers a specific immune response (e.g., production of antibodies or immunocompetent lymphocytes). An antigen normally has several antigenic determinants (specific surface structures called epitopes), and these react with the induced immune products (e.g., antigen–antibody reaction).

antioxidant: a substance that inhibits oxidation or the reactions promoted by oxygen or peroxides. Antioxidants are thought to protect cellular structures by preventing undesirable changes caused by oxidative processes.

antitoxins: neutralizing antibodies against toxins produced by microbes, plants, or animals (mostly immunoglobulins of the IgG class).

asepsis: freedom from infection. A method of wound treatment and wound care that avoids any touching of the wound with nonsterile material (instruments, dressing material). By contrast, antisepsis is a means of attempting to fight invading bacteria by chemical means.

AST: aspartate aminotransferase. Synonym: glutamic oxaloacetic transaminase (→ GOT).

asthma: a distressing disease characterized by sudden shortness of breath, wheezing, and bronchial muscle spasms. The recurrent attacks of respiratory obstruction are due to a chronically inflamed, hypersensitive bronchial system.

ataxia: failure of locomotor coordination; irregular movements.

atopy: a genetic predisposition to develop allergies.

atrophy: a reduction in the size of a cell, tissue, or organ. It may be caused by undernourishment, disturbed circulation, or endocrine dysfunction (hypophyseal insufficiency).

autohemotherapy: a nonspecific stimulation therapy that is used either on its own or in combination with naturopathic medicines for activating the immune system. It involves collecting blood from the patient's arm and injecting it directly into the gluteus muscle.

Ayurveda: the knowledge of life. A traditional system of East Indian medicine that addresses illness and its treatment. Earth, water, fire, air, and ether serve as metaphors for elementary states of the cosmic existence. The most important principles of the natural world are the three Doshas (forces that disturb); they are called Vata (air/ether; inconstant, cold, dry), Pitta (fire/water; light, hot, bright), and Kapha (water/earth; constant, cold, damp). The development of illness is interpreted as an imbalance of the Doshas or the deposition of waste products (Ama). The aim of treatment is to eliminate Ama and to achieve an allopathic balance of the Doshas. Herbal and mineral remedies, special diets, and various physiotherapeutic measures are used for this purpose.

bactericide: a term for microbicidal agents that kill bacteria. They include ethanol, phenols, soaps, and tensides, which destroy the bacterial cell membrane; other substances affect the bacterial metabolism.

basalioma: basal cell carcinoma, a semimalignant tumor of the skin derived from embryonic hair follicles. Slow infiltrative growth without metastases, mostly occurring at sites of chronic exposure to light.

bathmotropic: changing the stimulus threshold of the heart. *Positive bathmotropic effect:* reducing the threshold (increasing the excitability), *negative bathmotropic effect:* increasing the threshold (reducing the excitability).

behavior: a basic property of living organisms that aims at adjusting the body to the environment. It is controlled by a multitude of biochemical and electrophysiological functions in different organs and organ systems, such as the central nervous system.

BEI: biological exposure index. A reference value intended as a guideline for the evaluation of potential health hazards in the practice of industrial hygiene. It represents the level of a determinant that is most likely observed in specimens collected from healthy workers who have been exposed to chemicals to the same extent as workers with inhalation exposure at the threshold limit value (→ TLV).

benchmark concept: the estimation of a nontoxic dose range by means of the 95 % confidence interval.

bigeminy: an arrhythmia in which heartbeats occur in pairs with a pause between each pair. See also → trigemini.

bioaccumulation: the increase in the concentration of a substance in living organisms as they take in contaminated air, water, or food from the environment (→ exposure pathways).

bioactivation: the transformation of a → xenobiotic in living organisms (e.g., by enzymes) into a toxic or carcinogenic metabolite.

bioavailability: the degree and speed by which the active ingredient of a specific form of medication is absorbed and becomes available at the site of action, or the portion of a pharmaceutical that enters the systemic blood unchanged. The bioavailability of a substance is the ratio of the amount taken in by the organism to the amount absorbed. *Absolute b.:* bioavailability of a drug delivered by a specific form of medication, with IV administration as a reference. *Relative b.:* bioavailability of a drug delivered by a given form of medication, with administration of a similar form of medication as a reference.

biocatalyst: a substance that induces or accelerates a reaction in living organisms (e.g., enzymes, hormones, vitamins, growth factors, macrominerals, and trace elements).

biocenosis: the biotic community of organisms within a → biotope.

biological half-life: the time in which one-half of the originally administered dose of a substance is eliminated (degraded or discharged) by the body.

biological monitoring (biomonitoring): continuous or repeated measurement of potentially toxic substances, their metabolites or their biochemical effects in tissues, secretions, excretions, expired air, or any combination of these. Its purpose is to evaluate occupational or environmental exposure and health risk in individual persons by comparison with appropriate → reference values, which are based on knowledge of the probable relationship between ambient exposure and resultant adverse health effects. Related term: → environmental monitoring.

biotope: the abiotic (i.e., physically and chemically defined) habitat of a → biocenosis.

biotransformation: the enzymatic transformation of → a xenobiotic in a living organism.

Bq: becquerel. The SI unit of radioactivity.

bradycardia: slowing of the pulse rate to less than 60/min.

BW: body weight.

cacosmia: an unpleasant olfactory hallucination. See also → parosmia, → hyposmia, → hyperosmia, → anosmia.

cancer risk factors, chemical: chemical compounds, or mixtures thereof, which have been shown to be involved in human carcinogenesis. → carcinogenicity testing.

carcinogen: a substance that causes the formation of tumors in animals and humans.

carcinogenesis, chemical: the process of uncontrolled new formation (neoplasia) of tissues as the result of carcinogenic compounds. There are three stages of carcinogenesis: initiation, promotion, and progression.

carcinogenicity index (KI): the carcinogenicity index was introduced in Germany for product-oriented evaluation of various types of fiberglass. The index is based on data obtained from animal experiments on fiber carcinogenicity and on the chemical composition of the fiber. Dusts from fiberglass with KI < 30 are classified as carcinogenic substances (category 2, according to the hazardous substances regulations), those with KI > 30 but KI < 40 are suspected carcinogens based on evidence (category 3), and those with KI > 40 are noncarcinogenic. The evaluation scheme for dust from mineral fibers was approved in 1994 by the German hazardous substances committee (AGS) and published in the Technical Rules for Hazardous Substances (TRGS 905).

carcinogenicity testing: a special form of in-vivo → chronic toxicity testing; it is specifically directed toward detecting the carcinogenic effects of a substance. The test substance is administered to experimental animals five times a week for a period of 18–24 months, and the occurrence of tumors is recorded.

carcinoma: a malignant epithelial tumor characterized by rapid, destructive, and infiltrative growth and metastasis.

catalyst: a substance that increases the rate of a chemical reaction without itself participating in the overall equation and without changing its own composition. Small amounts of a catalyst are sufficient for having an effect on unlimited quantities of the reacting substances. Biocatalysts (enzymes) selectively influence very specific reactions or substances.

cell therapy: a controversial procedure in which animal cells (e.g., from unborn lambs) are injected to "rejuvenate" the human tissue.

CFCs: chlorofluorocarbons.

CFS: chronic fatigue syndrome.

CH: chlorinated hydrocarbons.

chamber test: the Duhring chamber test for skin tolerance. This closed → patch test involves testing under extreme conditions for establishing low irritation potentials of substances in topically applied products (e.g., tensides). The test substance is applied on cotton wool or filter paper by means of small aluminum chambers fixed to the forearm and left in place for 18 h (day 1), and again with fresh test substance for 6 h on each of the following 2–5 days. The skin reaction is then scored.

CHD: coronary heart disease.

chelates: from the Latin *chelae*, a crab's claw. Chemical compounds in which molecules possessing two or more free electron pairs (donor groups) simultaneously surround a central atom and form several bonds with it. A prerequisite is that these electron pairs are located sufficiently far apart. Very stable, water-soluble multidentate complexes (chelates) are formed in this way. Chelating agents include heterocyclic ring structures, such as aminocarboxylates, hydroxyaminocarboxylates, and hydroxycarboxylic acid, while the central ions are multivalent metallic ions. The process of chelation is used for binding water hardness elements (Ca^{2+} and Mg^{2+} ions), and also ions of copper, iron, nickel, manganese, arsenic, or mercury. Chelation is also used for chemotherapeutic treatment of metal poisoning.

chiropractic: a healing method based on manual techniques. The pain caused by dislocated vertebrae is eliminated through spinal adjustment.

chloasma (melasma): facial hyperpigmentation of the skin characterized by brown, expanding macules caused by hormones or drugs.

chloracne: severe skin disease with slow-healing, acne-like hyperkeratosis and scarring after exposure to chlorophenols or polychlorinated dibenzodioxins and dibenzofurans.

chronic toxicity testing: a toxicity test involving repeated administration of defined doses of a test substance over a period of at least 3 months.

chronotropic: affecting the course of time; in the narrow sense, affecting the heart rate; *positive c.* (e.g., sympathetic nervous system): the heart rate is increased; *negative c.* (e.g., parasympathetic nervous system): the heart rate is reduced.

clastogenic: giving rise to chromosome breaks.

clearance: a measure for the body's ability to eliminate a chemical substance. In addition to renal excretion, metabolic degradation of the substance in the liver as well as biliary and intestinal excretion lead to a decline of the substance in the body. Total body clearance (Cl_T) is defined as the sum of renal clearance (Cl_R) and nonrenal clearance (Cl_{NR}).

cocarcinogen: a substance that is active during the first phase of → carcinogenesis. It promotes DNA damage and the initiation of tumor cells without being a carcinogen itself (→ tumor promoter).

cohesion: the intermolecular attractive force that holds the particles of a material together. Cohesion plays a role in the dimensional stability of gels and in the surface tension of liquids.

colliquative necrosis: a type of necrosis in which necrotic cells and tissues are softened and liquefied. → necrosis, → gangrene.

combination effect: the intensification or weakening of an effect that occurs when several chemicals with comparable mechanisms of action are simultaneously present, with each affecting a particular organ or biochemical function in the body.

comorbidity: the simultaneous occurrence of several diseases in a person. It usually exists in individuals with → dysthymia. At least 60% of those with dysthymia show additional mood disorders during their lifetime.

compartment: a small enclosure within a larger space. In the narrow sense, a part of the total space in which a substance taken up by the body (e.g., pharmaceutical agent, radionuclide, toxin) is homogeneously distributed and therefore equally subjected to the laws of biokinetics. With the exception of the cardiovascular system, the volume of which can be assessed relatively accurately, the compartment is a theoretical space of hypothetical expansion and may consist of different body fluids or tissues depending on the substance in question. Various compartment models have been developed for the recording of kinetic processes related to pharmaceuticals, toxins, or tracers in biological systems; they represent a crude physiological approximation while simplifying the actual situation (one-, two-, and multicompartment models).

complete carcinogen: a substance that causes tumors in animal experiments when chronically administered without additional measures. According to the multistep concept of → carcinogenesis, these substances have both an initiating and a promoting effect. Synonym: solitary carcinogen.

composite: a synthetic resin used chiefly in dental restorative procedures. The tooth-colored plastic material is filled into the tooth cavity and then hardened chemically or by the application of light.

congeners: closely related chemical compounds, e.g., various polyhalogenated dibenzodioxins and dibenzofurans (→ dioxins). They may have different toxicological properties.

consistency: a collective name for the rheological properties of a substance. It includes the following properties: → viscosity, → thixotropy, and → cohesion, and it contributes to the characterization of a material (e.g., pasty or brittle consistency).

contamination: the unintended presence of any substance or organism that makes a preparation impure.

cross-allergy: the sensitization to biologically and chemically related substances with partly identical antigenic structures (→ allergen, → epitope). It may lead to allergic responses already at first contact. Cross-allergies occur to animals (e.g., domestic and wild cats, water fleas and mites), plants (e.g., pollen of ragweed, golden rod, sunflower, chamomile, and other members of the Compositae family), and medicines (e.g., penicillins and cephalosporins).

cross-reaction: the immunological reaction of specific antibodies or specifically sensitized T lymphocytes with substances that possess antigenic determinants similar or identical to the homologous antigen.

cross-resistance: the development of resistance to an antibiotic or chemotherapeutic agent in bacteria already resistant to a specific, chemically related antibiotic (e.g., kanamycin and neomycin).

cumulation: the accumulation of a substance in the body (associated with occurrence of the corresponding symptoms) caused by exceptional adhesive strength, insufficient degradation, and/or slow excretion. Cumulation occurs once the saturation dose is reached and more substance is continuously administered than is removed by degradation and/or excretion (subsidence rate).

cumulative poisons: toxic substances that accumulate in organisms at increasingly higher concentrations because of poor degradability or insufficient excretion (e.g., chlorinated hydrocarbons, DDT, cadmium or mercury compounds).

cyanosis: bluish discoloration of the skin and mucosae due to excessive concentration of deoxyhemoglobin in the blood.

cyclothymia: a mild affective disorder characterized by mood instability in the form of numerous alternating short cycles of mild depressive and hypomanic episodes over at least 2 years. None of the episodes is sufficiently severe or prolonged to fulfill the criteria for bipolar affective disorder or recurrent depressive disorder. See also → dysthymia.

cytochrome P450-dependent enzyme systems: a series of enzymes, each of which contains the protein cytochrome P450. The oxidized form of the cytochrome binds the substrate to be oxidized. The trivalent iron in the cytochrome is reduced to bivalent iron; this is the form which binds oxygen. However, it can also bind carbon monoxide by forming a complex with a characteristic UV peak at 450 nm (hence the name P450). This makes it possible to determine the cytochrome level in samples.

cytotoxic: damaging to cells.

dB: decibel. The standard unit for measuring sound.

DDT: dichlorodiphenyltrichloroethane (chlorophenotane). A contact insecticide. Because of its extraordinary persistence in the environment and bioaccumulation in the food chain, the use of DDT has been prohibited in the United States since 1973.

decomposers: heterotrophic organisms that break down dead organic matter. They play an important role in ecosystems.

decontamination: the removal of toxic substances from living or nonliving matter.

decorporation: the removal of toxic substances from the body (e.g., after accidental contamination with radionuclides).

delirium: a form of acute organic psychosis associated with disturbed consciousness or orientation, hallucination, disturbed autonomic functions, tremor, and motor restlessness.

dementia: a general term for changes in acquired intellectual abilities as a result of brain damage. It is associated with a general loss of cognitive abilities, including impairment of memory and perception, confabulation, impaired ability to think, disorientation, apraxia, stereotypy, and changes in personality.

depigmentation: removal or loss of pigment, causing a lighter than normal skin color.

deposition: sedimentation of solid, liquid, or gaseous molecules in the body.

depravation: a change for the worse; the aggravation of a disease.

dermatitis: inflammation of the skin, mostly in response to external damage.

dermatosis: any skin disease, especially one not characterized by inflammation.

desensitization: → hyposensitization.

detergent: a substance structurally consisting of hydrophilic as well as hydrophobic (i.e., lipophilic) groups. The groups reduce the surface tension of the water and thus increase or facilitate the wettability of surfaces.

detoxification: the removal of poison from the body. Procedures include those for the mechanical removal of exogenous poisons (e.g., cleansing of the blood) as well as methods for inactivating the poison (→ antidotes), reducing poison absorption, and forcing poison elimination. The term is also used for biological processes rendering endogenous toxic substances harmless through transformation into compounds that are easy to excrete. This transformation occurs mainly in the liver by degradation, conversion (e.g., oxidation, reduction), or coupling to other substances (e.g., glucuronic acid, sulfate).

dioxin(s): the generic term for a diunsaturated, six-membered ring system with two oxygen atoms in the ring. In colloquial speech, the term refers to the group of polychlorinated dibenzodioxins (→ PCDD) and sometimes also to polychlorinated dibenzofurans (→ PCDF). There are 75 PCDD isomers and 135 PCDF isomers. The most widely known dioxin is the one released at Seveso: 2,3,7,8-tetrachlorodibenzo[1,4,]dioxin (→ TCDD); it is far more toxic than all other → congeners.

disinfectant: a substance used for controlling pathogenic microorganisms.

disinfection procedure: any measure that is suitable for removing pathogens by mechanical means, or rendering them noninfectious by physical or chemical means.

dispersion: → distribution.

distribution: in pharmacology, the passage of a substance from one → compartment (e.g., blood, extracellular fluid) to another (e.g., fat tissue), tending to an equilibrium.

doping: in sports, an attempt to enhance performance in a nonphysiological way by intake or injection of a doping substance (e.g., stimulants, narcotics, anabolics, β-receptor blockers, diuretics, peptide hormones), administered either by the athlete or a helper (e.g., the trainer) before or during a competition or training.

dose: the amount of a substance administered to an organism (usually in mg/kg BW).

dose–response relationship: in toxicology, the quantitative relationship between the amount of exposure to a substance and the extent of toxic injury or disease produced.

Draize test: a skin test for checking the toxicity of a substance. Epicutaneous testing (→ patch test) is performed on the shaved skin of at least six rabbits, and the skin reaction is scored using a scale of 0–6: 0, no reaction; 1, mild erythema; 2, swelling, and so on.

dromotropic: influencing the conductivity of nerve fibers or heart muscle fibers; positively or negatively dromotropic means respectively increasing or decreasing the conductivity of the heart.

drug: originally, this term was used for dried substances of plant or animal origin that have softening, healing, anti-inflammatory, astringent, tonifying, or hallucinogenic properties. Today, the term is also used for chemically synthesized medicines and addictive substances.

dust: small, solid particles suspended in the air. Dust may consist of inorganic particles (e.g., rock dust, ash, sand, and clay) and/or organic particles (e.g., plant fragments, pollen, fungal spores, microorganisms, fragments of feathers and mammalian epithelia, parts of mites and insects, and soot). Dust particles smaller than 5 µm are able to pass into the lungs.

dyspepsia: indigestion. In infants, the course of an acute nutritional disorder not caused by impaired organ function. The most common cause is infectious gastroenteritis due to viruses or bacteria.

dysthymia: chronic mild depression. Continuous or regularly recurring depression over a period of at least 2 years. Intermittent periods of normal mood (euthymia) rarely last for more than a few weeks. Hypomanic episodes do not occur. See also → cyclothymia.

EC$_{50}$: median effective concentration. The concentration of an active ingredient that has a specified effect in 50 % of the exposed population.

eczema: a type of dermatitis caused by hypersensitivity of the epidermis and papillary body to repeatedly occurring stimuli. The acute state is characterized by redness, itching, and the outbreak of lesions that may discharge serous matter and become encrusted and scaly. The chronic state is characterized by lichenification, desquamation, hyperkeratosis, and rhagades.

ED$_{50}$: median effective dose. The dose of an active ingredient that has a specified effect in 50 % of the exposed population.

edema: the presence of abnormally large amounts of fluid in the intercellular tissue spaces of the body; e.g., swelling of the skin and mucosae caused by venous or lymphatic obstruction, or increased vascular permeability.

efflorescence: a rash or eruption of the skin.

ejection: in the context of toxicology and environmental medicine: the discharge of pollutants and poisons.

embryotoxicity: damage of the embryo during organogenesis (e.g., by chemicals). It leads to delayed development, disturbed organ function, malformation, or death.

emission: the release of a pollutant from a source (→ emitter) to the wider environment. → immission.

emitter: a source of ionizing radiation (α-, β-, γ-rays), nonionizing radiation (UV radiation, radio waves, microwaves), electromagnetic or mechanical waves, as well as particles, atoms, or chemical compounds. → emission, → immission.

emphysema: the pathological accumulation of gases in tissues and organs (e.g., putrefying emphysema due to gas-producing bacteria), or abnormal amounts of air in air-containing tissues (e.g., → pulmonary emphysema) or in tissues usually free of air (e.g., subcutaneous emphysema).

empirical medicine: the part of the practice of → medicine that is based more on experience than on scientifically accepted clinical evaluation and basic science. Its theoretical foundations include traditional models (e.g., → ethnic medicine, humoral pathology), the humanities (e.g., → anthroposophical medicine), and speculation (e.g., elimination therapy, stimulation therapy, irritation therapy).

endogenous: originating within the body.

environmental epidemiology: the science concerned with the frequency and distribution of diseases and their physical, chemical, emotional, as well as social determinants and consequences in the population.

environmental hygiene: the science concerned with the study of environmental effects on the population and with the identification of favorable and unfavorable factors.

environmental medicine: in contrast to environmental hygiene, it deals with individuals in the context of clinical medicine. If environmental injury is suspected, the patient's history is taken with special reference to occupational exposure, and the necessary therapeutic measures are initiated.

environmental monitoring: the use of living organisms to test the suitability of effluents for discharge into receiving waters and to test the quality of such waters downstream from the discharge.

environmental protection: the prevention or elimination of disturbances in ecosystems by means of social change and individual measures as well as changes in living conditions; e.g., promoting awareness of the environment through information, labeling environmentally friendly products, establishing and monitoring maximum limits for toxic substances and noise levels in production plants, prohibiting extremely toxic substances (e.g., asbestos, DDT), obligatory labeling of toxic compounds (e.g., formaldehyde), recycling, prohibiting or restricting the use of nonrecyclable packaging, reducing energy and water consumption, introducing environmentally acceptable sewage and waste management, restricting motor vehicle traffic and gasoline consumption, and adjusting traffic to optimum speed to reduce fuel consumption.

environmental toxicology: the scientific study of the effects of environmental factors (chemicals, radiation, noise) that disturb the ecological balance and endanger microorganisms, plants, animals, and humans. Environmental toxicology aims to detect and quantify the health risks caused by environmental factors present in air, water, and soil.

EPA: The US Environmental Protection Agency.

ephapse: electrical synapse. A nonphysiological contact between two nerve fibers at the site of a nerve lesion. Signal jumping results in abnormal impulse transmission (cross-talk), e.g., in the case of tonic facial spasm.

epicutaneous testing: → patch test.

epidemiology: the science concerned with the study of factors influencing the frequency and distribution of diseases as well as the physiological variables and social consequences in defined human populations.

epididymis: the elongated structure along the testis.

epitope: the defined antigenic site on the surface of a molecule that binds specifically to the → paratope of an antibody. Synonym: antigenic determinant (→ antigen).

epoxides: highly reactive metabolites mostly formed in the liver and able to react with cellular constituents. The formation of epoxides is responsible for toxic and carcinogenic effects (e. g., those of organic solvents).

erysipelas: an acute, contagious streptococcal inflammation of the skin and subcutaneous tissues that tends to spread through the lymphatic system.

erythema: inflammatory redness of the skin due to congestion of the capillaries. Often caused by a disease. There are many forms, some of which are infectious and require medical treatment and observation. Common erythemas include erythema autumnale (trombidiosis), erythema caloricum (heat erythema), erythema solare (sunburn).

esoteric: the hidden or deeper knowledge understood only by a few. Opposite: exoteric, knowledge that is publicly available and can be understood by all.

ethnic medicine: an anthropological discipline that deals with the concepts of health, illness, and healing in ethnic populations and cultural groups of any origin. In a wider sense, ethnic medicine compares the different systems of traditional healing and investigates the interaction of their proponents in contact situations. In addition to the collection and description of rem-

edies, methods and concepts, it points out the relationship between traditional healing methods and scientific medicine. Its special objectives are the analysis of conflict situations related to the transfer of medical knowledge and the evidence-based re-evaluation of various healing arts and folk remedies not covered by scientific concepts of academic conventional medicine. → Ayurveda, → shamanism, → traditional Chinese medicine.

evasion: the metabolic degradation and elimination of a toxic substance. Metabolic degradation (→ biotransformation) may lead to detoxification but may also make the toxic substance even more toxic (→ toxin generation).

exanthem: a skin eruption or rash that expands over large areas with multiple skin lesions. These eruptions are characterized by a defined course (beginning, peak, and end of the rash).

existential orientation: the emotional disposition and momentary state of a person. This state of mind may have emotional (e.g., anxiety), physical (e.g., pain), social (e.g., loneliness), or functional (e.g., ability to concentrate) dimensions. Disturbances in existential orientation are considered to be changes in the emotional state which the person in question experiences as interfering, or which deviate significantly in negative direction from the statistical distribution of emotional assessments in a reference group, or which lie above a critical threshold value. The emotional state of a person is the psychological equivalent to biological success; it can be measured with psychometric methods. The term *existential orientation* should be distinguished from the term → *annoyance*.

existing chemicals: a collective term for all chemicals that were on the market before 1981 and therefore did not undergo testing for hazardous properties. The European Council Regulation, adopted in 1993, empowers governments to test existing chemicals for environmental compatibility. All chemicals existing prior to 1981 are listed in a database called EINECS (European Inventory of Existing Commercial Chemical Substances).

exogenous: originating from outside the body.

exposure: short-term and long-term contact with a toxic substance or radiation without specification of the quantity.

exposure pathway: the route leading to the up-take of a → xenobiotic into the organism (→ load). Substances may be taken in from conta-minated air, food, water, or soil through inhala-tion, ingestion, or skin contact.

FAO: The Food and Agriculture Organization of the United Nations.

fetotoxicity: injury to the → fetus after organo-genesis is complete.

fetus: the unborn offspring in the postem-bryonic phase, i.e., after organogenesis. In hu-mans, from the 12th week of pregnancy.

fibrosis: the increased formation of fibrous tis-sue (e.g., in the lung or pancreas). See also → sclerosis.

first aid: emergency care given by medical per-sonnel or lay people before regular medical aid can be obtained.

first-pass effect: an important phenomenon of drug metabolism. After oral administration, the drug must pass through the liver before reach-ing the systemic circulation. Some drugs are so extensively metabolized by the liver that only a small amount of unchanged drug may enter the systemic circulation. The intestinal wall can also be a site of first-pass metabolism.

fissure: a cleft, crack, or rhagade. These lacera-tions develop when the elasticity of the skin changes and the skin becomes brittle.

flue ash: untreated flue ash may contain toxic compounds in high concentration depending on the combustion material (e.g., heavy metals, or-ganic compounds). Like filter dust, it must be removed by flue-gas purification and disposed of in an environmentally safe way.

food chain: the relationship between food pro-ducers and food consumers (e.g., forage plant–herbivore–carnivore). Energy is transferred from one organism to another through the food chain. Persistent, lipophilic toxic substan-ces accumulate over time by means of the food chain (→ bioaccumulation).

function: processes taking place in ecosystems (e.g., flow of energy, metabolic cycles).

GABA: gamma-aminobutyric acid (γ-aminobu-tyric acid).

gangrene: a form of ischemic → necrosis with autolysis of the tissue and discoloration through hemoglobin degradation. → colliquative ne-crosis.

genome: the complete gene complement of an organism.

genomics: the study of the entire → genome of an organism.

genotoxicity: toxic effects on the genetic mate-rial of cells or cellular constituents (e.g., damage to the DNA and the mitotic apparatus).

germicide: a compound that kills germs.

GIT: gastrointestinal tract.

glutathione conjugates: numerous → xenobiot-ics (e.g., paracetamol, organic halogen com-pounds) can react in the liver and other organs with the tripeptide glutathione and thus be-come transformed into nontoxic products that can be easily eliminated. Certain glutathione conjugates exhibit an increased toxicity in spe-cific organs (e.g., in the kidney). The consump-tion of glutathione (e.g., in case of drug over-dosage) may also have toxic effects.

GOT: glutamate oxaloacetate transaminase. Syn-onym: aspartate aminotransferase (→ AST).

GPT: glutamate pyruvate transaminase. Syno-nym: alanine aminotransferase (→ ALT).

GSH: glutathione.

guideline values: approximate values for evaluating the concentration of pollutants in soil, air, water, and food. They are derived from comparative measurements in polluted and unpolluted media and are used for orientation only; they are not legally binding.

Gy: gray. The SI unit for the absorbed radiation dose.

hazard: a source of danger; the potential for radiation, chemicals, or other pollutants to cause human illness or injury. Hazard identification of a given substance is an informed judgment based on verifiable toxicity data from animal models or human studies.

hazardous chemical: an → EPA designation for any hazardous material requiring an → MSDS under → OSHA's Hazard Communication Standard. Such substances are capable of producing fires and explosions or adverse health effects such as cancer and dermatitis. Hazardous chemicals are distinct from hazardous waste.

hazardous substance: 1. Any material that poses a threat to human health and/or the environment. Typical hazardous substances are toxic, corrosive, flammable, explosive, or chemically reactive. 2. Any substance designated by the → EPA to be reported if a designated quantity of the substance is spilled in the waters of the United States or is otherwise released into the environment.

hazardous waste: by-products of society that can pose a substantial or potential hazard to human health or the environment when improperly managed. Hazardous waste possesses at least one of four characteristics (ignitability, corrosivity, reactivity, or toxicity) or appears on special → EPA lists.

Hb: hemoglobin.

HBM values: → human biomonitoring values I and II.

HCB: hexachlorobenzene.

γ-HCH: γ-hexachlorocyclohexane → lindane.

HC value: hazardous concentration. The acceptable concentration limit based on ecotoxicology.

health: the state of complete physical, mental, and social well-being (WHO definition, 1998).

health risk: the probability that an adverse effect on human health occurs in a population exposed to a toxic factor. The risk depends on the dose and duration of exposure to a toxic substance or damaging factor, and on its activity.

hemangioma: a common benign tumor made up of blood vessels.

hemangiosarcoma: a rare malignant tumor of vascular origin.

hematopoiesis: the formation and development of blood cells, i. e., the formation of red blood cells (erythropoiesis), white blood cells (leukopoiesis), and platelets (thrombocytopoiesis).

hemoperfusion: an extracorporal procedure for the purification of blood, especially for the elimination of toxic substances by means of adsorbents (e.g., activated charcoal or nonionic resins).

holistic medicine: a system of medicine which considers a person as a functional unit and deals with all aspects of a human being and its environment; in the narrow sense, it is based on nonscientific medical systems (e.g., → Ayurveda, humoral pathology, → anthroposophical medicine, → shamanism, → traditional Chinese medicine) which assume that general realities are only accessible in the realm of ideas, although specific aspects are also accessible to scientific theories (→ empirical medicine).

Holland list: a listing of threshold contamination levels, or → reference values, for toxic substance concentrations in the soil. The list is used in the Netherlands for the assessment of contaminated sites.

homeopathy: a system of therapeutics founded by Samuel Hahnemann (1755–1843). It does not treat diseases by administration of substances directed against the symptoms (→ allopa-

315

thy); rather, it uses low doses of substances which, when given in high doses, cause symptoms similar to those of the disease (e.g., thallium in low doses is used for treating alopecia). In classical homeopathy, this principle of similarity (*similia similibus curentur*, Latin for "like cures like") is complemented by a complex system of assignments regarding both the patient's characteristics (constitutional type) and the medicines applied (which may be of plant, animal, or mineral origin). All this is taken into consideration when prescribing individual remedies. The medicines are thought to undergo energetic transformation (potentiation) by grinding or vigorous shaking. They are usually administered in extremely low doses, with the original material (→ mother tincture) being diluted on the decimal scale to create different potencies. The decimal exponent characterizes the level of dilution: 1 × or D 1 is a dilution of 1:10, 2 × or D 2 is a dilution of 1:100, and so on.

human biomonitoring values I and II (HBM I, HBM II): These are scientifically based threshold limits of biological exposure. They have been established by the Human Biomonitoring Commission of the German Federal Environmental Agency on the basis of toxicological studies in occupational medicine and environmental medicine. The HBM I value defines the border between ecologically safe values and those that need to be regulated. Once the HBM II value is surpassed, there is a considerable risk to human health; medical attention, measures to reduce exposure, and specific diagnostic procedures (monitoring of the effect) are therefore indicated.

human toxicity: the toxic effects of noxious substances on humans.

hyperemia: congestion. An increase of blood in organs and localized body areas, resulting from increased blood supply or reduced drainage.

hyperosmia: an increased sensitivity to smell. See also → anosmia, → cacosmia, → hyposmia, → parosmia.

hyperpigmentation: abnormally increased skin pigmentation resulting from increased melanin production.

hypersensitivity: 1. acquired h. (→ allergy); 2; inherited h. (→ idiosyncrasy; in most cases, unrecognized allergies); 3. insufficient protective function due to chemical damage.

hypopigmentation: abnormally diminished skin pigmentation resulting from decreased melanin production.

hyposensitization (desensitization): a form of immunotherapy by which a person is gradually desensitized against progressively larger doses of an offending allergen. The allergen-specific, IgE-mediated response is gradually reduced by treatment with subcutaneous injections or sublingual drops of the allergen at subliminal, slowly increasing concentrations at regular intervals over a long period of time.

hyposmia: a decreased sensitivity to smell. See also → anosmia, → cacosmia, → hyperosmia, → parosmia.

IARC: International Agency for Research on Cancer.

ICRP: International Commission on Radiological Protection.

idiosyncrasy: an inherited or acquired hypersensitivity to certain foods or drugs already upon first contact. It is most commonly caused by an enzyme defect (e.g., favism). It is not an → allergy.

IM: intramuscular; administration into a muscle.

immission: the concentration of a pollutant in the environment. The term is widely used for air pollution, noise, and radiation; it is often synonymous with → exposure. Immission is measured at the place where it may affect humans and/or the environment, unlike → emission which is measured at the place of origin.

immunosuppression: the weakening or suppression of immune responses. It may result in a diminished immune defense during infections.

immunotoxicity: any adverse effect on the immune system caused by exposure to chemical substances or other factors.

incidence: the number of new cases of a specific disease within a certain period of time. An epidemiological measure for characterizing the course of the disease in a given population.

incidence rate: the number of new cases of a disease per unit of time in relation to the number of people in the exposed population. → prevalence.

incorporation: the passage of a toxic substance into an organism or body compartment (e.g., lung, gastrointestinal tract).

in dubio pro aegroto: [Latin] "in cases of doubt, in favor of the impaired." This old legal principle cannot be used by a medical expert writing a report for compensation claims.

in dubio pro reo: [Latin] "in cases of doubt, in favor of the defendant." This old legal principle cannot be used by a medical expert writing a report for compensation claims.

infant enteritis: an early stage of → infant toxicosis.

infant toxicosis: a severe course of → dyspepsia with toxic symptoms, partly resulting from insufficient treatment at the initial stage. Synonym: acute encephaloenteritis.

infection: the invasion of the body by an infectious agent (e.g., parasite, bacterium, virus, prion).

inflammation: a protective response of the body and its tissues to various (damaging) stimuli.

initiator: a substance that causes irreversible damage to the DNA and may therefore initiate a tumor. → carcinogenesis.

injection: the introduction of a fluid into a body part by using a syringe.

inotropic: affecting the force or energy of muscular contraction (of the heart). A positive ino-tropic effect increases the strength of muscular contraction; a negative inotropic effect reduces it.

intake: the amount of a substance that is taken into the body, regardless of whether or not it is absorbed; the total daily intake is the sum of the daily intake by an individual from food, drinking water, and inhaled air. See also → uptake.

intertrigo: red, erosive, itching, and burning skin lesions occurring in body folds (e.g., beneath the breasts, in the armpits, at the perineum, between the thighs).

intervention value: a value discussed in connection with regulations for residues or contaminations found in foods that are below the guidance values. When the intervention limits are exceeded, suitable measures must be taken to minimize the introduction of the substance into the environment, thus minimizing the contamination of foods.

intolerance: medical incompatibility.

intoxication: poisoning. The effect of substances that are usually defined chemically. These substances originate from minerals, plants, animals, and microbes. They may enter the body through the gastrointestinal tract, the respiratory tract, intact skin, and also through wounds or by injection. The severity of the disease depends on the poisonous properties (toxicity) of the substance (poison), the quantity (dose), and the exposure time (duration). It also depends on the receptiveness (susceptibility) of the affected individual. The poisoned person usually shows characteristic symptoms.

intubation: the insertion of a special tube into the trachea or major bronchus.

inversion layer: a layer of warm, uniformly dense air in the atmosphere that prevents the rise of air from the ground and traps pollutants beneath it. Under certain meteorological conditions, this can lead to the formation of → smog in the layer close to the ground.

IP: intraperitoneal; administration into the abdominal cavity.

ipecac syrup: the syrup obtained from the roots of *Cephaelis ipecacuanha*, containing the alkaloids emetine and cephaeline. It is used as an expectorant because of its secretolytic and secretory properties and/or, at a higher dose, as an emetic in the case of poisoning.

isotonicity: the uniformity of osmotic pressure in the body fluids (e.g., blood plasma) of a healthy person. Isotonic solutions have the same osmotic pressure.

IV: intravenous; administration into the blood stream.

LC$_{50}$: median lethal concentration. The concentration of a chemical substance in the environment (in ambient air, or in the water in the case of aquatic organisms) that will kill 50% of the population exposed.

LCt$_{50}$: median lethal concentration time. The product of concentration and time (Ct) is a measure for the exposure to a chemical substance or poison. The LCt$_{50}$ (expressed in mg × min/m^3) is the exposure that will kill 50% of the population exposed.

LD$_{50}$: median lethal dose. The dose of a chemical substance (expressed in mg/kg BW) that will kill 50% of the population exposed.

leukemia: a → neoplasm of the blood-forming organs. Different clinical pictures are described on the basis of the acute or chronic course of this progressive, malignant disease.

lichen: any of several skin diseases in which the lesions are small, with firm papules set close together.

limit values: these have been established to limit the concentration of pollutants in the environment and thus protect humans and the environment from the toxic effects of chemicals or radiation. They are legally binding. Limit values based on toxicology are, for example, the maximum tolerated dose (→ MTD) for pesticides in food or the threshold limit values at the workplace (→ TLV).

lindane: γ-1,2,3,4,5,6-hexachlorocyclohexane (→ γ-HCH).

load: burden, exposure. *External l.:* Short-term or long-term exposure to toxic substances or radiation that affect the body from the outside. *Internal load:* Short-term or long-term exposure to toxic substances or radiation that affect the body from within. The internal load is a function of the concentration and retention time of the toxic agent or the source of radiation in the body. Any risk assessment for the individual person is based on the knowledge of the mechanism of action, toxicokinetics, dose–response relationship, and internal load.

LOAEL: lowest observed adverse effect level. The lowest dose of a substance at which harmful effects can still be detected.

LOC: level of concern. The threshold concentration in air of an extremely hazardous substance above which there may be serious immediate health effects to anyone exposed to it for short periods.

LOEC: lowest observed effect concentration. The lowest concentration of a substance at which harmful effects can still be observed.

maintenance dose: the dose providing a stable state over a long period. When given at a therapeutic concentration, it corresponds to the portion of the pharmaceutical that is eliminated during the dosage interval.

malignoma: a malignant tumor.

MATC: maximum acceptable toxic concentration. The MATC values mark the threshold between acceptable toxic concentrations and toxic exposure under defined conditions. Once a MATC value is reached, health safety regulations demand that measures be taken to clean up the soil. For a given ecological effects test, the range between → NOAEL and → LOAEL.

maximum acceptable toxic concentration: → MATC, → TSKB.

maximum residue level: → MRL.

maximum tolerated dose: → MTD.

MCS: multiple chemical sensitivity.

mechanism of action: the interpretation of elementary processes of pharmacological and toxicological effects on the biochemical, physical, and physiological levels. Each effect is based on a chemical mechanism. When the mechanisms are not sufficiently known, the term *mode of action* is used instead.

medicine: the science of human health and diseases. It deals with the causes and effects of diseases, and with their prevention and treatment.

MeHgX: methylmercury compounds. The letter X denotes a halide: chlorine, bromine, or iodine.

meiofauna: in ecology, the entirety of small animals (0.2–2 mm) that live in or on the ground.

melanoma: a malignant tumor of the skin, mucosae, or eyes. It is characterized by yellow to black melanin pigment and early metastasis.

metabolome: the collection of all metabolites in an organism, as the end products of gene expression. See also → metabolomics.

metabolomics: the systematic study of the unique chemical fingerprints that specific chemical processes leave behind (→ metabolome).

monograph: a detailed and documented treatise on a particular subject.

monopreparation: medicines that contain only one active ingredient.

morbidity: the → incidence and → prevalence of a disease in a population. See also → mortality.

mortality: the death rate. The ratio of the total number of deaths to the total population in a given time period.

mother tincture: the undiluted alcoholic extract of the original material, from which dilutions (potencies) are prepared by adding alcohol or water. → homeopathy.

MPL: maximum permissible level. It indicates the highest permissible limit for toxic substances in individual foods and is based on typical eating habits. It does not surpass the → ADI for these toxic substances.

MRL: maximum residue level. Comparable to a US tolerance level, the MRL is the enforceable limit on food pesticide levels in some countries. Levels are set by the Codex Alimentarius Commission, a United Nations agency managed and funded jointly by WHO and FAO.

MSDS: material safety data sheet.

MTD: The highest daily dose of a chemical that does not cause overt toxicity in a 90-day study in laboratory mice or rats. This dose is then used for longer-term safety assessment in the same species, usually lasting 2 years or a lifetime.

mutagenicity: the capacity to cause → mutation.

mutagenicity testing: test systems for studying the mutagenic properties of substances. These tests use bacteria (→ Ames test, salmonella mutagenicity test) and mammalian cells.

mutation: a permanent change in the genetic material of a cell, which is passed on to the daughter cells.

NAD: no abnormality detected. Without pathological findings.

necrosis: the localized death of tissues. The dying parts of a tissue or organ, while the surrounding cells survive. Necrosis develops as a result of injuries, oxygen deficiency, poisoning, burns, irradiation damage, etc. The dead tissue is replaced by granulation tissue, and scars are formed.

319

neoplasia: the formation of new tissue. 1. The result of regeneration (e.g., granulation tissue during wound healing); 2. the formation of a → neoplasm.

neoplasm: a new growth of tissue due to a loss in growth control rather than hyperplasia, hypertrophy, and regeneration. → tumor.

NET: no-effect threshold.

neural therapy: a form of treatment based on the idea that all vital processes are controlled by the autonomic nervous system. By injecting local anesthetics (e.g., lidocaine or procaine) into foci, or fields of disturbance (e.g., scars, focal inflammation), the disturbed self-regulation of the body can be influenced in a positive way.

NOAEL: no observed adverse effect level. The highest dose of a substance that does not have a noticeable harmful effect.

nocebo: a harmless substance or factor that is experienced as having an adverse effect on health as a result of negative expectations. See also → placebo.

nocebo effect: a phenomenon whereby a patient who believes that a treatment will cause harm actually experiences adverse effects. See also → placebo effect.

NOEC: no observed effect concentration. The highest concentration of a substance that does not have a noticeable effect.

normal value: the concentration of a substance, or mixture of substances, that occurs normally in organisms or in the environment.

nosology: the science of the classification of diseases.

noxa: a toxic factor or, in general, every damaging influence of a physical (noise, vibration, radiation) or chemical nature (toxic substances).

objectivity: an unprejudiced or open orientation to information about the nature of phenomena being studied. A quality criterion for test proce-

dures that indicates to what extent the results were changed by the investigator, or whether different analyzers obtained identical results.

occupational illness: the diseases qualifying as occupational illnesses are defined by government regulations and include those from which an insured person suffers as a result of certain working conditions as defined by the insurance coverage. According to current medical knowledge, these diseases are caused by specific factors to which certain groups of people are far more exposed during their work than the rest of the population.

occupational medicine: the branch of health sciences dealing with occupational diseases, workplace injuries, occupational hygiene, and occupational toxicology.

old hazardous sites: ground areas contaminated with substances that pose a health hazard (e.g., disused landfill sites, closed-down plants, abandoned industrial sites).

omics: a neologism referring to a field of study in biology ending in the suffix "omics" (e.g., → genomics, → metabolomics, → proteomics, → toxicogenomics).

organ toxicity: the property of a substance to induce organ damage.

OSHA: the US Occupational Safety and Health Administration.

ozone therapy: the ozone is diluted with regular oxygen and then either admixed to the blood of the patient (→ autohemotherapy) or injected directly into the body or into the cavity of the tooth.

PAH: polycyclic aromatic hydrocarbons.

paramedicine: a medical system with diagnostic and therapeutic principles and models of explanation that lie outside of commonly accepted, science-based conventional medicine.

paratope: the part of an antibody that is sterically complementary to the antigenic determinant (→ epitope) and is also the antigen-binding part of T-cell receptors. It consists of the hypervariable regions of the H and C chains of the Fab fragment. Synonym: antigen-binding site.

paresthesia: an abnormal skin sensation, such as burning or prickling, often in the absence of an external stimulus. → sensory disturbance.

parosmia: a distorted sense of olfaction. See also → anosmia, → cacosmia, → hyposmia, → hyperosmia.

patch test: an epicutaneous test for identifying allergic sensitivities. It shows whether a substance that comes into contact with the skin causes inflammation of the skin (contact dermatitis). The substance in question is applied under a piece of adhesive tape (1 cm^2) to healthy skin and left in place for 24 h. The patch is then removed, and the skin reaction is examined and scored after 10 min, 12 h, and 24 h. If the test is positive, the skin shows redness (+), papulovesicular lesions (++), or blistering (+++). It is essential that the substance to be tested is nontoxic; toxic substances almost always cause toxic dermatitis. To determine whether a substance may lead to sensitization, the patch test is repeated five times at intervals of 48 h and then again after 5 days.

PCB: polychlorinated biphenyls.

PCDD: a class of compounds called polychlorinated dibenzodioxins (→ dioxins) that includes 75 partly highly toxic chemicals. They originate from pentachlorophenol and are ubiquitous. Their best known representative is 2,3,7,8-tetrachlorodibenzo[1,4]dioxin.

PCDF: polychlorinated dibenzofurans. See also → PCDD; → dioxins

PCP: pentachlorophenol.

peak limitation: an exposure standard for certain working materials. Peak limitations are subdivided into categories 1–5 (e.g., category 1, locally irritating substances; category 5, substances of intense odor).

penetration: in pharmacokinetics, the passage of an administered substance into the circulation (blood and/or lymph circulation, → absorption) and its subsequent distribution and storage in the body.

permeation: the act of passing through, or penetrating, a tissue, cell, or cell membrane.

persistence: the stability of a substance against degradation in the environment or within an organism.

persorption: the passage of solid, undissolved particles (5–150 µm) through the intact epithelium of the intestine.

phobia: an excessive, irrational fear triggered by certain objects or situations. It is usually associated with the knowledge that it is unfounded.

photodermatosis: any skin disease that is induced by exposure to UV light (e.g., sunburn, solar urticaria, summer prurigo, farmer's or sailor's skin, pigmentation anomalies, connective tissue atrophies, cutaneous carcinoma).

phytotherapy: the therapeutic use of medicinal plants for the treatment and prophylaxis of diseases.

placebo: a dummy medical preparation without an active ingredient but resembling the true preparation (verum) in shape, color, taste, and appearance. Placebos are agents or factors that cause the experience of a health-promoting effect based on positive expectation. See also → nocebo.

placebo effect: the experience of a health-promoting effect based on positive expectation. See also → nocebo effect.

plasmapheresis: plasma exchange. The mechanical separation of plasma from drawn blood and retransfusion of the resuspended corpuscular elements (red and white blood cells, and platelets) into the donor.

PO: per os, administration by mouth.

poison: a substance that has toxic effects at a certain dose and causes death under certain circumstances because of its chemical or physical properties. Poisons are usually mixtures of different poisonous substances. Frequently, a poison is a mixture of secretion products (e.g., the poisons of bees and snakes) consisting of a multitude of individual components, some of which may represent → toxins and/or various enzymes.

poison categories: poisonous substances are classified according to their → LD_{50}. The German Chemicals Act distinguishes the following categories (doses for oral administration in rats, in mg/kg BW): highly poisonous, LD_{50} less than 25; poisonous, LD_{50} 25–200; less poisonous, LD_{50} 200–2000; not poisonous, LD_{50} more than 2000. A more detailed classification also considers the route of substance intake (SC, IV, etc.), the physical state of the substance (solid, liquid, gaseous), and the animal species.

pollutant: any substance that causes harm to the environment when it mixes with soil, water, or air. See also → toxic substance.

polyneuropathy: a disorder of the peripheral nerves that is not caused by trauma. Typical symptoms include distal paresthesia and reduced sensibility, followed later by flaccid paralysis, areflexia, possibly muscular atrophy and trophic disorder of the skin. Typical is the symmetrical distribution of symptoms.

porphyria: an inherited or acquired disturbance of the biosynthesis of heme that is associated with overproduction, accumulation, or increased excretion of porphyrins or their precursors.

ppb: parts per billion.

ppm: parts per million.

prevalence: the number of cases of a disease, or the frequency of a symptom, in a population at a specified point in time (point prevalence) or over a specified period of time (period prevalence). An epidemiological measure for characterizing the course of a disease in a population.

prevalence rate: the number of cases, or the frequency of a symptom, in relation to the number of persons examined. See also → incidence.

progression: the phase of increasing growth autonomy and malignancy during the development of a tumor (→ carcinogenesis).

promotion: the phase of proliferation of initiated cells during → carcinogenesis. → tumor promoter.

proteome: the complete set of proteins synthesized from the information encoded in the → genome.

proteomics: the study of the → proteome.

prurigo: an etiologically and morphologically heterogeneous group of skin lesions with itchy, partly urticarious papules, seropapules, or nodules.

pruritus: itching. An unpleasant cutaneous sensation that provokes the urge to scratch the skin. The following factors participate in inducing and processing this sensation: pain receptors, the autonomic nervous system, the cerebral cortex and emotions, certain mediators (e. g., histamine, trypsin, callicrein), the vascular system of the skin, and the internal organs. Pruritus may have numerous causes, such as internal diseases, nervousness, animal and plant parasites, hypersensitivity reactions, incompatibilities, and intoxication. Skin lesions caused by scratching include red streaks, crusts, hyperpigmentation, lichenification, and pyoderma.

PTWI: provisional tolerable weekly intake. The dose of a toxic substance that, according to current knowledge, does not lead to health problems even after weekly intake over a lifetime. (Note: intake is not the same as absorption). The PTWI value has been suggested by WHO for environmental contaminants in foods. See also → ADI.

pulmonary emphysema: the irreversible enlargement of the air spaces distal to the terminal bronchioles due to the destruction of alveoli and pulmonary septa. In patients under

40 years of age, it is mostly caused by α_1-antitrypsin deficiency, predominantly in smokers.

PVC: polyvinyl chloride.

pyrolysis products: substances that are formed predominantly during cooking of protein-containing foods and during the frying of meat or fish (e.g., aromatic and heterocyclic amines). Most of them have carcinogenic potential.

Quick's test: a test for detecting disturbances in the coagulation system, named after Armand J. Quick (a physician from Milwaukee, 1894–1978). A method for determining prothrombin concentrations in blood, based on the clotting time of citrated blood plasma in the presence of thromboplastin and calcium ions. The prothrombin time (Quick's value) is expressed in percent of the normal coagulation time; the reference interval is 70–125 %.

radicals: free radicals are atoms or molecules with unpaired electrons, i. e., a single unpaired electron occupies a molecular orbital. Radicals are therefore paramagnetic, i. e., they align themselves in a magnetic field. Radicals are generated through the uptake or loss of an electron, or by breaking up a covalent bond. They are characterized by extremely high reactivity. They are formed in all forms of life during (patho)physiological processes.

radiodermatitis: synonym for radiation dermatitis.

radioimmunoassay (RIA): an in-vitro procedure used in nuclear medicine and analytical immunochemistry for the quantitative determination of antigens and haptens, such as hormones, vitamins, and medicines, by means of specific antibodies (mostly monoclonal antibodies) and a radioactive marker.

RAST: radioallergosorbent test.

Raynaud disease: a syndrome first described by the Parisian physician Maurice Raynaud (1834–1881). Attacks of painful ischemic states caused by vasoconstriction (vasospasm), mostly in the fingers (digits 2–5). Induced by endogenous and exogenous noxae, various traumas (e.g., work-ing with compressed-air tools), and intoxication (e.g., heavy metals, vinyl chloride), as well as emotional stress.

reference dose: → RfD.

reference value: a value for quantifying the occurrence of a toxic substance in the population. It is based on the frequency distribution of concentrations measured in numerous samples and is usually the 95th percentile. It does not allow for any toxicological or epidemiological assessment about possible pathophysiological functions of a substance in the body. Values above the reference value only indicate an unusually high load. Synonym: background value.

reimbursement: the repayment of expenditure. In various countries, different regulations of governmental health departments and insurance companies (negative listing, flat fees) severely restrict the reimbursement of costs for prescribed naturopathic medicines. As the eligibility of medicines for reimbursement may change quickly due to pharmacopolitical regulations, it is recommended that one contacts the appropriate authorities early when having problems with claiming expenditures for naturopathic medicines.

reliability: a quality criterion for test procedures. It defines the extent to which a measurement gives the same result when repeated under identical conditions, i. e., how similar a measurement is when compared with measurements taken with other instruments.

reproductive toxicity: the effect of being toxic to the reproductive process (e.g., by drugs or environmental chemicals). It includes damage to fertility, embryonic and fetal phases, and perinatal and postnatal development.

RES: reticuloendothelial system.

resistance: a nonspecific protection of organisms against infection or poison. There are differences in the resistance of species (e.g., germs only pathogenic to humans), individuals (e.g., environmental injuries, age), organs (e.g., fungus of the skin), etc.

retention: the holding in place of substances, deposited particles, or gases in various organs of the body (e.g., in the respiratory tract).

reversion: the reversal of a mutation event by reverse mutation. The reversion rate is lower than the spontaneous mutation rate by at least a factor of 1000.

RF: risk factor.

RfD: reference dose, an estimate of a daily oral exposure to the human population, including sensitive subgroups such as children, that is not likely to cause harmful effects during a lifetime. RfD values are generally used for health effects that are thought to have a threshold or low dose limit for producing effects; they are not applicable to nonthreshold effects such as cancer. The RfD is operationally derived from the → NOAEL (from animal and human studies) by a consistent application of uncertainty factors (→ safety factor). It is more conservative than the older margin of safety (→ ADI).

rhabdomyolysis: myolysis of the striated muscles leading to muscle weakness, reduced deep tendon reflexes, muscle pain, and myoglobinuria.

rhagades: fissures, cracks, or chaps in the skin. They develop when the skin's elasticity changes and are most common at the transition from skin to mucosa (e.g., nose, lips).

RIA: → radioimmunoassay.

risk: *absolute risk* for a group of persons with similar exposure: the ratio of the number of disease cases to the total number of persons in the group. *Relative risk*: the ratio of the absolute risk of the exposed group to that of the unexposed group.

risk assessment: the quantitative determination of possible health hazards caused by chemicals or radiation depending on activity, dose, and exposure time.

risk evaluation: the rating of a risk according to aspects of social acceptability and health care policies.

RR: 1. The blood pressure measured according to Riva Rocci. 2. In environmental medicine: relative risk (→ risk).

safety factor: a factor taking into account that humans may be more sensitive to damaging factors (e.g., chemicals, radiation) than the most sensitive experimental animals, and that there may also be different sensitivities within the population. The highest ineffective dose identified in animal experiments (→ NOEL) is usually divided by a safety factor of 100 to establish the maximum limit (→ ADI). See also → uncertainty factor.

SAM: S-adenosyl-L-methionine.

sarcoma: a malignant tumor originating from mesenchymal tissue and characterized by early hematogenous metastasis. It is possible that an initially benign mesenchymal → tumor (e.g., meningeoma) develops into sarcoma.

SBS: sick building syndrome.

SC: subcutaneous; administration under the skin.

scleroderma: an autoimmune disease of the vascular system and connective tissues. There are systemic as well as localized forms.

sclerosis: the pathological hardening of an organ due to increased formation of connective tissue. See also → fibrosis.

screening: the examination of a group of individuals aimed at detecting a clinically symptom-free or premorbid stage of a certain disease (e.g., mass screenings for pulmonary tuberculosis, diabetes mellitus).

self-injurious behavior: self-harm; the deliberate injury to one's own body. It is caused by autoaggression and emotions, which themselves may be caused by disease or by personal, financial, or situational conflicts. In most cases, multiple factors contribute to this behavior.

self medication: the treatment of one's own diseases without consulting a therapist.

sensibility, sensory function: the ability to feel or perceive various stimuli. The stimuli are mediated by receptors, transmitted via afferent nerves and spinal pathways to the sensory cerebral cortex (sensory centers) while being modulated along this route. See also → sensory disturbance.

sensitivity: the ability of a diagnostic test to screen for persons with a certain disease. It is the ratio of individuals with positive test results to those who actually have the disease (the latter include false negatives).

sensitization: the (primary) immune response induced by first contact with an antigen, followed by an enhanced (secondary) immune response or hypersensitivity reaction of the body (→ allergy) on renewed contact with the antigen.

sensory disturbance: the altered perception of sensory stimuli. → paresthesia, → sensibility.

shamanism: a range of traditional therapeutic measures and spiritual practices and techniques (e.g., therapeutic touch). These are often associated with naive dilettantism, quackery, and deception (→ ethnic medicine, → placebo effect).

SHBG: sex hormone binding globulin.

side effects: all undesired or not primarily desired effects of the treatment with medicines. Known and foreseen side effects must be listed in the instructions for use (package insert).

silicosis: pneumoconiosis caused by deposition of inorganic (siliceous) dust in the lungs of exposed workers (e.g., miners, stone masons).

skin sensitization: sensitization responses are part of the immune defense of the body. Once sensitization has occurred, the immunological response to renewed exposure leads to skin lesions, such as reddening, edema, or scab.

smog: a mixture of smoke and fog. A severe form of air pollution that is dangerous to health. It occurs mainly over highly populated areas during weather conditions causing atmospheric inversion (→ inversion layer). When the maximum limits are surpassed, public smog warnings must be issued.

social deviance: forms of behavior that disagree with current norms and values of the social environment (e.g., alcoholism, drug abuse).

social medicine: the scientific discipline concerned with health problems caused by the social environment and with their prevention.

solitary carcinogen: an outdated term for → complete carcinogen.

somatization: The process by which psychological needs are expressed in physical symptoms that do not have a detectable or known organic basis. The resulting psychosomatic disorders are associated with vague physical symptoms, such as pain in the limbs, numbness, nausea, and amnesia.

specificity: in *immunology*, the selective reaction of an antibody or immunocompetent cells with a specific antigen. In *epidemiology*, the ability of a test to correctly recognize a person with the disease in question. The number of true negative results divided by the total number of those without the disease.

sterilization: the complete destruction of biological organisms, including their dormant stages, by physical and/or chemical means.

stimulus threshold: a quantitative measure for the sensitivity of nerves. The point at which a stimulus just produces a sensation.

subacute (subchronic) toxicity testing: a test involving repeated administration of a test substance over a period of 28–90 days.

sun protection factor (SPF): the quotient resulting from dividing the time leading to reddening of the skin *with* a sunscreen agent by the time leading to reddening of the skin *without* a sunscreen agent. Determination of the sunscreen factor is done by using a series of at least 20 test individuals with different skin types, either under artificial UV irradiation or under natural sunlight. For this purpose, individual fields of unexposed (i.e., not yet tanned) skin on the back are subjected to a stepwise increase in irradiation, and threshold times for the onset of erythema are then scored after 22–26 h for each test person. The SPF is calculated from the mean values of the results. It indicates how much longer the protected skin may be exposed to the sun than unprotected skin; for example, when using a sunscreen agent with a SPF of 6, one may stay in the sun 6 times longer than without sunscreen.

sunscreen: a sunscreen is an agent that should protect the skin from the damaging effect of the irradiation by the sun (UV-A, UV-B, and UV-C) without preventing pigment formation, the body's own natural protection. UV-B rays affect only the epidermis; when a certain radiation dose is reached, they cause erythema (sunburn) which is followed by indirect pigmentation as a result of melanin synthesis.

superadditive effects: synergistic effects; → synergism.

susceptibility: the state of being readily affected; predisposition.

Sv: sievert. The SI unit of radiation absorbed dose equivalent.

symptom: a sign of disease; a noticeable change in the patient's condition indicative of disease.

symptomatology: the systematic discussion of symptoms.

symptom complex: → syndrome.

syncarcinogenesis: the combined action of several carcinogenic substances. This is different from → cocarcinogenesis, in which the effect of a carcinogen is increased by the subsequent action of a noncarcinogenic substance (→ cocarcinogen, → tumor promoter).

syncope: the temporary loss of unconsciousness due to generalized cerebral ischemia (a faint). It can be induced by metabolic or toxic agents, or by psychogenic attacks (collapse, coma, shock). Sudden loss of strength combined with short-term loss of consciousness (a blackout lasting seconds to minutes) may have various causes:

1. heart problems (e.g., cardiac irregularity, cardiac insufficiency), 2. vascular problems (e.g., peripheral vasodilatation), 3. cerebrovascular problems (e.g., stenosis), or 4. cerebral problems (e.g., epilepsy, hysteria).

syndrome: [Greek: *syn*, together; *dromos*, course] a symptom complex. A set of → symptoms occurring together; the sum of signs characteristic for a specific disease of mainly diverse or unknown etiology or pathogenesis.

synergism, synergy: the combined action of several chemicals or factors, with the total effect being greater than the predicted sum of agents working together. The synergistic effect therefore surpasses the additive effect. According to another definition, the combined action is larger than the highest individual effect, and the synergistic effects are classified as multiplicative, additive, or potentiated.

T: tesla. The SI unit of magnetic flux density.

tachycardia: increase in heart rate to > 100/min.

TBG: thyroxine-binding globulin.

TCDD: trichlorodibenzo[1,4]dioxin(s) or tetrachlorodibenzo[1,4]dioxin(s); usually the abbreviation for 2,3,7,8-tetrachlorodibenzo[1,4]dioxin (2,3,7,8-TCDD); → dioxins.

TCDF: trichlorodibenzofuran(s) and tetrachlorodibenzofuran(s); → dioxins.

TDI: tolerable daily intake. The estimated amount of a → contaminant in air, food, or drinking water which can be taken in daily over a lifetime without appreciable health risk. Related term: → ADI.

TE: toxicity equivalent.

TEF: toxicity equivalency factor. This factor has been introduced for the toxicity assessment of certain mixtures: e.g., for polychlorinated dioxins and furans, the relative efficiency of individual compounds is established by comparing them to 2,3,7,8-tetrachlorodibenzodioxin (TEF = 1). Different toxic end products have different TEFs.

teleangiectasia: the permanent dilation of small, superficial blood vessels. The hereditary form is rare; acquired forms occur mostly in the face (caused by the weather), inside the nose (nose bleed), and after prolonged use of halogenated corticoid creams.

tenesmus: ineffective and painful straining during defecation or urination.

teratogen: a substance that causes congenital structural abnormalities in the developing embryo. The best-known example is thalidomide, which causes severe malformation of the inner organs and the limbs, in particular.

teratogenicity: the property of a substance to cause birth defects by disturbing the development of a fertilized egg into an embryo.

thixotropy: the property of a gel of becoming fluid when agitated and then semisolid again at rest. The opposite is rheopexy (negative thixotrophy).

threshold: the dose or exposure level below which a significant adverse effect is not expected.

threshold limit value: → TLV. The maximum permissible concentrations of air pollutants established for short-term and long-term exposures.

threshold of activity: → NOEL, → LOEL.

threshold value, threshold concentration: the dose or concentration at the threshold of activity, i.e., between the lowest observed effect level (→ LOEL) and the no observed effect level (→ NOEL).

thrombosis: the clotting of blood within an artery or a vein.

TLV: threshold limit value. The concentration of an airborne substance to which an average person can be repeatedly exposed without adverse effects. The TLVs are issued in the United States by the American Conference of Governmental Industrial Hygienists (ACGIH) for the protection of employees from health hazards. The time-weighted exposure limit (TLV-TWA) is the maximum average concentration of a chemical in air for a normal 8-h work day and 40-h work week to which nearly all workers may be exposed day after day without harmful effects.

In this list, the substances are classified in detail according to their fetotoxic, genotoxic, and carcinogenic properties:

Fetotoxic working material:
A: definitely fetotoxic,
B: probably not fetotoxic,
C: not fetotoxic,
D: classification not yet possible.
Genotoxic working material:
1: proven genotoxicity in humans,
2: proven genotoxicity in mammals (experimental animals),
3: damaging to the genetic material of germ cells in humans and in experimental animals.
Carcinogenic working material:
III: definitely carcinogenic,
III 1: definitely carcinogenic in humans,
III 2: definitely carcinogenic in experimental animals under conditions that may correspond to those of human exposure,
III 3: reasonably suspected to have carcinogenic potential,
III 4: carcinogenic substances with negligible or no genotoxic effects,
III 5: substances with carcinogenic or genotoxic effects, although their activity is probably very low.

total hydrocarbons: the sum of all hydrocarbons.

toxemia: the appearance of bacterial toxins in the blood, or changes in the blood count caused by toxins.

toxicity: the entirety of unwanted, unhealthy effects of an agent. The dose-dependent poisonous properties of chemical substances and physical factors that are damaging to health. Types of toxicity include → organ toxicity, → carcinogenicity, → mutagenicity, → embryotoxicity, and → teratogenicity.

toxicity equivalency factor: → TEF.

toxicity testing: the experimental study of adverse effects of a substance in living organisms.

It involves short-term or long-term exposure to defined doses of the test substance and studying the effects depending on dose and duration of exposure (→ acute, → subacute/subchronic, and → chronic toxicity testing).

toxicodynamics: the description of changes in the body caused by a toxic substance.

toxicogenomics: the study of the effects of toxic substances on the → genome.

toxicokinetics: a branch of toxicology with the objective of quantitatively recording the pathway and fate of a toxic substance in the body, i.e., uptake (absorption), dispersion (distribution), transformation (metabolism), and excretion (elimination).

toxicology: the scientific study of the harmful effects of toxic substances and factors on living organisms. It describes the types of dose-dependent effects (→ toxicity) as well as their cellular, biochemical, and molecular mechanisms and their kinetics.

toxicopy: the occurrence of apparent symptoms that resemble those of poisoning, although exposure to poison cannot be detected in the person affected.

toxicosis: a disease caused by endogenous or exogenous toxic substances.

toxic substance: Any substance that can cause acute or chronic injury to the human body (→ poison). See also → pollutant.

toxin: a poisonous substance produced by living cells or organisms for either predation or defense. Toxins are usually water-soluble, immunogenic proteins. They are produced by microorganisms (e.g., mycotoxins from fungi), plants (phytotoxins), or animals (venom) and show specific effects after various incubation times, as compared with chemically defined poisons (→ toxic substances).

toxin generation: the transformation of a substance in the organism (e.g., by enzymes) into a substance of higher toxicity than the original one.

toxinology: the science that deals with the → poisons of animal, plant, or microbial origin (→ toxin).

toxoid: resembling a poison; a → toxin that has been detoxified by treatment with formaldehyde and heat (e.g., incubation at 39–41 °C for 3–4 weeks). Toxoids retain their immunizing properties (the haptophoric group is preserved, while the toxophoric group is destroyed). They are used, for example, for active vaccination against diphtheria and tetanus.

traditional Chinese medicine (TCM): the ancient system of Chinese folk medicine. Developed since about 3000 BC, it has its philosophical roots in Buddhism and Taoism. Five major organ systems and their assigned metaphors are distinguished with respect to → nosology: spleen/stomach (earth), lung/large intestine (metal), kidney/bladder (water), liver/gallbladder (wood), and heart/small intestine (fire). The energy flows through these systems in channels (or meridians). The basic principles are Yin and Yang, and they have analogies in all aspects of life. Yin and Yang have opposite qualities which are also found in foods and medicines. Treatment is based on → acupuncture (to compensate for disturbances in the flow of energy), nutritional therapy, → phytotherapy, physiotherapeutic techniques (chi gong, shiatsu), and comprehensive rules for the general hygiene of body and soul.

transfer: in the context of environmental ecology: the transition of a → xenobiotic (e.g., cadmium) from an environmental medium (e.g., soil) into plants.

trigeminy: an arrhythmia in which a normal heart beat is followed by two extrasystolic beats. → bigeminy.

trophic level: in ecology, a feeding level in a food chain (plants, herbivores, carnivores) that is determined by the number of energy-transfer steps to that level.

tumor: [Latin for swelling] a circumscribed increase in the volume of a tissue. The new growth is spontaneous, uncontrolled, autonomous, irreversible, and excessive; it is usually associated with various degrees of loss in the specific functions of cells and tissues. → neoplasia, → neoplasm.

tumor promoter: a substance that promotes the development of initiated cells into a tumor without acting as a carcinogen itself. → carcinogenesis.

TWA: time-weighted average.

uncertainty factor: one of several → safety factors used in calculating the reference dose (→ RfD) from experimental data. These factors are intended to account for (1) the variation in sensitivity among humans; (2) the uncertainty in extrapolating animal data to humans; (3) the uncertainty in extrapolating data obtained in a study that covers less than the full life of the exposed animal or human; and (4) the uncertainty in using → LOAEL data rather than → NOAEL data.

unit risk estimate: a method of extrapolating the additional cancer risk from continuous exposure to a toxic substance at a certain concentration and over a lifetime of 70 years.

uptake: the → absorption and → incorporation of a substance by living tissues. The amount taken up is defined as the amount reaching the organ or tissue (e.g., lung, gastrointestinal tract).

validity: the quality criterion for test procedures that indicates how suitable a procedure is for demonstrating the features to be measured. The validity is examined by comparing the results with measurements of other features of the same individual or by examining the compatibility of the results with the underlying theoretical model.

virtually safe dose: a dose deduced from the → unit risk estimate. It is the concentration of a toxic substance that leads to one additional case of cancer per 1 million individuals exposed for a lifetime. It is a dose that is virtually nontoxic.

viscosity: the resistance to flow. The internal friction of a liquid depends primarily on the temperature, and it plays an important role for the flow behavior of liquids.

vitality: the ability to survive; the ability to multiply.

WHO: → World Health Organization.

World Health Organization (WHO): an independent organization of the United Nations. Its functions include, among others, the establishment of guide lines for toxic substances in air, water, and food, as well as issuing recommendations for the maximum uptake of toxic substances in foods (→ ADI; → PTWI).

xenobiotic: a chemical foreign to the biological system.

▪ Recommendations for Further Reading

Text Books

Hayes AW, ed. Principles and Methods of Toxicology. 5th ed. New York: CRC Press; 2007

Hodgson E. A Textbook of Modern Toxicology. 3rd ed. New York: Wiley 2004

Hulpke H, Koch RA, Nießner R, eds. Römpp Lexikon Umwelt. 2nd ed. Stuttgart: Thieme; 2000

Marquardt H, Schäfer S, McClellan RO, Welsch F, eds. Toxicology. New York: Academic Press; 1999

Marquardt H, Schäfer S. Lehrbuch der Toxikologie, Wissenschaftliche Verlagsgesellschaft, Mannheim, 2004

Tischendorf FW, ed. Der diagnostische Blick. Stuttgart: Schattauer; 1998

Reference Books

Dart RC. Medical Toxicology. 3rd ed. Philadelphia: Lippincott Williams & Wilkins; 2004

Barceloux DG. Medical Toxicology of Natural Substances. New Jersey: Wiley & Sons Inc.; 2008

Ellenhorn MJ. Ellenhorn's Medical Toxicology: Diagnosis and Treatment of Human Poisoning. 2nd ed. Baltimore: Williams & Wilkins; 1997

Hardman JL, Limbird LE, Gilman AG, eds. Goodman and Gilman's: The Pharmacological Basis of Therapeutics. 10th ed. New York: McGraw-Hill Professional; 2001

Kimbrough RD, Jensen AA. Halogenated Biphenyls, Terphenyls, Naphthalenes, Dibenzodioxins and Related Products. 2nd ed. Amsterdam, New York, Oxford: Elsevier; 1989

Klimmek R, Szinicz L, Weger N. Chemische Gifte und Kampfstoffe – Wirkung und Therapie. Stuttgart: Hippokrates; 1983

Mebs D. Gifttiere. Stuttgart: Wissenschaftliche Verlagsgesellschaft; 2000

Reichl FX, Mohr K, Hein L, Hickel R. Taschenatlas der Pharmakologie und Toxikologie für Zahnmediziner. Stuttgart: Thieme; 2007

Wichmann HE, Schlipköter HW, Fülgraff G. Handbuch der Umweltmedizin. Landsberg/Lech: Ecomed Verlagsgesellschaft; 2002

Periodicals

Archives of Toxicology (official journal of EUROTOX), Springer, Heidelberg, Germany

Ecotoxicology and Environmental Safety (official journal of the International Society of Ecotoxicology and Environmental Safety), Academic Press, Orlando, USA

Environmental Toxicology and Pharmacology (an international review journal), Elsevier, New York, USA

Fundamental and Applied Toxicology (official journal of the Society of Toxicology), Academic Press, Orlando, USA

Human and Experimental Toxicology (official journal of the British Toxicology Society), Stockton Press, Hampshire, UK

Naunyn-Schmiedeberg's Archives of Pharmacology (official journal of the German Society of Experimental and Clinical Pharmacology and Toxicology, DGPT), Springer, Heidelberg, Germany

Pharmacology and Therapeutics (an international review journal), Elsevier Science Inc., New York, USA

Science (official journal of the American Association for the Advancement of Science, AAAS), Washington, USA

Toxicology and Applied Pharmacology (official journal of the Society of Toxicology), Academic Press, Orlando, USA

Toxicology in Vitro (an international journal), Elsevier Science Ltd. (Pergamon), Oxford, UK

Toxicon (official journal of the International Society on Toxinology). An interdisciplinary journal on the toxins from animals, plants, and microorganisms. Elsevier Science (Pergamon), Oxford, UK

Online Information Systems

UN database: www.chem.unep.ch (UNEP: United Nations Environmental Programme)

European database: www.oshweb.com (Environmental Chemicals Data Information Network)

German database: www.dimdi.de (DIMDI: Deutsches Institut für Medizinische Dokumentation und Information)

General toxicology information: www.toxikologie.de (German Society of Toxicology) [in German]

■ General Index

Page numbers in *italics* refer to illustrations or tables

A

ABC rule 30, *31*
abdominal pain *73, 77, 79, 81,*
    201, 275
    see also colic
abscesses *83*
absorption 12, *13*, 38, 304
    facilitators 304
Acanthaster planci 258, *259*
acaricides 192, *193*
acceptable daily intake (ADI) 46,
    304
accumulation 36, 304
    bioaccumulation *63*, 307
    interference with transport
        processes 46, *47*
accuracy 18, *19*
ACE inhibitors 90
acetaminophen 80, *81*
acetone 234
2-acetylaminofluorene *29*
    as no-threshold carcinogen
        28, *29*
acetylation *15*
acid cleaning products 234, *235*
acid rain 134, *135*
acid smog 134, *135*
acidosis *75, 77, 81, 141*
    respiratory *139*
acne 304
    chloracne *113, 115*, 116, *117,*
        308
aconitine 266, *267*
Aconitum napellus 266, *267*
acrodynia 176, *177*
acrolein 136
activated charcoal 32, *33*
acupuncture 304
acute toxicity class (ATC) test 20,
    21, 304
adaptation 304
adder 262, *263*
addictive substances 82–93, *83*
adenoma 304
administration 304
Adonis vernalis 272, *273*
adonitoxin 272, *273*

ADP-ribosyl transferases 288,
    289
Aethusa cynapium 274, *275*
aethusin 274, *275*
aflatoxins 210, *211*
    aflatoxin B1 lethal dose *5*
Agaricus arvensis 284, *285*
Agaricus augustus 284
Agaricus campestris 284, *285*
Agaricus xanthoderma 284
aggression 45
agitation *75*
agonist 304
Agricola, Georgius 2
air
    airborne emissions 48
    clean air control 50, *51*
    composition 48, *49*
    lifespan of organic com-
        pounds 48, *49*
    pollution 48–51, 134, *135*
        concentrations 48, *49*
        epidemiology 50
        guidance values 48, *49*
        particulate 122, *123*
        preventive measures 50,
            51
        threshold concentrations
            50
        toxicology 50, *51*
    quality standards 48
airway irritation *95, 99, 113, 117,*
    135, 137, 209, 237, 245
    lung irritants 238, *239*, 246
ALARA (as low as reasonably
    achievable) 304–305
alcohol 84, *85*, 94
    chronic alcoholism 86, *87*
        secondary diseases 86, *87*
    metabolism 84, *85*
    smoking and 156
    withdrawal symptoms 86, *87*
aldehydes 136
aldrin 194, *195*
alginates 220, *221*
alicyclic hydrocarbons 94
aliphatic hydrocarbons 94
alkaline cleaning products 234,
    235

alkaloids 68–73, 266–*271*
alkoxy radicals 146, *147*
alkylating agents 242, *243*
allergens 305
    contact allergens 222, *223*
allergic contact dermatitis 222,
    223, 253
allergic reactions *51, 95, 171,*
    173, 175, 259, 261, 265, 285,
    305
    contact allergens 222, *223*
    cosmetics 222
    cross-allergy 309
    food allergies 212
    plastics 188, *189*
allopathy 305
alpenrose 278
α-solanine 270, *271*
α-tocopherol 148, *149*
alternative health care 34
alternative hypothesis 18
aluminium 160, *161*
alveolitis *209*
amalgam 254, *255*
Amanita citrina 282, *283*
Amanita muscaria 282, *283*
Amanita pantherina 282
Amanita phalloides 280, *281*
Amanita virosa 280, *281*
amaryllis 268
amatoxins 280, *281*
amblyopia 87
Amenonia sulcata 256, *257*
Ames test 22, *23*, 305
amidosulfuric acid *235*
2-amino-1-methyl-6-phenylimi-
    dazol[4,5-*b*]pyridine (PhIP)
    132, *133*
2-amino-3-methyl-9 H-pyrido
    [2,3-*b*]indole (MeAαC) 132,
    133
aminoacetylation *15*
4-aminodiphenyl 130, *131*
aminophenazone 124
amphetamines 90, *91*
amphibians 262, *263*
amygdalin 62, *63*, 272
anatoxin A 62, *63*